TINY
BUT
MIGHTY

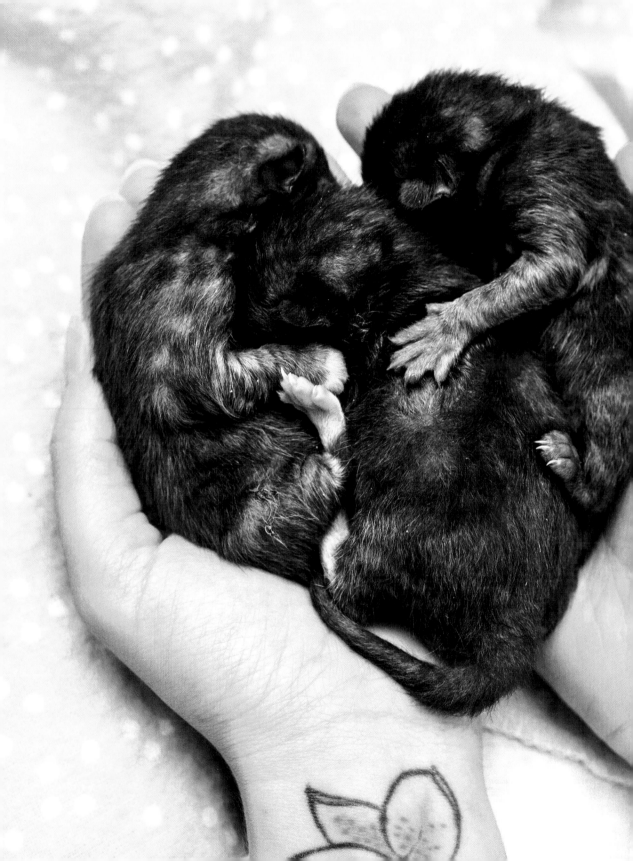

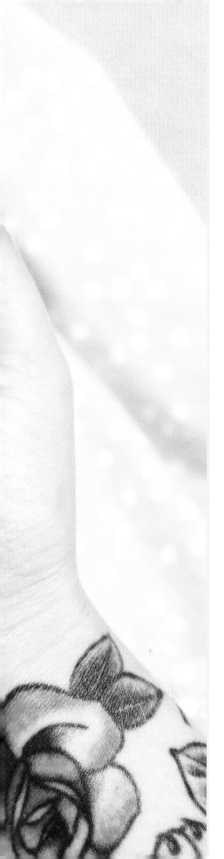

TINY
BUT
MIGHTY

Kitten Lady's Guide
to Saving the
Most Vulnerable Felines

HANNAH SHAW

Photographs by
Hannah Shaw and Andrew Marttila

PLUME

PLUME

An imprint of Penguin Random House LLC
penguinrandomhouse.com

Photograph on page 209 taken by Alexandra Keen; photograph on page 225 taken by Kim Adams; all other photographs courtesy of Hannah Shaw or Andrew Marttila.

LIBRARY OF CONGRESS CATALOGING-IN-PUBLICATION DATA
Names: Shaw, Hannah René, 1987- author.
Title: Tiny but mighty: kitten lady's guide to saving the most
vulnerable felines / Hannah Shaw.
Description: New York: Plume, [2019] | Includes bibliographical references and index.
Identifiers: LCCN 2018049630 | ISBN 9781524744069 (hardcover) |
ISBN 9781524744076 (ebook)
Subjects: LCSH: Kittens. | Cat rescue. | Animal welfare.
Classification: LCC SF447 .S46 2019 | DDC 636.8/07—dc23
LC record available at https://lccn.loc.gov/2018049630

Printed in the United States of America
10 9 8 7 6 5 4 3 2 1

Book design by Nancy Resnick

For Coco

CONTENTS

TINY BUT MIGHTY

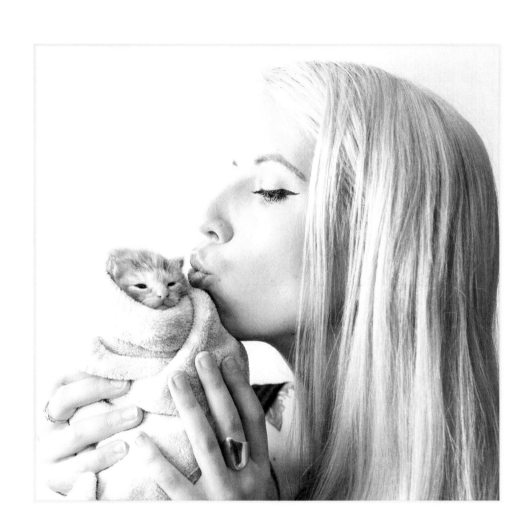

INTRODUCTION

TINY

My name is Hannah Shaw, but most people know me as Kitten Lady. I'm a professional animal rescuer, a humane educator, and a fierce advocate for the protection of kittens. My life is dedicated to saving young kittens, and I've spent my career teaching people all around the world to do the same. I am on a mission to change the world for the smallest and most vulnerable felines.

Everything I do is structured around saving little lives. I live in a home with a built-in kitten nursery that is tailored to meet the needs of orphans, helping them to recover, blossom, and thrive. Once a motherless kitten enters my home, she is safe here; this is where the cold become warm, the sick become well, and the hungry get a bellyful of nutritious food. Over the years, I've saved hundreds of babies. The transformations I witness here are profound, and it is absolutely life-changing to watch as some of the tiniest and most hopeless kittens grow into robust, mighty cats.

I'm so immersed in rescue that I sometimes forget how unique it is to be a kitten mom. Once I was at a grocery store, purchasing human baby food for a sickly orphan, when a chatty employee started asking me about my child.

"Do you have a baby at home?" asked the clerk.

"Yes, I do!" I replied.

"Oh, how wonderful. Boy or girl?"

"She's a little girl."

"Lovely! How old?"

"She's five weeks old."

"Wow! Only five weeks old? You look great!"

". . . Why thank you!" I laughed.

"And what's the little girl's name?"

"Earthworm."

Her face went pale and she stopped talking to me. Hey, she didn't ask what species!

Being a surrogate caregiver to baby cats is a unique and fulfilling experience. My work as a kitten advocate has taken me to some pretty wild places: whether I find myself on an international train with a secret kitten hidden in my hoodie, on an overnight road trip in a van with dozens of kittens, or crawling in the dirt on my hands and knees to find the source of a tiny "meow," it's *always* an adventure! Kitten rescue has taught me that true compassion is spontaneous and unconditional, and that even though I'm just one tiny person, if I bear witness to suffering, I have the power to do something about it.

A life of kitten rescue wasn't something I actively sought out—in fact, quite the contrary! Kittens came into my life like a whirlwind and made their presence impossible to ignore. A lifelong animal advocate, I knew I had it in my heart to help— but as one individual, how could I possibly make a difference?

I quickly learned the hard way that there are very few resources available to young kittens. I discovered that if unweaned kittens entered an animal shelter, they were considered too young to be viable, and they were typically euthanized. Everywhere I turned for help, there seemed to be a gap in resources when it came to the littlest lives. I found that even if I wanted to help them myself, there was almost no reliable information available about what I could personally do to give them a chance. Ultimately, I determined that if these resources didn't exist, I could take small steps to be a part of the solution. And so the day I found my first kitten outside, my journey began.

COCO, THE KITTEN WHO STARTED IT ALL

It was a day like any other day. I was twenty-one years old, working for a summer camp that served children with special needs, and we had taken the campers to a public park for some fun afternoon activities. As I sat on a bench next to a coworker, I looked up into the tall trees above, which were speckled with bright sunshine. I noticed a small, curious silhouette that looked out of place . . . and I could swear I saw a tiny eye among the leaves.

I rubbed my eyes, squinting to get a better look, and gasped. There she was: a little black kitten was looking back at me with one eye crusted shut. She was at least fifteen feet high, lying on a branch like the littlest leopard. My mind was racing: *How did she get up there? Where is her family? What happens if I leave her there? What should I do?* I looked down at my shoes: in flip-flops, I was in no shape to be climbing a tree. And suppose I did climb the tree . . . then what?

It was only a matter of minutes before I found myself with my feet stuffed into a coworker's sneakers, testing my strength as I shimmied my way up the bark. My colleagues gathered the children, who watched for what I would do next. A crowd started forming, and soon total strangers were cheering me on. Suddenly the world around me disappeared and I was fixated on a singular goal: I had to get this dang kitten out of the tree.

Clumsily, I climbed the tree to the branch where the kitten lay, scrawny and lethargic. I reached out, grasped my hand around her skinny body, plopped her into my shirt, and shimmied back down. The children squealed and the strangers clapped. For about one minute, I felt triumphant in my achievement, and shocked that I was now holding a small, furry individual. But the feeling of accomplishment was immedi-

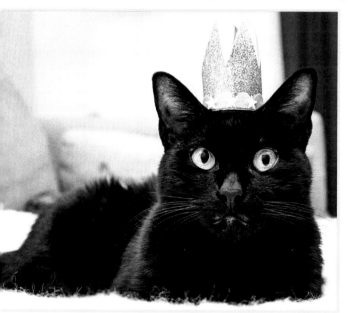

ately overshadowed by the panicked question: ". . . So what do I do now?"

That was the day I unexpectedly became the mother to a tiny, meowing carnivore. The moment I first wrapped my hand around her five-week-old body, I felt an immediate responsibility to ensure that she had what she needed, though admittedly I had no idea what that was. It's embarrassing, but I distinctly remember carrying her back to the office at the summer camp, opening the fridge, and thinking, *She can probably eat a hot dog, right?* I emptied a box of children's building blocks, and that became her first temporary home. As scared and clueless as I was, I felt determined to give her a good life. I named her Coconut—Coco for short—because I'd shimmied up a tree to pluck her like the sweet fruit.

It didn't take long for me to fall in love. Coco became my lil' sidekick, and I became her family. Since I rescued her, hundreds of other kittens have passed through my home, but only she (and my cat Eloise!) have stayed. She sleeps beside me at night, greets me every morning, and sits in my lap while I work, her purrs deep and therapeutic against my legs. Coco is my ride-or-die, my right-hand cat, my inspiration, and my very best friend.

SAVING KITTENS' LIVES

After I rescued Coco, a veil was lifted, and I started finding kittens absolutely everywhere. By dumpsters. Beneath backyard grills. Under parked cars. Admittedly, the more kittens started finding me, the more I started looking for them. Every time I took in a new kitten, I gained a little more knowledge and experience with their care, and a little more of a reputation, too. Soon, I became known among friends and colleagues as the person to call if you found a kitten, and boy, did the calls start coming: "I heard you're a kitten lady."

Coco was the gateway kitten who opened my eyes to the plight of kittens, setting into motion a journey that led me to discover that kittens are one of the most at-risk and misunderstood populations in the United States. For as loved as kittens are by our culture, they are also killed by the hundreds of thousands due to a complex and interrelated set of factors, including resource scarcity and lack of public awareness. This means that without the intervention of animal rescuers and an active community of foster homes, kittens too young for adoption—particularly newborns, known as neonatal kittens—face a ticking clock, and often an untimely death. These forgotten felines need an advocate more than anyone.

My journey wasn't always easy—I had a big learning curve. For years I was totally overwhelmed by the act of saving kittens' lives, whether due to the confusing illnesses and mystery poops, the challenges of knowing what supplies to use and

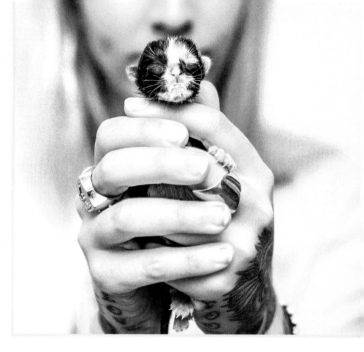

how to use them, or the perplexing process of finding a kitten a forever home. I've experienced the challenges of fostering orphans while working full-time or living in a studio apartment, the emotional hurdles of saying good-bye to kittens I've loved, and even the heavy burden of taking on too much and having to learn how to balance being compassionate to others with being kind to myself.

I've learned, one tiny step at a time, how to provide a caring, supportive, enriching experience that sets kittens up for a lifetime of health and happiness. What I know now came through many late nights of research, through collaboration with other rescuers, and through the trial and error that comes with the heartbreak of loss—and the triumph of success. All along, my goal has been to do the greatest good that I possibly can, and to do it in a way that is sustainable, impactful, and fun.

Having been through it all, I became passionate about sharing what I know regarding the protection and care of kittens so that other people can save lives, too. I began to create the resources I wish I'd had when I was getting started, and something incredible began to happen: people started listening! I made it my mission to be a source of support to those who want to help kittens, by providing them with helpful information, empowerment, and the inspiration to know that they can make a big difference, too.

Since beginning my project, Kitten Lady, I've taught millions of people how to get active for kittens. I've created dozens of free educational videos, hosted over a hundred live workshops, and given out tens of thousands of instructional booklets to foster parents. I've partnered as a consultant with shelters all across the country and abroad to help improve their programs for kittens, collaborated with animal control to increase their impact with cats and kittens in the field, and worked hard to influence policies that impact kittens at the local, state, and federal levels. I've even created a 501(c)(3) nonprofit organization, Orphan Kitten Club, which saves kittens' lives by providing lifesaving care and resources to sick, injured, and or-phaned kittens in need.

I'm passionate about sharing my life as a kitten advocate because ultimately my goal is to self-replicate. To that end, I openly document the fun, ridiculous, and adorable adventures that I have as a kitten rescuer, oversharing in hopes of helping others discover that rescue is for everyone. I'm grateful to do this work alongside my partner, Andrew Marttila, who is a professional cat photographer and whose beautiful photos (many of which are on the pages to come!) capture the essence of these precious little lives in crisp perfection. Together, we've amassed the most fantastic following of compassionate cat-lovers and budding activists, and built a community that I love with all my heart. Helping others realize the impact they can make and welcoming them into the wonderful world of rescue fills me with enthusiasm and hope.

As one person, I can do only so much, but as a community, I truly believe we can change the world for kittens. This book is an invitation for readers to join me on this journey and to add their own piece to the puzzle. In the pages to come, you will learn all about why kittens need your help, and I'll give you all the tools you need to help them. You'll learn about the physical and behavioral development of kittens, how to feed and care for them, and how to help them find a loving home. I'll show you how to save lives in ways complementary to who you are. You'll see hundreds of beautiful photos of kittens I've rescued, and read uplifting tales of their triumph and transformation. I'll give you ideas for helping kittens no matter who you are—whether your contribution is through fostering, adopting, volunteering, educating, or simply becoming a more informed voice for cats. My hope is that you will see yourself in these pages, and feel supported in your own rescue journey.

"Tiny but mighty" is a phrase I use to describe the kittens I save, because even when they're as tiny as a packing peanut, they have such a mighty spirit and so much capacity to flourish if we just give them a hand. All the constituent parts of a pocket panther are jam-packed into each furry seedling, and with proper care, they can bloom into a glorious, independent cat. "Tiny but mighty," to me, encap-sulates the essence of the fragile feline's potential.

But that isn't the only reason I love the phrase. It's also a reminder that we, as rescuers, create major changes through *small* acts of kindness. After years of trying to untangle the impossibly gnarled knot of animal suffering, I've come to find that change actually doesn't typically happen through massive, sweeping action. On the contrary, most change comes from an accumulation of tiny actions: a bowl of food, a warm bed, a temporary refuge for the homeless, a momentary extension of a compassionate hand. Movements are made up of individuals, and our small individual actions have the power to change everything.

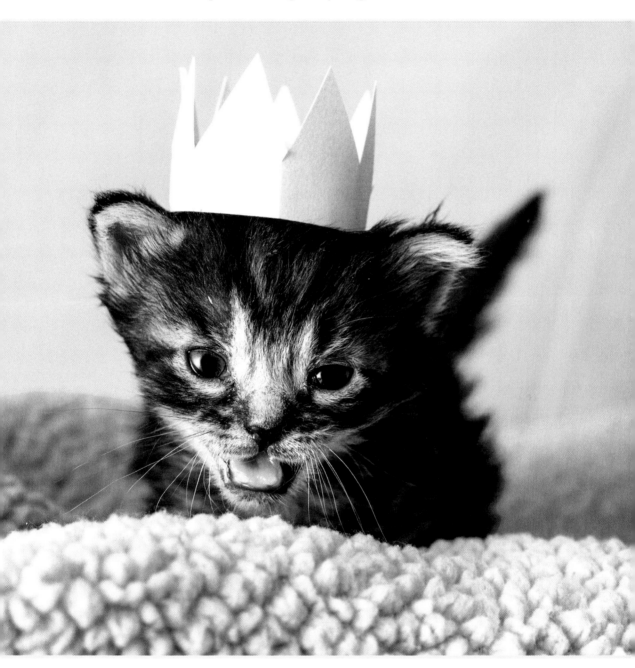

CHAPTER ONE

STATE OF THE KITTEN

EVERYONE LOVES KITTENS

I spend a lot of time in transit.

Working in so many different communities, I've become accustomed to the monotony of travel: the long hours, the rigorous TSA inspection of my supplies (seriously, who travels with this much cat food?), and the small talk that occurs between strangers in airports and hotel lobbies. The question people always want to ask is, of course, "What do you do?"

When I tell people I'm an animal advocate who specializes in kittens, the response is almost always the same. First, a facial expression falling somewhere on the spectrum between utter confusion and absolute delight. Second, a comment about how I have the most adorable job ever. Third, some variation of the following inquiry:

"Do kittens really need advocates? I thought everyone loved kittens already."

I do my best to summarize with a smile, but the truth is that to fully explain the magnitude of suffering that kittens face and the importance of our efforts to save them would take an entire book. And so here we are.

In many ways, working with kittens *is* absolutely adorable. I'm surrounded by fluffy little bobbleheaded dinguses every day of my life. I get to watch innocent beings grow and flourish. From the serene satisfaction of a baby's first gentle purr to the bellyaching hilarity of a room full of pouncing micro-predators, working with kittens is truly an enjoyable calling. But it isn't their charming nature that inspires me to do what I do. To me, kitten advocacy has very little to do with cuteness, and everything to do with a great need for tangible change in the way we view, understand, and treat the tiniest and most vulnerable felines.

The truth is that kittens are universally loved in our culture, yet we kill them in epidemic numbers. Unweaned kittens make up a large proportion of feline euthanasias nationally; for many shelters, their deaths account for the majority of euthanasias. The general public is completely unaware that kittens under eight weeks old are one of the most at-risk populations in the US shelter system. Without public knowledge of these issues, we cannot empower people to get active and save kittens' lives. We must start with a basic understanding of

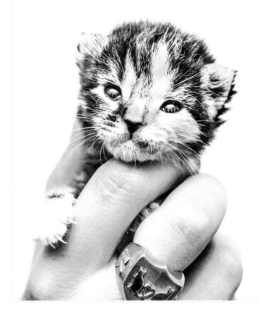

not just what is happening, but also *why* it is happening, and how each of us can take tiny steps to help solve this problem. We must unravel and examine this complex issue, rally the troops, and forge ahead toward a day when no kitten must die due to lack of resources or of community awareness.

THE UNADOPTABLES

For decades, millions of cats were being euthanized each year. I'll never forget when the 2016 national data was published and, for the first time in my rescue career, the number of cats dying in US shelters annually was fewer than one million.

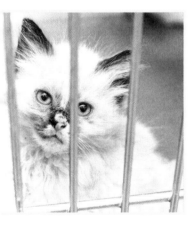

I wept with happiness to learn that we presently have national euthanasia rates of roughly 860,000 cats per year.[1] Maybe it seems odd to celebrate that hundreds of thousands of cats are still dying in shelters, but seeing the number drop so dramatically over the course of my career has certainly given me reason to feel optimistic about a brighter future for cats, and to push ahead.

It's an exciting time to be an advocate, as things are truly getting better for cats all the time. Having rightfully won the adoration of the general public, cats are now being adopted in higher numbers than ever before. Roughly 37 percent of US households are now home to a cat, and while I obviously think that number should be higher (seriously, have you met cats? they're pretty great), this is a huge achievement. More people than ever are discovering the joy of sharing life with a feline, resulting in a steady rise of cat companionship. As adoption rates rise, there is, in turn, a marked decrease in euthanasia.

It's easy to see why increased adoption would mean decreased euthanasia. Adoption is a solution to euthanasia, and the two variables are thus inversely correlated; as adoption goes up, euthanasia goes down. But this is not a one-to-one correlation, as adoption is only one of several variables necessary to get euthanasia to zero—it is not a full solution. Adoption, of course, only helps cats who are adoptable. If you examine the data, you'll quickly find that the cats who are dying in shelters tend not to be cats for whom adoption would have been a solution. The populations that are most at risk in modern-day animal shelters are the *unadoptables*.

Unadoptable animals are those who are not candidates for an adoption program. For felines, this comprises two main populations: cats who are feral and cats who are under eight weeks old. Many people don't realize that while a two-month-old kitten is the likeliest to find a home in a shelter, a two-week-old kitten is the likeliest to be killed. You simply can't go to an animal shelter and adopt a neonatal kitten or a fractious cat who doesn't tolerate touch. But that doesn't mean those animals aren't there, or that they don't deserve our help. Feral cats and unweaned kittens are the two biggest populations comprising the 860,000 feline deaths in shelters each year, which is why these are the two populations I've dedicated my life to understanding and saving.

Just because an animal isn't a candidate for adoption doesn't mean her life is without value; it simply means she needs a different solution than an adoption program. For feral cats, this means providing them with a solution that allows them to live their full lives outdoors, where they are most at home, without bringing more kittens into the world (read more about feral cats in Chapter Two). For kittens, it means providing a solution that keeps them alive until they are old enough to be adopted into a home. There are a number of programs that aim to protect unadoptable populations, including trap-neuter-return, on-site nurseries, and foster care. The result of these strategies is that we are able to reduce the number of kittens being born, while shepherding those kittens who *are* born through the vulnerable period of unadoptability. We are able to create hope where there otherwise would be none.

STAY STUBBORN, HAVE HOPE

What is hope? To me, hope is more than a cheesy motivational poster or a platitude embossed on a charm bracelet. It is the defiant resistance against suffering, and the relentless insistence that a positive outcome is possible. It is the shifting tide that occurs when we refuse to accept needless death as an inevitability. From this stubborn love, miraculous things can occur! When it comes to the euthanasia epidemic, I've always been stubborn . . . and I've always had hope.

Euthanasia is, by definition, "the act or practice of killing or permitting the death of hopelessly sick or injured individuals."[2] But is a kitten hopeless just because she is three weeks old? Heck no! Having raised hundreds of thriving babies, I hardly consider them beyond hope. The fact is that they are only hopeless if we fail to provide them with opportunities to stay alive. When we intervene with love and hands-on support, we find that they are, in fact, bursting with the capacity to grow, to heal, and to become wonderful companions. We must simply give them the chance.

The process of raising kittens is as close to actual magic as I'll ever get. The moment I bring home a new batch of filthy, hungry wiggle worms, it's like I suddenly grow five extra hearts. Over the next several weeks I pour pure love into each individual, and it makes them transform from "hopelessly" scrawny into pudgy, strong-boned, affectionate little creatures who return the love tenfold. When it's time for adoption, I get to give this tremendous gift of companionship to total strangers, brightening their world and giving a lifetime of happiness to the cats. It feels totally silly to say, but the love we give has ripple effects that we may never even know.

As heavy as it can feel to examine the state of the kitten, the beautiful thing is that each of us is capable of creating tangible hope that actively shifts the future for both the individual animal and sheltering as we know it. Every tiny moment of kindness, every small act of compassion adds up to create a safer world. At the end of the day, my time with each kitten is just a blip—a small moment of stubborn hope. But to a being whose entire future is dependent on surviving for a few short weeks, these tiny moments make all the difference.

So if euthanasia is meant for hopeless animals, and kittens aren't hopeless, why are so many kittens killed in shelters? Before examining these heartbreaking issues, it's important to note that most shelters are doing the very best they can with the resources available to them, and that their success and the success of the animals in their care is dependent on our ability to approach them with compassion and support. Sadly, though, for a myriad of reasons, most US shelters are not set up to save the little guys, who are therefore being killed in epidemic numbers.

Neonatal kitten care is a niche skill that requires specialized training and supplies—neither of which are a given in your average animal shelter. When I train shelter staff, I always ask how many people have ever bottle-fed a kitten, and I typically find that few or no employees have been trained in providing this care. In addition to the lack of training, essential items such as kitten formula or bottles often aren't kept in stock; there simply aren't sufficient supplies or staffing to provide the care. With hundreds of other animals to feed and support, resources tend to be focused around saving the adoptable populations; kitten care is thus not a main priority for most shelter management.

It makes sense that neonatal care is traditionally not a top concern, as many shelters will not be able to keep a neonate alive on-site for even twenty-four hours. Most organizations have limited operating hours and are unable to provide overnight care; it would therefore be quite unethical to leave an unweaned baby with no assistance while the facility is closed for the night. For this reason, young kittens generally meet their fate within hours of entering the shelter doors: either they make it out the door to a foster home before the shelter closes, or they don't make it out at all.

Even for facilities that do have overnight care, space is an issue. When you consider that shelters have limited housing, it's easy to see why it is more responsible to give kennel space to an animal who can be quickly adopted than to an animal who will require that space for eight weeks. There simply isn't adequate space to house every kitten in every community for the duration of her upbringing until she is old enough to be adopted. Moreover, kennels aren't optimal for socializing kittens during these critical early weeks.

In addition to the challenges of providing feeding, care, and space to young kittens, most shelters also struggle to meet the medical needs of neonates. Kittens are immunocompromised (read more about immune systems on page 161) and are extremely susceptible to illness in a high-volume setting such as an animal rescue facility; even an hour in a shelter can expose a neonate to viruses or parasites that can be life-threatening. To safely accommodate kittens requires strict quarantine protocol and specially designated nursery units, which is not possible for many shelters operating with limited space.

Shelters can find the treatment of sick neonates to be a challenge. Young kittens are likely to become ill, but treatment can be difficult when veterinarians don't have experience with the specific needs of neonates. For instance, many prescription drugs are only officially labeled for use in kittens over eight weeks, and even if they are demonstrably safe for use in neonates, some veterinarians are not comfortable prescribing off-label for these little young'uns. Many veterinary professionals are hesitant to provide effective treatment options such as antibiotics or other necessary medications to help save a kitten's life due to the limited knowledge base around feline pediatrics. And when we fail to act swiftly and aggressively against illness, many kittens fall progressively more ill, and either die in care or are euthanized.

It's plain to see that due to their special care requirements, kittens often will not find a suitable environment in their local animal shelter. Brick-and-mortar shelters are well suited to finding homes for adoptable animals, but these unadoptable babies can only thrive in an environment that can provide more individualized and special care. We must find creative solutions that meet the needs of these tiny lives.

PAINT BY NUMBERS

It isn't exactly a secret that kittens under eight weeks old are dying in large numbers, but it's obscured in a way that prevents public awareness and programmatic change. In order for the public to care and to take action, we need to be aware that there is a problem to begin with; we can't do better until we know better. But from the language we use in the sheltering industry to the way we track intakes and outcomes, we often fail to represent what is happening to kittens in shelters. How can we even begin to unpack the issue for the public when we have no figures with which to quantify it? We simply cannot paint an accurate picture of the state of the kitten when we fail to represent how deeply at risk they are.

One of the major problems is our data reporting in animal shelters. There is no national requirement for tracking and reporting animal data, which makes it a challenge to share how dire the situation is. While several states do require shelters to report their numbers, it's uncommon for them to specifically track kittens under eight weeks old. The industry standard is to track the status of cats at five months or younger and five months or older, noting whether they are adopted, are euthanized, or have another outcome. This skews the data dramatically, as kittens two to five months old are highly adoptable, while those less than two months old are not adoptable at all.

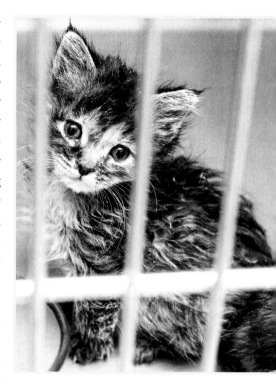

Shelters also often fail to count each kitten as an individual, as database software allows the input of kittens as a litter as opposed to counting them as separate animals. This means six neonatal kittens can be counted as one litter. When this happens, they aren't considered individual lives; they are a unit—unless they are candidates for adoption, in which case they become individuals, each with his own profile. The result is that we don't have precise numbers for this unadoptable population, either in terms of how their age impacts the likelihood of euthanasia, or in terms of how many are being killed versus how many are saved. We count their successes individually, but not their suffering. This makes it a challenge to demonstrate to policy makers, administrators, and members of the public the great need for programs that specifically target neonates.

The truth is that the early death of the neonatal kitten is a foregone conclusion written into the very DNA of the US shelter system, even through the language we use. While no governing body oversees animal sheltering as a whole, an industry standard called the Asilomar Accords provides recommended protocol for definitions and reporting shelter statistics. Taken directly from these standards: "The mission of those involved in creating the Asilomar Accords is to work together to save the lives of all healthy and treatable companion animals." The document continues: "The term 'healthy' means and includes all dogs and cats *eight weeks of age or older* that . . . have manifested no sign of a behavioral or temperamental characteristic that could . . . make the animal *unsuitable for placement as a pet . . .*" (emphasis my own). This text, while created in the spirit of lifesaving, has the unintended consequence of obscuring public perception around who lives and who dies in shelters. Using this industry definition, shelters can report that they've saved all healthy and treatable animals, even if they have, in fact, euthanized thousands of neonates and feral cats.

While most shelters don't track unweaned kittens, there are some that do, such as Los Angeles Animal Services. Between July 2012 and June 2013, the City of Los Angeles saw more than nine thousand unweaned kittens enter the doors of its shelters, and 65 percent of those were euthanized. Through public reporting of these numbers, the demand for help increased. Kitten nurseries were opened; transfers to rescue organizations increased; foster homes increased. The city's open reporting, though upsetting, allows us to paint a picture of what is happening to kittens, what factors are helping them get out alive, and what further help is needed. We can then measure our successes and continue on the correct path. Euthanasia has now dropped substantially; between July 2017 and June 2018, just 20 percent of LA's unweaned kittens—roughly 1,500 kittens—were killed. While there is still a great need, things are getting better. By acknowledging and talking about the issue, the community has been more capable of working together to solve it.

It's a challenge to raise awareness about the plight of kittens, or to create strategic programs to save them, when we can't track their status through data or understand what's happening to them with precision. My belief is that if we want to be able to change something, we have to be willing to analyze it and discuss it publicly. We cannot keep ourselves and our communities in the dark; we have to bring this information into the light, no matter how painful it is to know the truth. We must paint an accurate picture and give the public the tools to change it.

TO KILL OR NOT TO KILL

I've been fortunate to work with countless shelters throughout the country, from large city shelters to small rural facilities, from "no-kill" shelters to shelters with high euthanasia rates. I've found that the organizations that need the greatest help also tend to receive the most vitriol from the public—a sort of backlash against killing that is understandable enough, but very much misplaced. Many people simply hear "kittens are killed" and get out their pitchforks before they can even attempt to understand the complexities of the situation. The truth is that it's complicated: no animal shelter desires to kill cats, yet they collectively kill more than 2,300 every single day in the United States.

I'll admit that when I first got involved in rescue, I had no idea why some shelters killed while others did not, and I felt furious at those that did. It's often human nature to turn to anger before turning to empathy, and shelters are thus routinely targeted by angry but well-meaning animal-lovers. Knowing what I do now, I recognize how naive and unproductive those feelings were. My position is that we must approach shelters in the spirit of cooperation and collaboration. A shelter that kills is quite simply a shelter that needs more support from the community, and this support is hard to recruit when judgment stands in the way.

Shelters that kill are often referred to by the general public as "kill shelters," a term that I comprehend but simultaneously find deeply problematic. While accurate in nature, this term scares away would-be adopters, volunteers, and donors, who proudly proclaim that they'd *never* support a "kill shelter." Simultaneously, many members of the public claim to only support "no-kill shelters" without fully understanding what these shelters' policies are. I believe one of the very first steps to being an effective advocate is to understand the structure of the movement; from this starting point, we can begin to see where we fit in as part of the solution. We must understand what kinds of shelters exist, how each one operates, and what support they need.

In general, there are two kinds of shelters: *municipal* shelters, which are typically *open admission*, and *private* shelters, which are typically *limited admission*. Most communities have at least one municipal shelter and perhaps one or even several private shelters.

A municipal shelter is run by the local government, usually a city or a county. These facilities are part of the government just like the police department or the fire department. As part of a governmental body, these organizations receive funding from their municipality, and they are contractually obligated to serve the public as a whole using their allotted budget. That means that they have to accept every single animal that is brought to them from within their contracted region—no matter what. That includes every owner-surrendered cat, dog, guinea pig, or snake; animals from hoarding situations or cruelty cases; stray and free-roaming animals from outside; sick and dying animals; and, yes, tons and tons of neonatal kittens who are way too young to be adopted.

When a shelter is contractually obligated to take in every animal, that's called being an *open-admission* animal shelter—they have an open door to everyone within the municipality. These are the shelters we tend to be talking about when we refer to "kill shelters," as they must continue to take in animals even if their resources are exhausted. When there aren't enough resources to save every animal in their care, those resources must be focused where they can do the most good, leaving more vulnerable populations such as neonatal kittens susceptible to euthanasia.

A private shelter, on the other hand, is a nonprofit organization; it is not run by the government. Private shelters can be open admission if contracted with the local government in a public-private partnership, but more commonly these organizations are *limited admission*, meaning they are under no obligation to take in every animal. A private organization is just that: it's private. They take on what they are able to take on, and no more. This means that if they're full, or if someone brings them an animal like a neonatal kitten whom they do not have the resources to care for, they can turn the animal away.

Because of this, limited-admission shelters are almost always going to be "no-kill." Makes sense, right? Rather than take in animals they don't have the ability to help, they simply don't accept them into the program. These organizations can determine exactly what they have the budget, space, and manpower to do, and then set out to do it, without taking on more than they can handle.

Understanding this core difference between open-admission and limited-admission shelter models is critical to understanding the killing of cats and kittens in shelters. One model is not better or worse than the other; they are simply different—and equally important. Open-admission municipal shelters are critical because without them, many animals are left without anywhere to go. Limited-admission shelters are essential, too, as they can take in overflow animals from the municipal shelters and have the flexibility to choose which populations they want to focus on. For instance, some private shelters have neonatal kitten nurseries, and others focus on special-needs animals. These groups are both completely essential for saving animals' lives.

The challenge is when we dichotomize "kill shelters" and "no-kill shelters," because this juxtaposition creates a judgment zone. "Kill" and "no-kill" are not perfect opposites; our success as a national movement is, in fact, interdependent. We must all work together and develop a more nuanced understanding of where we are and where we need to go—*together*.

In order to not kill, a shelter must have either fewer animals coming through its doors or sufficient support to save every animal who does. This means that while limited-admission shelters can achieve "no-kill" by focusing only on the lives they *can* save, open-admission shelters can only save every animal if they have enough support from the community.

It's important to note that "no-kill" does not even necessarily mean that kittens will be saved. The goal of the movement is to reach a day where every healthy or treatable animal is saved—but we have to keep in mind that even many leading organizations do not consider kittens under eight weeks old "healthy and treatable." While I am a massive supporter of the movement, I also think it's important to be honest with the public about what we mean when we say "no-kill." My hope is that as we develop a greater awareness of the numbers of kittens dying in shelters, the public will respond with support, and the movement will be inspired to expand its definition to include neonatal kittens as well.

FOR THE KITTENS, FOR THE HUMANS

I'll never forget one of the most devastating and beautiful conversations I've ever had at an event. A woman approached me with tears in her eyes, sharing that she'd been employed by her local open-admission shelter for years and had been made to euthanize hundreds of kittens in that time due to lack of resources. As she hugged me, we both cried. My heart broke for her—a brave, compassionate, and hurting person. She told me that the increase in community awareness is having a real impact on the number of kittens being saved in her shelter through foster care. She asked me to keep advocating, and told me that she will be pushing ahead, too, as hard as it might be. With a lump in my throat, it hit me that kitten advocacy doesn't just save animals . . . it saves people, too. I will never forget her words.

When we buy into the rhetoric that people who work in open-admission shelters enjoy killing animals, we are spitting in the faces of some of the bravest people in our movement. It takes a bold, loving, selfless person to stand at the center of the storm, doing triage. Those of us on the sidelines must bring compassion and awareness to the animal-loving community, and learn to extend a helpful and gentle hand to our courageous friends working in shelters. We must all find it in ourselves to do our tiny part toward a day when shelters are sufficiently supported so that they are safer spaces for animals and humans alike.

A truly no-kill nation is not far away, and we can each do our part to make it happen. In order to achieve a safer future for felines, there are three essential components: policies, programs, and participants. First, the shelter administration and local government have a duty to develop ordinances and organizational *policies* that create opportunities to save lives. Then, the shelter has to take the next step by creating *programs* that serve each vulnerable population, such as a TNR program for community cats and a foster program for kittens. Finally, and most important, the community must supply *participants*. Even a shelter with progressive policies and programs still cannot succeed without us—the community. A foster program is nothing without foster parents; a TNR program does not exist without trappers.

With this understanding, we can start to see that killing is not a shelter problem; it's a community problem with a community solution. It's the responsibility of the shelter to create these policies and programs, but it's ultimately the responsibility of the public to participate in them. When kittens are coming through the doors in boxes and buckets, their fate is not in the hands of the shelter employee; it's in *our* hands. By participating in community-based programs like fostering, we enable a shelter's lifesaving capacity to expand exponentially—stretching out beyond the limited square footage of four concrete walls and into the safe haven of our homes.

While it can be distressing to peel back the curtain and begin to understand how many cards are stacked against kittens, doing so is our first step to being part of the solution. Knowing where we stand today enables us to be aspirational in the actions that lead to tomorrow, and to keep the wheel in motion. My belief is that animal welfare is at an exciting turning point, and that we have a tremendous opportunity to do good by extending our awareness and efforts to the *unadoptable* populations. In the next chapters, we'll take a deep dive into the lifesaving actions we can take for these vulnerable kittens through prevention programs and fostering.

CHAPTER TWO

IT'S RAINING KITTENS:
HOW TO STOP THE FLOOD

RIDDLE ME THIS

Here's a riddle for you. What can you love with your whole heart, but simultaneously not want more of?

Pizza and kittens.

Turns out it *is* possible to have too much of a good thing! Just like an overstuffed belly can't accommodate another slice, an overpopulated community can't save more kittens than it has the capacity to help. Whether we're talking full stomachs or full shelters—full is full. I love kittens, but we certainly don't need more of them! That's why one of the primary ways to

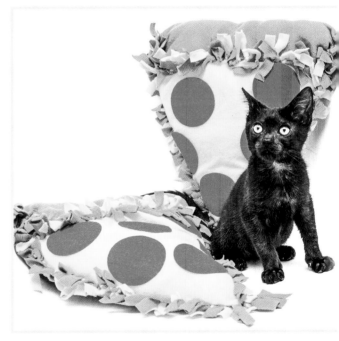

save kittens is to actively prevent more of them from being born. When we decrease the number of kittens being born each year, we get closer to a day when every kitten has a safe place to thrive.

You know what they say: April showers bring May kittens! Okay, maybe that's not what *everyone* says, but it's certainly true. Kitten season is a phenomenon wherein breeding occurs rampantly during the warm seasons, flooding animal shelters with an often unmanageable number of litters. Kitten season hits at different times depending on the location's weather and sunlight; for instance, many mid-Atlantic caregivers see very few kittens between October and March, but in the sunny South, kitten season can be nearly year-round. As it turns out, humans aren't the only species that get spring fever.

So why does kitten season occur? It has a lot to do with cats' heat cycles, which occur most frequently in a warm and sunny climate. Female cats' heat cycles are dependent on the presence of abundant daylight due to the impact of the sun on the body's hormones. During the darker, shorter days of winter, cats' melatonin levels increase and they are less likely to breed, but as the days become longer and melatonin decreases, cats are more likely to be on the prowl for a mate. This means kitten caregivers are typically swamped with babies during the summer, but get a nice winter break. Heat cycles and cold weather don't mix!

Kitten season is a perfect storm. Cats reach sexual maturity very young, and are able to become pregnant as young as four months of age. They have short gestation periods, with an average of roughly sixty-three days, and large litter sizes, with an average of five kittens. This means that cats breed young, often, and in high numbers. Oy vey.

Cats are amazingly adaptive creatures, and it makes sense that they have evolved to reproduce seasonally so that their offspring are more likely

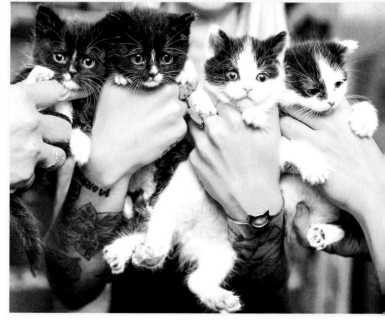

Kitten season is a handful for animal shelters.

to survive the outdoor conditions. Tragically, while they may be more likely to survive outdoors in the sunshine than in a snowstorm, the rapid increase in reproduction means that they're also entering shelters at a dangerous rate during the warm months. The major spike in the population can severely wear on shelters' resources, making it a challenge to find placement for every animal. That's why fostering is truly a perfect spring/summer activity.

I CAME TO SPAY

With hundreds of thousands of cats and kittens being killed annually, prevention programs are paramount. Spay/neuter efforts have long been a top priority for the animal welfare community, and for good reason: sterilization programs are proven to play a significant role in decreasing the intake and euthanasia of cats and dogs in animal shelters.[1] But while we may have come a long way in spay/neuter awareness, when it comes to decreasing the kitten population, we've still got a long, long way to go.

Over the past decade, there has been tremendous effort put into decreasing the number of feline pregnancies through sterilization. Advances in veterinary medicine have resulted in the rise of pediatric spay/neuter, allowing veterinarians to perform surgery on kittens at two pounds and two months of age, eliminating the risk of accidental pregnancy (read more about pediatric sterilization on page 237). Low-cost spay/neuter clinics are popping up across the country, making services more accessible than ever to rescue groups and members of the public. As spay/neuter surgeries have become more affordable and expanded toward pediatric patients, sterilization has become an essential component of adoption programs. While it used to be fairly common for organizations to adopt out cats who were intact, it is now a standard policy for all animals in a shelter to be sterilized prior to adoption. Millions of dollars in funds are granted to sterilization programs every year in hopes of reducing the number of animals who need homes.

In spite of this fantastic progress, many people still fail to have cats and kittens sterilized due to lack of funds, transportation, or awareness, or even due to delayed surgery that results in an accidental pregnancy. Every day I receive messages about pregnant pet cats, or read comments from people who are thrilled to share that their companion cat has just given birth to kittens. While cat-lovers may be excited to experience "the miracle of life," the truth is that increasing the number of kittens in need is anything but miraculous. We must continue to respectfully educate the community about the urgent need to reduce the number of cats born each year.

But as important as it is to help pet cats get sterilized, by far the largest obstacle we have to overcome is the lack of awareness about the importance of sterilizing outdoor community cats. While many people do understand the responsibility of spaying and neutering the cats in their home, the average cat-lover does not grasp the importance of actively extending that support to the unowned cats living outside in their neighborhood. But whether the cat is a cuddly companion or a feral feline, spaying and neutering is critical, because sterilizing pet cats actually addresses only a small sliver of the feline population. Spend just a season rescuing kittens, and you'll have no question that our efforts need to extend beyond our doorstep and into the great outdoors.

FROM THE STREETS

Kittens come from the darnedest places, I tell ya. Over the years, I've rescued kittens from some of the most bizarre, unexpected origins. Kittens like Scraps, a tiny tuxedo I found curled up in a compost bin in my friend's garden. Kittens like Kiwi, a little tortie I pulled from a bush in front of a busy restaurant. Kittens like Gadzooks, a teeny tabby who was living underneath the hood of a car. I used to joke that if you want to find a kitten, all you have to do is step outside, open your eyes, and pivot.

For years, I offered these kittens refuge and care, never understanding how so many were wandering outside alone. Looking back, it's unbelievable to me that it took me so long to make the connection. Here I was, managing what felt like a constant flood of kittens, without taking a moment to consider the source of the flow. As advocates, we must not only find better ways to save the lives of those in need, but also trace their stories to their sources in order to understand how to change the future.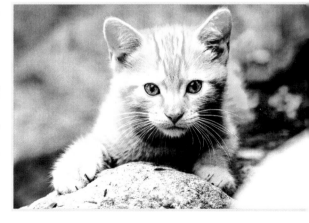

And their beginnings are almost always identical: they are coming from the streets.

Every time I rescue a kitten from outside, people want to know what kind of horrible person would have abandoned the kitten under a porch or in a trash can. Yet the answer is simple. Who would put a kitten outside? Her mother would! Porches, bushes, compost bins, and even dumpsters make great shelter for cats, so it's common to find that nursing moms have placed their kittens in these makeshift hideaways. The vast majority of kittens found outdoors aren't abandoned—they are simply there because that's where they were born. Research suggests that roughly 80 percent of new kittens born each year are born outdoors to free-roaming cats.[2] Their mothers are typically unowned, unsterilized cats who may be right around the corner, roaming the neighborhood in search of their daily meal.

NEW KITTENS BORN ANNUALLY

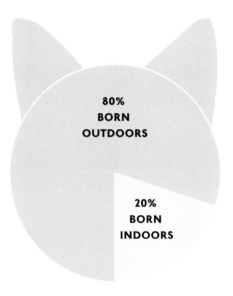

80%
BORN
OUTDOORS

20%
BORN
INDOORS

Unfortunately, it's all too common for Good Samaritans to stumble upon kittens outdoors and, assuming they've been abandoned, pick them up and take them away from their mother. What happens next depends on the individual who found them. They may try to care for the kittens themselves, either successfully or unsuccessfully. They may bring the kittens to an animal shelter, a veterinary clinic, or a pet store, all of which are often unable to provide the care the kittens need. It's tragically ironic that those who think they have saved an abandoned animal are often responsible for setting into motion a series of events that ultimately leads to the kitten's untimely death.

Even when orphaned kittens end up in the care of a rescuer like me, they are at a disadvantage. The fact is that while I may be a pro at working with orphans, I will never be able to raise a kitten like a mama cat can. When a kitten is separated from her mother, it requires immense resources and energy to keep her alive. After eight weeks of pouring my heart and soul into these motherless babies, it always hurts me to know that as I work so hard to save their lives, their mothers and fathers are often still out there on the street . . . procreating more and more. This is why I believe we have a duty to educate our communities about why so many kittens are outside to begin with, and why it is so important to decrease the kitten population by spaying and neutering community cats.

TRAILER PARK GIRLS: BANJO AND FIDDLE

It was a winding and beautiful drive through the West Virginia mountains to get to the county animal shelter. I'd been brought in to teach the local animal control officers a hands-on workshop about how to trap outdoor community cats for sterilization, and I traveled in a car full of trapping supplies. The officers had identified a trailer park that was a major source of problems for their community—for years, kittens and cats had been surrendered from that location, and neighbor complaints about the cats were frequent. I couldn't wait to help them solve the problem.

After teaching the classroom portion of the workshop, we drove caravan-style past luscious green trees, over creeks and streams, deep into the hills. Nestled in the forest was a community of about twenty trailers, and the moment we pulled up, I knew it was going to be an intense afternoon. Cats darted across the road, lay sprawled on the grass, and hid in the shade of cars. Within just one minute of arriving I saw half a dozen cats pop in and out of the open windows of one trailer, coming and going as they pleased. "Yep. That's the lady who puts out all the food," an animal control officer said with a sigh.

I knocked on the door, and it slowly opened with a creak. An elderly woman in a pink muumuu and thick glasses emerged, and at her bare feet two young cats chased each other out into the yard. "Hi there, my name is Hannah, and I'm here to help your cats."

I talked with her for several minutes, reassuring her that we didn't want to take her cats away—that, in fact, I loved her compassionate heart and simply wanted to help her have a better experience and to get the population under control by getting everyone spayed and neutered. The situation was clearly out of hand, but fortunately the county was willing to work with her as long as the animals were sterilized. The officers and I set out traps throughout the property next to the trailers, in the woods, in driveways, and under porches. One by one, the cats went into the traps and we loaded them into the officers' vehicles in preparation for surgery. As the sun was setting, we felt confident that we'd gotten as many as we could that day and began to pack up. And that's when I heard a tiny muffled noise.

Meowww!

"Do you hear that?" I wondered if I had made it up. "I swear, I think I just heard a little meow." I stood still and waited.

Meowww! Meowww!

"Where on earth could that be coming from?" I ducked down, looking under the porch. Nothing. Under the car. Nothing. Still, more little meows came.

I got on my hands and knees and pressed my ear against the bottom of the trailer, which had a vinyl covering that wrapped over its base.

MEOWWW!

"Oh my god. I think there is a kitten trapped underneath the house." Before I knew it, I was prying back the vinyl and peeking my head inside. The underbelly of the trailer was about two and a half feet high and pitch-black, but my flashlight revealed a dirt floor crawling with bugs and fuzzy pink insulation above. I moved my light from side to side until it illuminated a small stack of cinder blocks, and inside one I spotted a tiny black-and-white kitten, meowing her head off.

"I see you! I'm coming!"

Of course, where there are unsterilized cats, there will be kittens. The act of feeding cats is a compassionate one, but without additionally spaying and neutering the population, this cat colony had been enabled to grow and grow. Although the officers and I were there to put an end to that, the fact remained that in the moment, kittens were there—and they needed help.

Hunched over, I slowly crawled across the dirt floor, holding my flashlight in one hand and batting away cobwebs with the other. *Oh my god, this is so gross*, I thought, but I knew I wanted to get that little kitten. Spiders ran over my shoes and jumped onto my arms. *Just look straight ahead. Get the kitten and get out.* The meows got louder and louder as I shuffled closer.

"Oh no! There's another one!" I looked up into the insulation and saw that a mama cat and her calico kitten had made themselves a bed. I sighed. This wasn't going to be easy. Approaching the kitten in the cinder block, I cautiously extended a hand. She was surprisingly unafraid. I picked her up, held her against my chest, and shuffled my way back out. She was about five weeks old—the perfect age to be weaned and socialized for adoption. I knew I'd be able to get her a great home in due time.

By this point, the sun had set and everyone was ready to leave . . . except me. I was so determined to get the mama cat and the other kitten that I didn't want to return to my hotel. I went back under the trailer, but to my frustration couldn't get anywhere near the pair—the mama wouldn't budge, and the little calico just kept running deeper and deeper into the insulation. The day was over and I knew I had to let it go. The officers made a plan to come back and trap the mama and the other baby, so I reluctantly packed up to leave. At least I'd gotten the one.

But as I walked to the car, I just felt more and more angry at myself for not getting the second kitten out of there. She was right at the age where she could be socialized, and I knew that by leaving her behind I risked having her grow past socialization age. I couldn't get myself to leave. *I am getting that darn kitten.* So after the officers had left, there I was, underneath this elderly woman's house, late at night, covered in bugs and filth, still trying to get this little calico. The harder I tried, the less I cared about the spiders in my hair. I had my eyes on the prize.

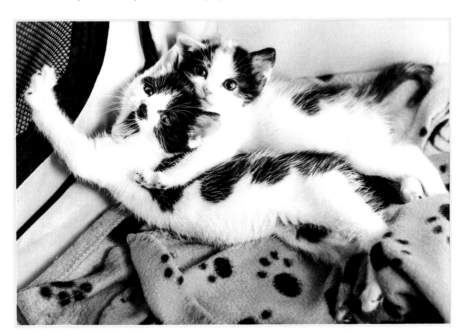

By the time I emerged with the calico, I was covered head to toe in dirt and cobwebs, and laughing hysterically in the moonlight. Unlike her sister, this kitten was tense and not amused by me. "Oh my god, little one. I can't believe I got you. You're going to have such a good life, I promise. Trust me."

I got back to my hotel and set them up in the bathroom with some food and water, which they gobbled up right away. I sat with them, gently talking and offering little scritches to their heads and cheeks. Though they were skeptical at first, their tension slowly melted into trust, and soon we were all fast friends. I named them Banjo and Fiddle, and the three of us returned to Washington, DC, together, where they spent the next few weeks being prepared for adoption.

Banjo and Fiddle's home colony was sterilized, and their feral mama was spayed so that no more kittens would be born under the trailer in the future. Now that the population was stable, the sweet woman in the muumuu could keep feeding her feline friends without sending the shelter an unending stream of kittens from the trailer park. Case closed!

As for Banjo and Fiddle, they made it out at the perfect age: old enough to leave mom, but young enough to become acquainted with human affection. By the time Banjo and Fiddle made it to adoption age, they were the cuddliest kittens on the planet, and they were adopted into a loving home by a man who adores them. Inspired by their story, their adopter became involved in not just kitten rescue but also kitten *prevention*. He is now active in fostering and sterilizing all the would-be kitten parents in his community.

MEET THE PAWRENTS

So who are all these cats giving birth under trailers and in the bushes, and where did they come from? Before getting active in kitten rescue, I had no idea that so many unowned outdoor cats populated the streets of the United States. But after years of working to end kitten euthanasia, I now know that this is a classic case of the chicken and the egg; we can't understand how to help kittens without first understanding how to help their parents. I now dedicate a large portion of my work to raising awareness about these free-roaming felines: community cats.

Community cats are unowned outdoor cats who live in family groups called colonies. While some refer to them as feral cats, I find that the term "community cat" is a much more accurate descriptor for the population of cats who live out-doors. "Feral" describes behavior that not every free-roaming cat exhibits, while "community cat" refers to the place where these cats live and is thus an all-encompassing description: they are part of the community, just like you and me. Some research suggests that roughly half the cats living in the United States are community cats, though an accurate number is impossible to estimate at this time.

Community cats are incredibly resourceful animals, and they may have one, two, or even ten food sources, including caregivers in the neighborhood, refuse, and even small rodents. They tend to congregate around densely populated urban areas due to the abundance of resources available, such as shelter and human food waste, but they are also commonly found in rural areas near farms and in suburban areas near businesses and housing developments. Simply put, wherever there are people, there are bound to be community cats. And where there are unsterilized commu-nity cats, there are bound to be kittens!

While community cats can exhibit a wide range of social behaviors, many of them are undersocialized to humans because they have had limited interaction with us, up close and personal. They may be friendly, feral, or somewhere in the middle, but the less early exposure they had to human touch, the more likely they are to be on the feral end of the spectrum. Don't fear these cats—while the term "feral" can call to mind a negative connotation, most community cats aren't fero-cious to humans unless cornered. Feral cat behavior tends to be avoidant rather than aggressive! As stealthy and sleek as cats are, they can make themselves scarce if they don't want to be seen. That's why when you find kittens outside, it's common that no mother is in sight; she's probably hiding from you!

While some may be surprised to find that there are so many community cats outdoors, their presence in our lives is anything but new. I like to think of commu-nity cats as the original cat, as our relationship with them can be traced back all the way to the advent of agriculture in the Fertile Crescent, over ten thousand years ago! As humans began successfully growing and storing grains, farms be-came a haven for rodents seeking food. And who did the rodents attract? You guessed it. All cats we know today are descendants of the wildcats, *Felis silvestris lybica*, that lived alongside early human civilizations. In a fascinating 2017 paleoge-netics study, researchers found that cats initially spread from their home in the Near East along the pathways of the farming and trade movements, being utilized for rodent abatement on ships and eventually settling throughout nearly every corner of the world. These untamed mousers weren't considered domesticated pets for the majority of our shared history. That is, until the 1947 invention of cat litter became popularized in the late 1950s and 1960s, bringing these community cats indoors . . . and changing our relationship with felines forever.

If you look at our 10,000-plus years of history living alongside cats, it's only within the blink of an eye that we've been keeping them as indoor pets. Yet as a few generations have passed, we've forgotten where cats originally came from. Today, cats are still living in large numbers the way they always have: outdoors, in symbiosis with human populations. While the goal might be to change the future of cats, we can't strategize about where we are headed if we don't acknowledge where they come from, and where they currently stand. I believe it's critical for us to recognize that we're not standing at the end of the domestication timeline—if anything, we're only halfway there.

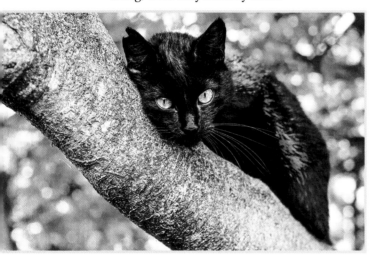

Tragically, we often fail to meet the needs of this population. In the absence of a community cat program, these cats are frequently killed in shelters because they are not candidates for adoption. In many cases, they may be picked up by caring individuals who believe they are lost cats and bring them to a shelter in an attempt to help them. In other scenarios, they may be dropped off by complainants, or they may even be picked up by animal control officers. In any case, once they make it to the animal shelter, the majority aren't suitable for an adoptive home because they are so often undersocialized. If no program exists to save their lives, many shelters have no solution for these cats aside from euthanasia.

Because of their unique needs, which are distinct from those of the pet cats we see in adoption programs, community cats and neonatal kittens make up the two largest feline populations killed in shelters. If you're an advocate for kittens, it's essential that you're an advocate for their parents, community cats, too. After all, community cats and kittens are two sides of the same coin, and their fates are intertwined. We must fight for them simultaneously.

Like kittens, community cats are a deeply misunderstood population, and that misunderstanding prevents the public from knowing how to help. It's therefore critically important to increase public awareness about who community cats are, why there are so many kittens outside, and what to do when you find a feline. I believe that a large reason we don't understand community cats is the narrative we construct around them.

If you look at the language we use to talk about cats who are found outdoors, it's almost always presumptive of prior habitation in a human home. We refer to them as "stray," implying that they are lost and have wandered away from a guardian, or as "homeless," falsely portraying them as being without a home base of their own. But community cats are not lost or homeless; the outdoors is their home. They have deep connections with their surrounding habitats, forming relationships with other cats in their colonies and establishing routines and patterns just like we do. When we fail to understand community cats, it becomes much more confusing for the public to understand why there are so many kittens outside. This results in another misused term: many people will call kittens from outside "abandoned," implying that the kitten has been cruelly discarded by a human, when in reality outdoor kittens are almost always there because they were *born* there—in a community cat colony!

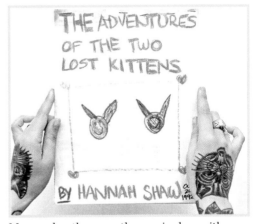

This misuse of language is detrimental in a number of ways. For starters, lack of public awareness about community cats causes people to assume that any kitten found outside will be motherless. This results in kittens becoming orphaned simply because our society does not realize that their parents—community cats—are living all around us. Additionally, our assumption that outdoor cats are lost pets causes us to look upon them with pity that they don't get a warm lap to sit on or a windowsill from which to observe the world. This pity erases the cat's own desires, which may have nothing to do with

My grandmother recently surprised me with a funny creation from my childhood: a story I had written on construction paper in 1992, titled "The Adventures of the Two Lost Kittens." Growing up, I shared the common assumption that any kittens outside must be lost. Now I know that they are typically born to community cats!

a human home. Consequently, staggering numbers of community cats are killed in shelters every year because they have been surrendered by people who were trying to give them a better life, thus robbing them of the good life they already had. But perhaps the most damaging effect of the lack of awareness of community cats is the hindering of our ability to do widespread, impactful work for them and their kittens. After all, we can't change what we don't understand.

We also use this harmful language within the animal sheltering industry, much to the detriment of the cats we are tasked with saving. When keeping data on cats who enter animal shelters, we tend to have five options for the origin of the animal:

- Stray/at large (found outdoors)
- Relinquished by owner (surrendered to be put up for adoption)
- Owner-requested euthanasia (surrendered to be euthanized)
- Transferred in (coming from another shelter or agency)
- Other intakes (miscellaneous)

More than half of all cats entering US animal shelters are classified in the system as "stray," but unlike stray dogs, who are often truly lost or abandoned, the vast majority of these "stray" cats aren't lost at all; they are simply unowned.[3] This accounts for the major difference in owner reclamation with cats and dogs: while 33.9 percent of lost dogs were reclaimed in 2016, only 4.7 percent of "lost" cats are reunited with an owner, according to Shelter Animals Count. These cats often are not reclaimed because they never had a home to begin with. When the animal welfare industry itself offers no option for quantifying the number of animals coming into shelters who are not lost but are, in fact, community cats and kittens, it becomes immeasurably more difficult to make impactful policies and to change public awareness of issues affecting these animals. Policies are built on data, and our data is skewed by misleading criteria; we are measuring the wrong things. Community cats need their own language just as much as they need their own programs.

None of this is to say that cats shouldn't be indoor companions; my personal cats are indoor-only (aside from the occasional walk on a harness!), and my entire career is spent bringing kittens *off* the streets and placing them into indoor homes. Rather, this is to suggest that on a small scale, we must meet cats where they are in order to save their lives, and on a larger scale, we have to be realistic and honest about our starting point if we want to be pragmatic about achieving change. Like it or not, we are starting with the reality that tens of millions of cats live outdoors in the United States, and without a cultural shift and a plan of action, we will be dealing with orphaned kittens and high euthanasia rates for years to come.

With so many community cats living in close proximity to humans, people are going to be finding a lot of kittens—and we have the option of making a big difference in their lives through our kind actions. But we must start at an understanding of their context, recognizing first that not all cats who wander are lost.

STARTING AT THE SOURCE

Anyone who works in cat welfare knows that the source of kittens is community cats, but in order to create effective policies and programs, it's essential to examine the data. Time and time again, research shows that kittens are coming primarily from the outdoors. "The sheer numbers and high reproductive capacity of community cats combine to make them the leading source of new kitten births," according to a study led by Dr. Julie Levy, a renowned veterinary scientist and professor of shelter medicine.[4]

Perhaps the best national statistics available at this time come from Shelter Animals Count, an initiative that compiles data from more than three thousand organizations to demonstrate trends in intakes and outcomes for cats and dogs in the United States. Upon examining their 2017 intake records of more than 1.5 million cats, it's plain to see that the single largest population entering shelters is kittens (up to five months in age) who are found outside (stray/at large).

CAT INTAKES 2017				
	Adult	Up to 5 Months	Age Unknown	Total
Stray/At Large	300,926	369,179	141,929	812,034
Relinquished by Owner	199,676	134,194	41,919	375,789
Owner-Intended Euthanasia	21,128	2,071	3,662	26,861
Transferred from Another Agency	81,864	100,206	23,457	205,527
Other	41,109	30,565	10,836	82,510
Total	644,703	636,215	221,803	1,502,721

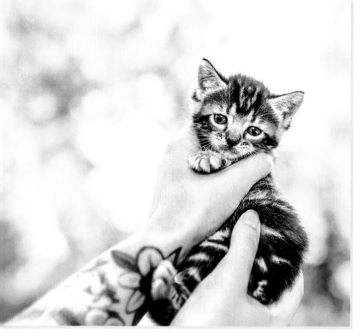

Awareness that cats from outdoors—and particularly their kittens—comprise the majority of animals entering shelters should be enough to stop all animal welfare advocates in their tracks. We absolutely must be directing attention to these free-roaming kittens and their abundant source: community cats. It raises the question: If kitten season is a flood, do we spend all our time mopping the floor, or do we try to plug the leak?

TNR: A KITTEN-PREVENTION PROGRAM

Sterilizing community cats is the number one way to prevent kittens and to save the lives of community cats. This is done through a process called TNR, or trap-neuter-return.

Trap-neuter-return is a process through which community cats are humanely trapped, brought to a veterinarian for spay/neuter and vaccination, eartipped, held overnight for recovery, and then returned to their outdoor home. This gives cats the ability to continue living out their natural lives in their colonies, while stabilizing the population so no new kittens can be born. Over time, populations naturally decline. This decreases the life span of the colony while increasing the life span of the individual cat—a win-win for everyone.

The most beautiful thing about TNR is that it lowers the number of animals both entering animal shelters and being killed there. Levy's 2014 study at the University of Florida found that after targeting one region with community cat spay/neuter, 66 percent fewer cats from the target zone came into the animal shelter, and euthanasia for cats from that region decreased by a whopping 95 percent.[5] Similarly, the Fairfax County Animal Shelter in Fairfax, Virginia, saw a 41 percent decrease in their orphaned kitten intake after three years of TNR, which makes sense, because outdoor cats were no longer breeding rampantly![6] By integrating a community cat program into their work, this shelter was able to decrease the number of cats in the shelter, making it possible to find all the remaining cats and kittens foster homes and adopters. Bravo!

TNR and kitten rescue go hand in hand; think of TNR as a kitten-prevention plan. If you've rescued a kitten from outside, you should also be ensuring that the remaining colony is sterilized. Conversely, if you're sterilizing community cats, you should make sure you have a plan for any kittens who are found. One thing is sure: once you get out there on the streets, you'll be able to make a world of difference for the felines in your community. A trap and a spay keep the kittens away!

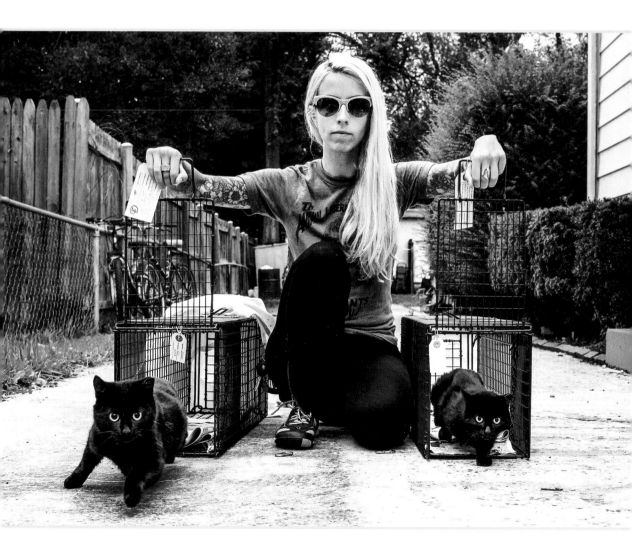

An eartip is the universal sign that a community cat has been sterilized. If you see a cat outside, the first thing you'll want to do is identify whether she has an eartip so

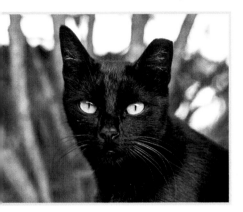

you can determine if she needs to be TNR'd or not. An eartip is the removal of the top three-eighths of an inch of the cat's ear, which is done while under anesthesia. It doesn't cause cats any pain or loss of function, but it does gain them a world of protections. Eartips help caregivers like you and me identify that a cat has already been sterilized, so if we see him outside, we know not to trap him again. Many municipalities are even enacting eartip protection laws to prevent the unnecessary impoundment of cats who have been through the TNR program. Eartips save lives!

DOUGIE FROM THE BLOCK

The DC summer heat is sticky and sweltering, so on a hot July afternoon my friend Katherine and I were hiding out in her air-conditioned apartment, drinking cold seltzers and catching up. "You know, there are a few cats living in the bushes outside my place, and I'm positive they're not sterilized. In fact, I think one might be a kitten," she told me. I hadn't noticed them when I came over, but my curiosity was piqued, so we put our shoes on and headed downstairs to take a look. As we stepped outdoors, a wave of humidity hit my face.

I looked to the left and gasped. She was right: not only were a mom and a large kitten sitting right outside of the bushes, but the kitten was nursing! The mom tensed up and stared me down, and the kitten scooted sideways so he could watch me out of one skeptical eye, but he never took his mouth off his mama's breast. There we stood, getting the stink-eye from this huge kitten, who seemed way too old to be breast-feeding, and his mama, who was clearly a well-fed community cat who had never been spayed.

As I kneeled down to greet them, they both darted off down the block. The kitten was what I call a "cusp kitten." At about eleven weeks old, he was just on the verge of being too old to socialize for adoption. I knew that if I waited even a week, the window for socialization would close—maybe it already had. So I hopped in my car, drove home to pick up traps and bait, and came back with all the gear I needed to catch the cats.

I set my traps with stinky tuna and sardines, hid them under the bushes, and waited. My friend and I watched from about fifteen feet away as the mama cat, a black beauty, stepped cautiously into the trap. One little step at a time, she inched toward the back of the trap until . . . *click!* She stepped on the trip plate and the door closed. As I approached to cover the trap with a blanket, she hissed and rammed the side of the trap. She was not a happy mama.

Next, I needed to catch the kitten. Without his mama around, he was more skittish than ever. He ran back and forth, bopping around the block, unsure about entering the trap. I moved it several times, trying to place it somewhere that felt stable and natural to walk into. "Little kitten, I have delicious snacks! Come and get 'em!" I said in a singsongy voice, laughing at myself. For a while it was like we were doing a dance together, but as the sun set, I finally started to get in sync with him. I placed the trap against a brick wall and walked off out of sight. We waited, and waited, and finally heard the sound every trapper waits for: *click!* The door was shut and the kitten was caught. I looked up at the sign on the corner, which read DOUGLAS ST NE. "Nice to meet you, Douglas," I said, and loaded the kitten and his mama into my car.

That night, I put the two traps in my bathroom in preparation for the TNR clinic the following day. The mom was clearly going to be eartipped, but I wasn't so sure about the kitten—I needed to assess him and see if he was a candidate for socialization. After a few hours of settling in, I lifted the cover from his trap and he sat there, still as a statue, looking at me. As I spoke with him, he cocked his head to the side like a confused puppy dog. He took a baby step toward me, then two steps back. One more toward me, then back again. While he was scared, he seemed open to the idea of human interaction.

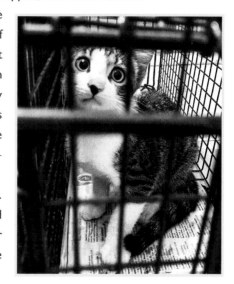

The following morning the two went in for surgery. The mama was sterilized, vaccinated, and eartipped, and after she recovered, she was returned to her outdoor home, where she still lives (and thrives!) today. The little boy was neutered, but instead of being returned to the block, I brought him home to recover in a playpen. Cautiously curious, he would allow me to scratch his head, but would gently hiss as if to say, "I like this, but I also hate this." For days the only sound I heard from Douglas was a hiss, but every time I worked with him, he got a little more comfortable, until he was eventually leaning into my pets. I knew it would be only a matter of time before I had him eating from the palm of my hand . . . literally.

Just like we'd done our trapping dance, we now did a dance of socialization. I'd move in with chin rubs and wet food, and he'd slowly get more and more comfortable with the idea that I was safe. I'd hold his food in my hand, and he'd nibble on it but keep his distance. Four days passed of actively talking to him, hand-feeding him, and teaching him physical affection, and when the fifth morning came, I couldn't believe my ears.

Meow! Meow! Meow! Douglas' little vocalizations were suddenly reverberating throughout my home, high-pitched and constant. I ran into the room to see why he was crying, as I'd never heard him make a single peep (aside from hissing!). To my surprise, when I walked in, he jumped into my lap and let out a long "meoooooooow." Seemingly overnight, he'd transformed from a cautious kitty to a needy sweetie! I

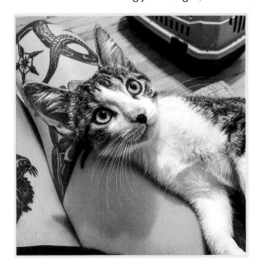

cracked up. This tough street kitty who had started out so hissy was now completely obsessed with me—following me around, meowing, and begging for me to pay attention to him.

Douglas was adopted just one week after he was trapped, setting the record for one of the quickest kitten adoptions I've ever done. I still see his mama on Douglas Street, where she has a daily caregiver who feeds and shelters her. When I see her eartip, it puts a smile on my face to know that I was able to stop the cycle of reproduction so that Douglas is the last kitten I'll ever have to lure from the bushes on that block.

When you work with kittens outdoors, knowing how to humanely trap a cat is essential. Most of the time trapping is done using a humane box trap, which is a metal box that encloses the cat safely and harmlessly. Inside the box trap, a small trip plate is set, which triggers the door to close when the cat walks to the back of the trap to eat the bait.

Trapping can sound overwhelming, but it's a simple, impactful, and really fun activity that anyone can learn to do. Here's a step-by-step guide to get you out there!

Plan

🐱 **Get to know the colony.** First things first, you'll want to know how many cats and kittens are in the colony in order to properly prepare. By setting out food at the same time each day and observing from a distance, you can track how many cats and kittens are present. Get to know where the cats spend their time, who they are, and when they like to come around. Note if there are kittens, cats with eartips, etc. Plan to trap every cat or kitten without an eartip in the colony.

🐱 **Communicate with the neighborhood.** Determine if the area where you want to trap is on private property, and talk with the owners of the property, as well as the surrounding neighbors, to obtain permission before trapping. A little communication goes a long way, and can help people understand what you're doing and why it's so important. Talking with neighbors will also help you determine if any of the cats in the neighborhood are in fact pets, and other people in the neighborhood might even be able to tip you off to the location of kittens, other caregivers, and more!

🐱 **Make a spay/neuter appointment with a vet clinic.** You'll need to have an appointment at a clinic in order to start trapping. Note that many private practice vets do not accept community cats for surgery, so you'll need to find a spay/neuter clinic that offers TNR services. Once you have your appointment, you can make your trapping plan!

- 🐱 **Prep their bellies!** Feeding the cats at the same time every day will get them on a routine. You can feed them in a dish, or if you have the traps ahead of time, you can slowly get them used to eating from the trap (just don't set the trip plate until you're ready to catch them, and keep the door locked open with a clip!). On the day before you trap, withhold food—you want them to be hungry enough to be willing to go into the trap.

- 🐱 **Gather supplies.** Most of the supplies you'll need are cheap or free, but since most of us don't have a cat trap at home, that's the one piece you'll likely need to borrow or buy. Many animal shelters or TNR groups have trap loan programs, so call around and see if you can borrow what you need. Otherwise, you can purchase a trap online or at many hardware or feed stores. To trap a cat, you'll need the following supplies:

  - 🐱 A humane box trap (preferably enough traps for every cat in the colony)
  - 🐱 Newspaper or cardboard (to line the trap)
  - 🐱 Bait (I prefer tuna in oil, mackerel, or stinky wet food)
  - 🐱 A trap cover (a sheet or large towel)
  - 🐱 Tarp (to line your vehicle and overnight space)

Trap

- 🐱 **Pick a time and place.** Plan to trap on the day before your vet appointment, during the time of day that the cats are used to eating. Make sure you're putting the trap on a level surface in an area that the cat or kitten is likely to go. Most cats will feel safest going into a trap that is in a covered or partially contained area, such as behind a bush, under a porch, or alongside a building.

- 🐱 **Count your traps.** Make sure you know exactly how many traps you put out, and where, so you can collect them all and ensure you haven't left any behind. Don't miss this crucial step!

- 🐱 **Prep your traps.** Line the base of the trap with a folded piece of newspaper or a flat piece of cardboard. Ensure that it is smooth across the bottom so the cat can comfortably walk into the trap. Place a large spoonful of bait on the back end of the trap, behind the trip plate. Place one or two pea-sized bites at the front to entice the cat. Partially cover the trap with your trap cover. Set the trap and exit the area.

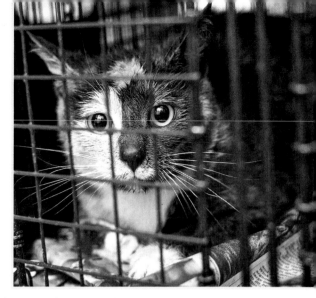

Bait 'n wait. Once the traps are set, stay close enough to see if the cats go into the trap, but far enough away to allow them to comfortably explore. Hang out in your car, listen to some music or a podcast, and watch from a distance until the cats start entering the traps.

Peek and cover. Once a cat enters the trap, take a quick peek to ensure you know who you got. Is the cat eartipped or wearing a collar? If so, release her. Is the cat actually a raccoon? If so, release her. If you've caught the cat or kitten you've intended to catch, cover the trap completely with a blanket to help calm him down.

Hold overnight. If you can't go straight to the clinic and must hold the cat overnight, choose a safe, climate-controlled holding area such as a spare room or bathroom. Line the floor with a tarp and keep the cat inside the covered trap. Never touch, bother, or take the cat out of the trap before surgery.

Spay/Neuter

Drop 'em off. To transport the cats to the clinic, place a layer of tarp down in the car to protect the vehicle, then place the covered traps over it. Once at the clinic, fill out the paperwork and indicate the services you would like. You'll always want a spay/neuter, FVRCP and rabies vaccines, pain medication, and an eartip, but you may also decide to include a microchip, flea treatment, or other services.

Pick 'em up. After surgery, cats may be groggy from anesthesia. Read the discharge paperwork and ask any questions you have.

Hold overnight. If the clinic will hold them overnight for you, great! If not, you'll need to hold them for recovery in your climate-controlled holding area. Monitor the cat for any signs of lethargy, vomiting, or bleeding. If you're concerned about the cat's recovery, call the clinic.

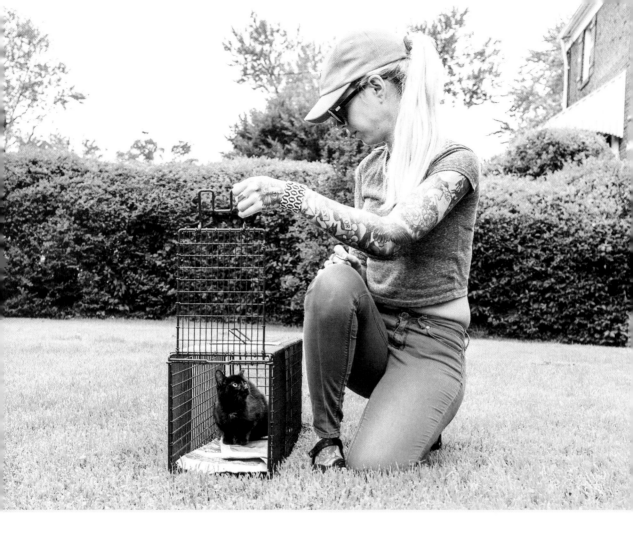

Return

🐈 **Rise and shine!** In the morning, check on the cat. If he is bright-eyed and alert, then you can return him to his outdoor home.

🐈 **Return to the exact home.** Make sure you're returning the cat precisely where you trapped him. Cats are bonded with their homes, and it's important to ensure that they're returned appropriately. You wouldn't want to wake up from surgery in another state—so never release a cat to a place that is unfamiliar to him.

🐈 **Let 'em fly!** This is the most fun part! Unlatch the lock, pull the door upward, and let the cat run free. He'll be so thrilled to be back home!

🐈‍⬛ **Feed and monitor.** After TNR, it's compassionate to continue giving support to the colony as much as you are able. Ongoing colony care can involve providing daily food and water, providing winter shelter, and monitoring the site. If you weren't able to trap every cat, keep trying and don't give up! If any new cats without an eartip show up, now you know to get them TNR'd, too.

CATCHING KITTENS

Don't let their cute faces fool you—kittens can be feisty. For your own safety and for the safety of the animal, you should never attempt to physically pick up a kitten on the street with your bare hands. Although they might be tiny, they can (and often do!) fight back when they feel threatened. If you're bitten by a kitten outdoors, it can result in a lot of pain—and not just for your skin. Kittens who have bitten a

human are typically required to be quarantined by the local government, which is far from ideal. Protect yourself and the kittens by using a humane trap to catch them, or if they're young enough to simply scoop up, wear protective gloves to ensure a safe rescue for everyone.

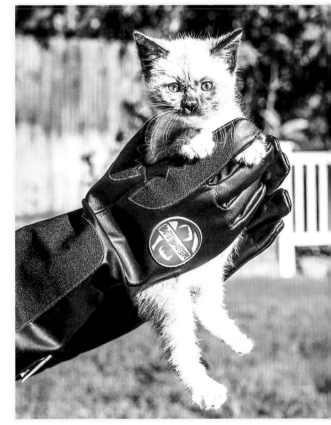

Sometimes, you may find yourself in a position where a kitten is in need and you don't have time to get the proper tools to save her, such as a trap or gloves. In these situations, you should act with caution and compassion, taking as many steps as possible to reduce the risk of harm to either yourself or the kitten. In some scenarios, it will be best for you to leave the kitten where he is until you can return with proper equipment. In other cases, you may find that the situation is urgent and that rescue cannot be delayed. If this is the case, you can either call upon your local animal control to assist, or you can cautiously take matters into your own hands, understanding that there is always a risk associated with rescuing kittens without proper equipment.

In the absence of proper equipment, I have been able to catch injured and critical kittens using available materials such as blankets and sweaters, which provide a protective layer between myself and the animal. While it's always preferable to use proper trapping equipment with kittens, the reality is that if a person is going to do without, it's better to do it with a spirit of harm reduction and a little creativity.

TO CATCH A PIGEON

It was almost midnight, and the neighborhood was illuminated by yellow streetlights. Having just come from teaching a kitten-care workshop across town, I was walking through Brooklyn in a striped dress, accessorized by a massive travel carrier where my foster kitten, Tidbit, sat on a soft bed like a little prince. As I made my way up the block toward my friend's apartment where I'd be sleeping that night, I noticed a young woman crouching on the ground, clearly distressed. A small silver can glimmered in her hand and stopped me in my tracks.

"Are you trying to help a cat?" I asked instinctively.

"How did you know?" she responded. "There's a little kitten I'm trying to catch. Her eyes are all messed up and I don't know what to do. I've been out here all night."

I gestured toward the little orphan in my carrier. "I'm a kitten rescuer—I had a hunch. Do you want a hand?" She couldn't believe I had a kitten by my side already! She showed me where the kitten was hiding out, under a dumpster behind a large metal gate. Next thing I knew, I was lying with my white dress pressed firmly against the dirty sidewalk, with my cheek against the ground. Sure enough, a tiny tabby was under the fence, seemingly blinded with swollen, red eyes.

I agreed to put my things down at my friend Candace's place and come back quickly to help. I silently opened the door to the apartment, tiptoeing so I wouldn't wake anyone. I set my kitten carrier down and looked around, trying to quickly come up with a plan. Fortunately, I had an entire tool kit of animal care supplies and cat food with me . . . but what I didn't have was a trap or gloves. *Darn.* I'd need to make do with what I had. *I wonder if Candace would be okay with me using her bedding to catch a kitten on the sidewalk?* She was going to have to be.

I rushed back out to the sidewalk with a can of cat food and a big blanket. "Here's what I think we need to do. We need to be completely quiet so she will come out and eat. Then I will try to scoop her up with the blanket." For about twenty minutes, we sat quietly, gesturing but not making a peep. Finally, a tiny nose cautiously poked out from under the fence . . . then whiskers . . . then ears. The little kitten sniffed at the bowl of food and soon she was chowing down, unaware that I was just a foot away from her, hovering with a blanket and waiting in silence.

My heart pounded in my chest. I knew I had only one shot to get this right, or she might run off and not return. I waited . . . and waited . . . and waited . . . and . . . whoosh! I dropped the blanket over the kitten and quickly wrapped it around her. "It's okay. It's okay. You're okay. I got you. It's okay."

I couldn't believe it—I'd caught her! But now what?

The young woman suggested I come inside. We walked up the steep steps into her small apartment, where we took a first look at the kitten in the light. One eye was crusted shut, while the other was swollen open. The kitten shivered as I cleaned her up using a warm compress and some eye meds I serendipitously had in my bag. She was clearly pretty petrified of people, but at about seven weeks old, she was young enough that I knew she'd warm up quickly. "Are you able to foster her?" I asked, and the woman replied that she wasn't able to and hoped she'd find someone who could. I looked down at the kitten and sighed. "She can come with me. She'll get better in no time."

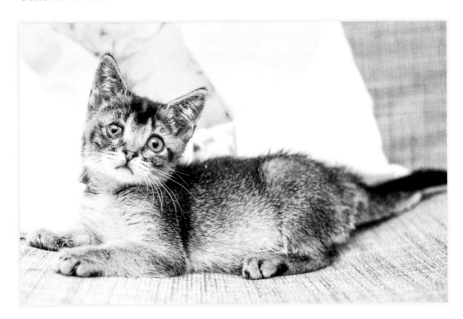

Tiptoeing back into my friend's apartment, I tried my best to stay silent as I set the kitten up in the bathroom for the night. By this point it was nearly 2 a.m., I was covered in filth, and I was stowing away a secret street cat, so I must have made a bit more noise than I'd intended, because pretty soon my friend was standing in front of me.

"You all right?" Candace whispered as she came out of her bedroom in her pajamas, rubbing her eyes.

"Hi! Okay. I can explain. So, don't get mad . . . but there's a feral kitten in your bathroom."

Candace erupted with laughter. "Of course there is."

"Oh, and I used your blanket to catch her, so now I have nothing to sleep with."

"Of course you did." Candace chuckled again. This is why we are friends—we are both massive animal advocates, and neither of us would expect any less from one another.

The next morning I drove back to DC with my new foster kitten, and while I wasn't able to stay behind and address the breeding population on the block, I'm happy to share that the woman I'd met that night ended up being able to catch the mom and have her spayed. As for the baby, I decided to name her Pigeon, after the birds that live in the city; like them, this kitten was a little grimy, but very beautiful. She was a tough little New Yorker.

Pigeon flourished in my nursery, and as her eyes healed, so did her spirit. She became a trusting, playful little cat who loved climbing cat trees, hiding in her cat tunnel, and getting her belly rubbed. She was promptly adopted after a friend of mine visited and decided that she couldn't live without her. I can't blame her . . . Pigeon was quite a catch!

WHAT TO DO IF YOU FIND A KITTEN OUTSIDE

Every kitten season, thousands of kittens are scooped up from the streets by compassionate people trying to lend a hand. Yet without knowledge of what the kitten needs, sometimes these good intentions can do more harm than good. Each scenario is different, so you'll want to use your best judgment based on the specific situation, such as the kitten's age, the presence of a mother, the sociability of the kitten, and the availability of a foster home.

Don't forget that if there are kittens present, it means there is also a breeding population—so try to get everyone sterilized. While it's wonderful to help individual kittens, we must simultaneously fix the leak in order to stop the flood!

In this section, I'll teach you everything you need to know about assessing kitten scenarios so you know how to respond effectively if you find a kitten outside. In order to accurately assess the situation, you'll need to know how old the kitten is, so make sure you check out "Act Your Age!" on page 73 to learn about determining age. Let's look at the various situations you might encounter, and how to decide the best course of action.

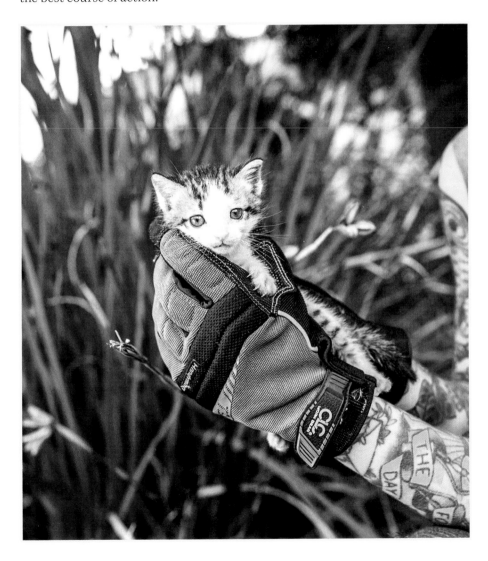

Kittens fewer than five weeks old will still be nursing, and will not be eating independently. No one is better at caring for these babies than their mother, so they should be kept with her whenever possible. If you've found unweaned newborns, the first step should be determining if they have a mother, and making every attempt to keep them safe with her.

If no mother is present, you'll want to wait and see if a mother does return. If the kittens are alive, clean, and appear to be in healthy condition, they are almost certainly being cared for by someone . . . and it isn't the friendly neighborhood opossum, it's their mom. In many cases, the mother is right around the corner looking for food, or may simply not be there because *you are!* If no mother returns after an attempted reunion, you'll need to intervene quickly and take them into your care. Saving orphaned neonatal kittens requires specialized knowledge and supplies, so check out Chapter Four to learn how to act as a surrogate caregiver to unweaned kittens who have been separated from their mothers.

If a mother is present, the very best option is to trap and place the entire family into foster care together. Friendly moms can be cared for in a loving foster home, and once the babies have reached eight weeks of age, the entire family can be spayed or neutered and placed for adoption. If the mother is unfriendly, she can still

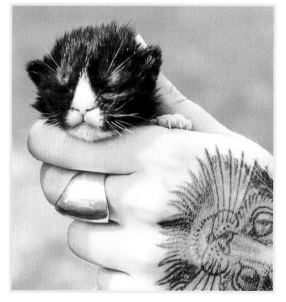

go into foster care—she'll just need someone who is willing to care for an unsocialized cat. Feral or undersocialized moms can be kept in a covered kennel with a comfortable hideaway where they can avoid human interaction and nurse their young. As soon as the kittens are weaned, the mother can be spayed and returned to her colony.

It's important to recognize that not all situations are the same, and that helping kittens outdoors is a matter of balancing the specific circumstances and the available resources. Use your best judgment, know your local resources, and offer as much support as you are able.

At five to twelve weeks of age, kittens are becoming much more mobile and independent. Improved eyesight and coordination allow them to explore their surroundings, and with their sharp baby teeth present, they're learning to eat on their own and relying less on nursing. During this period of time, kittens are forming their impressions of the world and are adaptive to new surroundings such as a foster home. These characteristics make the five-to-twelve-week range an ideal age to rescue kittens from the outdoors.

The earlier you rescue kittens in this age range, the more quickly they will adapt to life indoors. Think about it like learning a new language: if you're introduced to a language at an early age, it's easy to pick it up, but as you get older it becomes much more challenging. Thus, six-week-old kittens may adapt to a new routine within hours, but ten-week-olds may take a week or even longer (read about the socialization window on pages 152–154). Intervening early during this critical socialization period will allow the kittens to have a smooth transition, to obtain necessary veterinary care, and to prepare for a loving home.

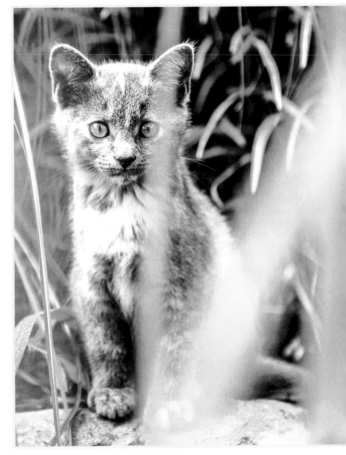

It's important to make decisions based on the specific situation and the resources available; there is no one-size-fits-all method to rescuing kittens. For instance, if a kitten is nearing twelve weeks old and unsocialized, and no foster home is available, it may be more suitable to TNR the kitten than to keep her in a shelter setting where she may not receive effective socialization. Use your best judgment to help during each individual situation.

As they approach twelve weeks, kittens are becoming highly independent, resourceful, and more set in their ways. Around this time, the window for socialization is closing. While kittens who are already social toward humans at this age can often be successfully transitioned into a human home, those who have not been exposed to humans will likely be quite averse to the idea of interaction. It becomes exponentially more challenging to socialize kittens for adoption as they age, so if a kitten exhibits feral behaviors and is more than twelve weeks of age, the best outcome will typically be TNR.

While some may attempt socialization with feral kittens over twelve weeks of age, I will caution that this strategy can sometimes backfire and result in a kitten who is suited for neither a home nor a colony. It's all too common for an animal shelter or rescuer to take in a feral kitten, fail to appropriately socialize him over a period of many weeks, and then be stuck with a cat whom they can neither safely return to the colony nor place in a home. For this reason, it's critically important to be realistic about what we can and cannot achieve depending on the specific circumstances. TNR is always a more humane outcome for healthy unsocialized kittens than euthanasia, and with love and colony management these kittens can grow up and become quite successful members of their outdoor communities! There are many different ways to be a cat, and it's up to us to help make the best judgment calls about how to meet kittens where they are and help them achieve the best outcome possible.

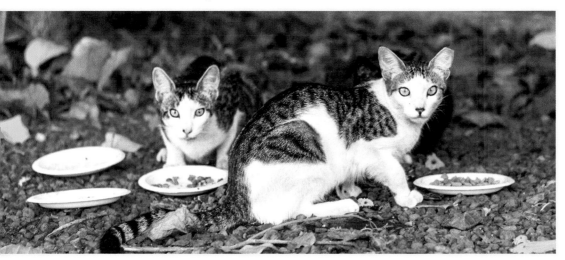

When we remove young kittens from the outdoors without getting the mama, we put the kittens' health at risk and we fail to address the breeding population. But when we leave the kittens outdoors in their colonies, we put them at risk, too. Even with their mama, neonatal kitten mortality on the street is high, and their fragile bodies can be threatened with exposure to the elements, fleabite anemia, or even predation. Nearly half of all kittens born outdoors die within their first year.[7] The best way to ensure that the kittens will be safe and that the cycle will end is to reunite the entire family in foster care.

When to wait for mom

- Kittens are unweaned and will not be able to eat on their own.
- Kittens look bright-eyed, clean, and alert.
- Kittens appear healthy and well-fed.
- Someone is able to monitor and provide help if the mother does not return.

When not to wait for mom

- Kittens are lethargic, unresponsive, or seriously ill.
- Kittens are filthy or emaciated.
- Kittens are in immediate danger, such as during a snowstorm or hurricane.
- You're certain that the mother has died or is not present.

How to determine if mom is present

- Line a shallow box with a blanket, ensuring that the kitten is still easily visible. If the outside temperature is less than 90 degrees, provide a heat source, such as disposable hand warmers.
- Place the kitten in a safe area away from direct sunlight, rain, traffic, and other potential hazards. Ensure that she is still within ten feet of where she was discovered.
- Observe from a reasonable distance. The amount of time you wait is entirely dependent on the situation; I generally suggest waiting no more than three to four hours to determine if the mother returns.

- Can't wait around? Create a thick ring of flour around the kitten box. If there are paw prints when you return, you'll know there's a mom.
- If you find a mom, make all attempts to trap and reunite her with the kittens. If no mom is found, care for the kittens—but return to the colony to TNR the remaining cats as soon as possible.

How to trap mom using kittens

- Place the babies in a closed carrier lined with a blanket and a heat source, and press it against the back side of your humane box trap.
- Cover the back of the box trap and the carrier with a blanket or trap cover. This will create the illusion of an entryway for the mother cat to walk into to retrieve her kittens.
- Set your trap and wait. The mother cat is likely to hear her young and walk into the trap to be with them.
- Cover the trap completely, then bring the whole family unit to be placed in foster care.
- Once the kittens are weaned, the mom can be spayed, vaccinated, eartipped, and returned to the colony.
- Don't forget to TNR the rest of the colony so no more babies are born!

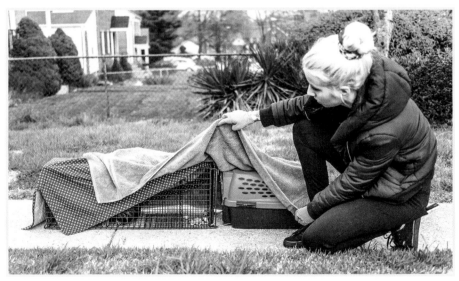

Using babies to trap a mama.

"There are three newborn baby kittens in a bush in my front yard. Where should I take them?" read a comment on my social media.

I clicked the profile, saw that she lived in my city, and responded instantly: "Please do not take them anywhere! Send me your address and I'll be right there." I grabbed a few supplies, hopped in my car, and headed over to assess the situation. I know this scenario all too well: People find kittens outdoors and, meaning well, remove them without attempting to reunite them with their mothers. The babies are put at risk, and the mothers are left behind to continue procreating. This time, I wanted it to be different.

I pulled up to the house and was pointed toward the prickly palmetto bush where the woman had last seen the babies. As I approached, the spiky shrub trembled with low, threatening growls. I ducked down to take a peek, and as I did, a feral cat quickly shot a warning hiss in my direction, lunging toward me like a bolt of lightning. I jolted back, so shocked that I nearly lost my footing! Just as I suspected, there was a mama . . . and she was *not* pleased. I couldn't help my nervous laughter over the scare she'd given me. If her intention was to scare me off, she'd done about as good a job as any cat could ever hope to do—but I don't frighten that easily.

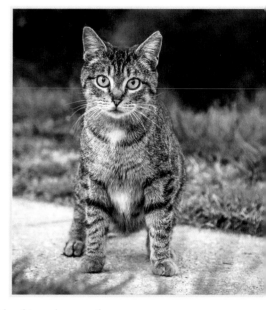

Looking around, I realized the yard was suddenly crawling with other cats. A black fluffball emerged from a hedge. A gray tabby peeked around the side of the house to check out the commotion. A juvenile brown tabby skipped across the grass. I looked over at the caregivers, perplexed—*who are all these cats?* I quickly learned that there were actually about fourteen cats living in the neighborhood, and that almost all of them had been born from the mama who had just hissed at me. She was the matriarch—the queen of the neighborhood, if you will. None of her prior kittens had been sterilized, so there were constant births in the yard, and the colony was expanding exponentially. "She's a kitten factory!" I said to the family.

Now I was even more determined. This wasn't just a rescue . . . This was a whole project!

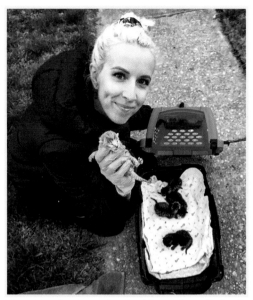
Moments after removing five kittens from the bush.

The mama exited the scene, and I quickly got on my knees and pressed my face against the bristly bush to peer around with a flashlight. I counted not three but *five* little wiggly babies, all about one day old. Their eyes were closed, their umbilical cords were attached, and they were writhing around in a small nest of mulch and twigs. When I picked them up one by one, they were lighter than air, but louder than a fire engine! I shook my head, wondering how many kittens she'd reared in that very spot. Their cries persisted as I placed them each into a carrier prepped with a heating pad. They wanted their mama, and I was determined to reunite them and to ensure that this would be the last litter she would ever have to raise.

I typically trap community cats using enticing meaty foods as bait, but in this case, I knew that the best bait would be the kittens' cries. I placed the kitten carrier against the back end of a humane trap and covered the whole setup in a large towel, creating the visual effect of a long dark tunnel. I set the trap, walked across the street to observe, and stood with my jaw tight and my fists clenched, hoping that the mama would walk inside.

The mama finally emerged. She peeked into the bush, and once she found that it was empty, she began to look around frantically for her babies. The kittens mewed from the trap, and the mama hurried over, circling in search of an access point. The moment she noticed the entrance, she rushed in. *Click!* The trapdoor shut behind her and I exhaled with relief. I got her!

Once everyone was in the foster room, I set up the mesh kennel that would be the nursing den. I was eager to reunite everyone, as they'd been separated for more than an hour at this point. But the mama was less focused on greeting her babies and more focused on getting the heck away from me. She bolted around, slamming against the mesh and hissing furiously! It was clear that the best way to calm her was to cover the kennel in a light blanket and give her space and silence, so I exited and hoped that she would calm down as she adjusted to her new digs. After half an hour,

I poked my head back in, and although she was lying on her side to feed her babies, her body language was very clear. Ears flat, teeth bared, claws out—she was telling me, "STAY AWAY."

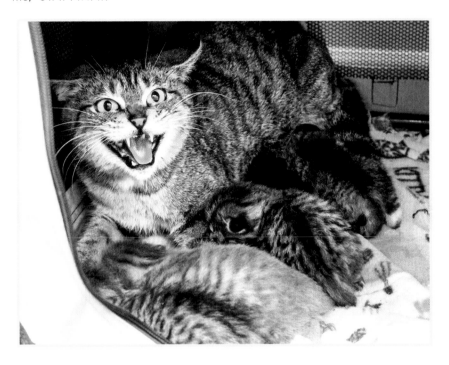

And so I did. She was a wonderful mother, but wanted nothing to do with humans. Once a day I would check in on her babies to weigh them and ensure that they were healthy and progressing, but because I couldn't safely reach for them, I had to access the kittens in what can only be described as a hilariously unique method: with a *spatula*! I would slowly approach the family, extend the arm of the extra-long cookout tool, and gently glide each kitten across the wood floor toward me. Because I could only handle the kittens using a grilling utensil, I named them after cookout items. The kittens were Patty, Teeny Weenie, Shish Kebab, Smoky Mesquite, and Coleslaw. Since the mama was the one who held the family together, she was easy to name: Bun.

For six weeks, Mama Bun raised her babies, and not a day went by where she didn't hiss and growl. As comfy as her home away from home was, it felt to her like she had been kidnapped and taken from the colony where she reigned. I think if she had the ability to leave a review for her B&B experience, she would probably say:

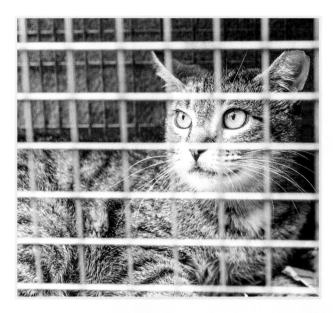

"Hated it. Would not stay here again. Was poked with a cooking utensil! Couldn't wait to go home. One star."

Knowing that her kittens were being weaned and that she'd soon be returning to her kingdom, I set out to ensure that all the remaining cats at the site were sterilized. A friend and I geared up with traps, trap covers, and bait, and headed over to the colony to scoop up as many cats as we possibly could. I've always greatly enjoyed trapping with friends—it feels like we're secret agents on a mission to save lives. We silently wait in the shadows as the cats approach the traps, and suddenly—*aha!*—we've got our guys. Once we'd trapped all the cats we could find, we brought them to the clinic for sterilization and returned them to the colony so that they could continue their lives without bringing any further kittens to the cat party.

The colony was still missing its queen, but not for long! Mama Bun was spayed, vaccinated, and received her honorary eartip: a sign that in the future, she'd never have to experience pregnancy again. The morning of her return, I placed the trap in the cool grass, lifted the sheet, and told her how happy I was for her. She responded by hissing and batting violently at the bars with her claws out, in her typical fashion. I smiled anyway, knowing she was about to be surprised with exactly what she hoped for: an open door to return to her kingdom. Mama Bun leapt from the trap, and my heart overflowed with joy for her. She was finally home.

Back at my house, the babies were all eating independently and preparing for adoption. Because they had always been with humans, they were social and friendly (well, except Shish, who was mostly sweet but would let out the occasional tiny hiss, y'know, to let you know she was still her mother's daughter). The kittens cuddled at my side, pounced on plush toys, and played in cardboard boxes just like your every-day house cat—and when it was time for adoption, you'd never have known they were born in a bush to a feral, hissy mother. The woman who had originally called me about the kittens in the bush became so passionate about what had transpired that she actually became inspired to get active in TNR as well. Best of all, she sent me the most precious updates of Bun, who was unrecognizably happy as she rolled in the grass and soaked up the sun.

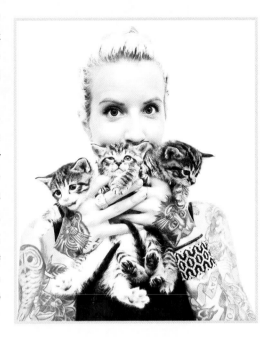

To me, this is the happiest story in the book. Mama Bun, in her fierce feral glory, was able to continue a life of lounging in the sunshine with her colony, her babies were kept safe and healthy until adoption, and the entire extended family was now sterilized, ending the cycle of reproduction. So often my rescue stories end with a cliff-hanger, not knowing where the parents are or if they're still out there popping out babies in the bushes. But this story ends with a period: there will be no more buns in Bun's oven again.

SPOTLIGHT: RESCUED IS THE BEST BREED

With so many kittens dying in shelters and on the streets, we don't need to be creating more of them—but that's exactly what some people are doing through the unfortunate trend of commercial cat breeding. Popular cat culture continues to perpetuate the idea that it is acceptable to breed cats for certain physical qualities, such as coat pattern, folded ears, or even shortened limbs. Many breeds are the result of selecting for genetic defects that are actually damaging to the cats' physical well-being, such as Manx and Munchkin cats. The commodification of the cat is deeply troubling to me, as cats are living individuals, not inanimate products to be bought and sold. We should not have the luxury of custom-designing kittens while so many die without homes.

When I speak with people who have purchased cats from breeders, it's always clear that they do love their cats, but that there's a substantial disconnect between the love they feel for their companions and their comprehension of the consequences of breeding. They may see their purchase as harmless, but they have typically never stood inside a municipal shelter that reverberated with the cries of cats on death's door through no fault of their own. These cats are literally dying for the home that is instead being filled with a designer cat.

When we throw our trash on the ground, it may feel like an innocuous act, but our litter doesn't disappear—it floats downstream. Somewhere someone is suffering the consequences of our actions. Somewhere there is an island of garbage accumulating, whether we see it or not. Having spent years trying to clean up the unimaginably monolithic tragedy of overpopulation, I am struck by the fact that the average cat fan might not know that to purchase from a breeder is to add another life to the pile. When it comes to bringing home a cat, we have the option of being part of the solution or part of the problem. We must challenge the notion that certain cats are more worthy than others, and encourage would-be cat guardians to open their homes to a feline in need.

SHUTTING DOWN THE KITTEN FACTORY

Sterilization is all about decreasing the supply to meet the demand. We must focus on both ends of the equation: decreasing the number of kittens in need, and increasing the resources available for those who do need assistance. It is the complex work of cat advocates to simultaneously shut down the kitten factory *and* find a safe haven for all our feline inventory! Now that we've talked about the state of the kitten and the significance of kitten-prevention programs, it's time to dive into the main course: saving the littlest lives.

CHAPTER THREE

WHAT TO EXPECT (WHEN YOU'RE EXPECTING KITTENS)

EVERYDAY SUPERHEROES

Saving kittens requires community-based solutions in which everyday people like you and me step up and lend a hand. By offering our homes to vulnerable animals, we provide a solution where there would otherwise be none. We are the answer to the cries of the tiny tabby; we swoop in like superheroes and literally save the day! Foster parents are the difference between life and death for the little ones. Ordinary people can transform into extraordinary lifesavers by simply opening their doors and their hearts.

Fostering saves lives in a number of ways. We are able to provide a safe haven where kittens will not be exposed to illness; we can provide them with individualized attention that meets their unique needs; we can even be there for their midnight feedings! We can help the weak become strong and the tiny become triumphant. Most important, we can provide them with affection in a home environment, preparing them beautifully for a loving life ahead. With a little bit of know-how and a lot of love, anyone can save lives.

SAY YES

"We are overflowing with kittens who need rescue."

Shelters' pleas for help during kitten season are constant—there are simply far more kittens in need than there are people willing to provide them with care. Most of us are far removed from the reality that kittens face at the animal shelter. We aren't hearing their high-pitched cries or looking into their tiny faces as their eyes scan the room between the bars, aching for a source of comfort. It's easy to be unaware of animal suffering when it's occurring behind closed doors, but harder when the animal in need is sitting at your feet. That's why when the average person finds a kitten outside, they actually *do* want to intervene and lend a hand.

In a 2018 survey I conducted of more than 14,000 current kitten foster parents, an overwhelming 76 percent reported that they first became active in kitten rescue because they found a kitten outside—not because they signed up to foster at a shelter. Of course, that's how I got started, too: had I not found Coco up in that tree, it never would have occurred to me that these little lives were suffering, and that I could actually do something to prevent that. Looking at her frail body clinging to a branch, I had to decide if I was a person who sees an animal in need and says *no*, or a person who says *yes*. By saying yes to my first kitten, I discovered that I have the power to create lifesaving change for countless vulnerable beings just like her.

You may not know it yet, but you have what it takes to save lives, too. Kittens need advocates who become aware of their plight and make the decision to be a person who says yes. If you walked outside today and saw an orphaned kitten on your doorstep, would you help her? If you're someone who believes in saying yes, then don't delay—kittens are already waiting for a superhero like you. While there are many ways to help save little lives (see page 293, "Find Your Feline Superpower"), fostering is the very best way to directly make an impact in the life of a kitten. In this chapter, I'll walk you through the basics of preparing for kitten fostering. I'll dismantle some of the perceived obstacles, teach you the building blocks of kitten development, and welcome you into the wonderful world of rescue. You've got this!

CROSSING GUARDS

With all the bottle-feeding and butt-wiping I do, it's reasonable to consider my role in a kitten's life a parental one. "Foster parents" are responsible for the well-being of their little ones just like a mother or father, but sometimes I think the term carries a connotation of parental commitment that intimidates and scares away would-be rescuers. The truth is that rather than being like parents, a more fitting comparison would be that kitten rescuers are like *crossing guards*—we simply provide temporary protection. Like crossing guards, we place ourselves in a dangerous intersection, see that someone is standing in harm's way, and volunteer our time to escort them to safety. Once they've arrived at their destination, we wish them well and return to our post, knowing there are always more who need assistance.

Kittens stand at the intersection between vulnerability and viability, and it's up to us to be their crossing guards. For them, making it across the road—to adoption age—is a matter of life and death. The pathway can be eight weeks or just eight short days, but either course is perilous without a hand to hold. As beloved as cats and kittens are, we just can't seem to find enough people who are willing to volunteer their time escorting kittens to the safety of the sidewalk—to help bridge the gap between homeless and home.

People often wish they could lend a hand, but believe that they can't due to some barrier such as not having enough space or time to dedicate to the cause. As someone who has helped many cat-lovers take the leap into fostering, I'm happy to report that these obstacles often exist only in our perception, not in reality. Just about anyone can save kittens, and we certainly need as many people as we can get! You don't have to be a stay-at-home parent or a millionaire to help out. On the contrary, all you need are a little knowledge, a bit of time, and a whole lot of love.

MAKING TIME

If you've heard the saying "they grow up so fast" to describe human babies, just wait until you meet a newborn kitten. Kittens develop at lightning speed, and they only require specialized care for a few weeks before they're prepared for a forever home. Over the course of just eight weeks, the kitten transforms from a defenseless jelly bean into an independent little lion cub! Fostering is therefore a short-term commitment with a lifelong impact.

The length of the commitment depends entirely on how far from adoption age the kittens are when they arrive in your care. While kittens may be unadoptable as newborns, finding forever homes can be a piece of cake once they reach eight weeks. This means you'll be in a great position to plan your time commitment from the start. Subtract the kitten's age from two months, and you'll have an estimated length of commitment, which will help you to plan accordingly!

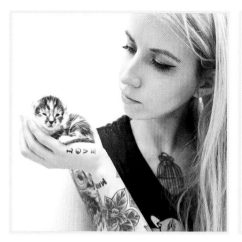
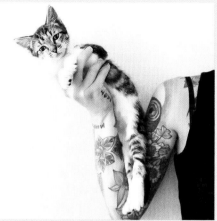

Keep in mind that kittens have different needs at different stages of development, so you can choose which age range works best with your lifestyle and availability. For instance, a six-day-old kitten requires overnight feedings, but by six weeks old, most kittens are weaned and able to be left alone during working hours and overnight. If you don't have time to help newborns, you may still be able to help weaned kittens, feral kittens, or moms with babies! Find the population that works with your schedule and needs.

Finally, remember that you don't have to do it all alone. Having friends who can occasionally kitten-sit is a helpful way to ensure you can fulfill the time commitment of fostering. Kitten-sitters and co-parents allow you to make it to your business meeting, attend that out-of-state wedding, or just take a weekend off. Talk to your friends, family, and other community members about the possibility of collaborative kitten care, and you'll find that there are many people who will jump at the opportunity to kitten-sit!

I'm a busy bee, so no one knows better than I do what it's like to balance the time commitment of animal care with the rest of life's responsibilities. When I know I'll be home for several weeks, I take on more complicated cases or younger kittens, but if I know I've got a hectic schedule or travel planned, I'll take on older kittens who require less of a commitment and can be placed for adoption more quickly. Your life doesn't have to stop in order for theirs to continue—it's all about finding the balance that works for you.

At the end of the day, we only *have* time to do what we *make* time to do. When just a few minutes every few hours can save a life, it's up to us to make those minutes count. If we have time to scroll through social media or take a coffee break, we can absolutely find a moment to feed a hungry animal—it's all about how we prioritize. The clock is ticking for kittens, and by giving them a little bit of our time, we can stop their time from running out.

PURRMANENT RESIDENTS

Many people are afraid to get involved with rescue work because they already have animals at home, but this doesn't have to stop you from saving lives. Believe it or not, my cats, Coco and Eloise, are not fans of kittens at all! They prefer to be the queens of the castle (and rightfully so), so they don't take too kindly to newcomers. Regardless, I've been able to raise hundreds of kittens without my grumpy girls having to bat an eyelash. Whether you have a pack of pups or a crew of cats, you can still safely foster kittens without causing stress to your animal family. Here are some tips for managing your permanent residents while fostering:

- Keep them separate. The easiest way to keep the peace in your home is to keep your foster kittens separate from your personal pets. A room with a door that can close is your best bet, but if you don't have a spare room, you can always keep kittens in an enclosed playpen on the floor or table.

- Use different supplies. Don't allow your pets to share water dishes, litter boxes, blankets—anything the kitten has had contact with—until you know the kitten is healthy. Certain parasites and viruses can travel via feces and saliva, so it's best to keep separate supplies when first introducing a kitten into your home.

- Know your pet. As a pet parent, you'll know your furry friend's personality better than anyone. When presented with a new animal, your cat or dog may be anything from interested to aggressive to avoidant. The important thing is to keep a barrier between the animals that is appropriate given the circumstances, and not to put either party in harm's way.

- Give your cats vertical space. Introducing some new wall perches, cat trees, and platforms can help your cats expand their space, allowing them to feel less cramped and giving them more confidence. It's great to do this for your cats anytime, but especially when bringing foster kittens into your home.

Give your kittens a boost. If you've got a dog in the house, keeping the kittens up on a high table or counter may be the safest way to keep them out of reach of the pup.

Practice good preventative care. Cats should be kept up-to-date on the FVRCP vaccine to protect them against common viruses. Double-check with your vet to make sure your personal pets' vaccines are up-to-date before allowing any contact with foster kittens.

THERE'S ALWAYS ROOM FOR KITTENS!

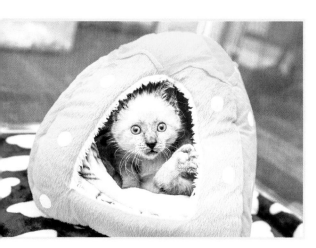

If you're concerned that you don't have enough space for kittens, fret not! Kittens are very small and don't need much space. Swaddle a neonatal kitten in a baby blanket, and he'll be about the size of a cannoli. If you've got room for a cannoli in your home . . . you've got room for a kitten! Whether you live in a five-bedroom house or a studio apartment, you can save kittens' lives. Here's what you need to know about preparing your home for your foster babies.

PREPARING YOUR SPACE FOR KITTENS 0 TO 3 WEEKS OLD

Kittens under three weeks old are not big explorers. In fact, they spend most of the day asleep when they aren't eating! During the first weeks of life, the most important thing is that they are safe and contained as they hibernate through their most vulnerable developmental stage. At this age, kittens should be kept in a top-opening nesting box that can be easily sanitized or disposed of, such as a plastic tub, a lidless aquarium, or a cardboard carrier that is at least twelve inches tall. A top-opening carrier allows you to easily see and access the kittens, and because the neonates are so small, they will not be able to jump over and out. Avoid front-opening carriers, as the metal grates can be hazardous for tiny limbs.

Inside their carrier, you'll want:

🐱 A heat source. Place your heat
source at one end of the kittens'
space, leaving ample room for
them to choose whether they
want to use the heat source or
move away from it.

🐱 A soft baby blanket. Cover the
heated and nonheated areas.
You'll want to get several blankets and change them out as
needed, typically every few days
or any time they are dirty. Make
sure that the blanket is flat
enough that they are not smoth-
ered and can breathe easily.

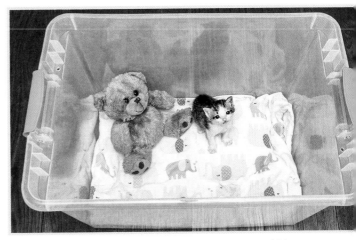

A lidless plastic tote is just enough space for a neonatal kitten.

🐱 A stuffed animal. I highly recommend providing a soft teddy bear for the kitten
to cuddle, which can provide a wonderful source of comfort, especially for solo
kittens.

🐱 No litter box is needed for neonates under three weeks old, as you will need to
stimulate them to pee and poo.

PREPARING YOUR SPACE FOR KITTENS OVER 3 WEEKS OLD

By three weeks old, kittens are becoming coordinated enough to start slowly exploring their surroundings. This also means that they'll be curious about popping
over the top of their top-opening carrier. This is a great time to expand their world
and upgrade them to a covered playpen! Playpens are an affordable way to keep
kittens safely contained while allowing them to navigate their environment. Even
if your space is limited, you can foster kittens all the way to adoption age inside the
safety of a playpen.

Inside their playpen, you'll want:

- 🐱 A heat source. The heat source is no longer necessary after four weeks old if the kitten is healthy and the ambient room temperature is at least 70 degrees.

- 🐱 Soft baby blankets and a stuffed animal. Kittens of all ages appreciate a soft place to snuggle.

- 🐱 A shallow litter box. At three weeks, kittens will start exploring the litter box. Use a nonclumping litter with a very shallow box so that they can get in and out easily. A cardboard tray from a case of wet food makes an excellent disposable training box!

- 🐱 Toys. It's important to start introducing play as kittens become more coordinated, and toys will help bring out their natural predatory instincts, keeping them happy, healthy, and enriched. Choose jingly balls, soft mice, and other kitten-safe toys (see pages 135–136 to learn about kitten-safe toys).

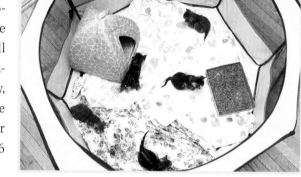

- 🐱 A hideaway. Kittens love having a comfy place to get away from it all, such as a small plush tent!

KITTEN-PROOFING YOUR HOME

If you plan to have kittens loose in a room, or if you'll be integrating kittens into your whole home, be sure the space is kitten-proofed. Kittens, by nature, are curious, impulsive, pint-sized mischief-makers, which means if there is any potential to get into trouble, they will. I'll never forget the day I came back into my office after a meeting and found one of my kittens screaming from the bottom of my recycling bin after climbing inside! I've seen kittens get into everything from the trash can to the toilet, which has taught me that you always want to consider your space carefully before letting the little guys loose. Here are some tips for kitten-proofing your home:

- Avoid long, dangling strings on blinds or curtains, which can easily wrap around a leg or neck.
- Close up any holes in the wall such as areas behind appliances.
- Don't leave dresser drawers open.
- Check your dryer, dishwasher, refrigerator, and other household appliances for kittens before closing them.
- Keep your bathroom curtain on the inside of the bath so the kitten cannot climb up and fall into the bathtub.
- Keep curtains away from the floor to deter kittens from climbing them.
- Be mindful of all electric cables and cords, including laptop and phone cords.
- Many common houseplants, including azaleas, English ivy, and lilies, are toxic to cats. Make sure to keep toxic plants out of reach of curious (and climbing) kittens.
- Avoid leaving trash cans open or with bags draped down the side, which kittens can use to climb up and into the can.
- Keep kittens away from couches with open bottoms, where they may get stuck. Furniture with accessible springs, like pull-out couches, or other sharp infrastructure can be dangerous or even lethal to tiny kittens.
- Don't leave open beverages, especially glasses of water, unattended. Curious kittens will stick their heads and paws into glasses, drink from your water, and then knock/head-butt/swipe the glass off the table!

CUTEST COWORKER EVER

Young, unweaned kittens need care throughout the day, so when I rescued my first neonate, I was petrified that my employer wouldn't accept his presence. Too scared to ask permission, I snuck him into work every day in my scarf, slipping out of the room every few hours like a covert operative to sneakily bottle-feed in a bathroom stall. Once he got a bit older I decided it was time to fess up, and when I did, I was astonished to find out that it wasn't the end of the world after all! Young kittens fit discreetly in a small carrier and spend most of the day silently sleeping, and I found that my employer was very understanding. Ever since then, I've never had an issue bringing a kitten with me to work once I've had a simple conversation.

Talk to your employer about fostering neonates in the office—you'll be surprised to find that once they understand the request, they may say yes. Depending on their age, kittens can sleep up to twenty-two hours a day, so their presence beneath your desk will barely be noticeable. Assure your supervisor that the kittens will be nonintrusive, and suggest a short test run. Apart from being unbearably cute, kittens cause minimal distraction and can even go completely unnoticed. If your office has a firm no-pet policy, there's always the option of co-parenting with a friend or a loved one! If you can't make it work, you can always rescue weaned kittens or moms and babies, who don't need supervision at all hours.

WHEN YOUR PLUS-ONE IS A KITTEN

I used to worry that I'd cause an inconvenience by bringing little ones with me to gatherings and social events. Over the years, I've brought kittens to dinner parties, potlucks, picnics, business meetings, cafés, movie nights, bowl-a-thons, and even a number of weddings. What I've learned is that no one resents the presence of kittens, and moreover, everyone appreciates a compassionate act. I've also found that it's astonishingly easy to bring kittens along without strangers noticing—probably because no one expects to see a kitten! This means that most of the time, those who don't need to know don't have to, and those who need to know don't mind. I no longer worry about whether I can incorporate rescue work into my day-to-day life; instead I figure out how to do what needs to get done.

The first priority should always be the kitten's well-being. Kittens should not be brought into any environment where they will be exposed to loud noises or extreme temperatures, and should not be left unsupervised in unfamiliar places. The care schedule should remain constant, and the kitten should be kept in a warm, comfortable carrier. Physical contact with humans aside from the caregiver should be limited for a neonate. If others are to touch the kitten, hand washing should be required before contact.

The second priority is discretion. If I'm going somewhere it isn't common to bring a cat, I prefer to use a well-ventilated puppy purse that looks like a handbag. Before bringing a kitten as a plus-one, I try to determine if I will have access to a refrigerator for my supplies, and if there will be a discreet place to feed. This sometimes means feeding in a bathroom at a wedding reception, or excusing myself to a guest room at a friend's holiday party. It can feel a little sneaky and silly, but I can't even begin to count the times I've shaken hands with a fellow partygoer who had no idea that they were just inches away from a few napping babies in my bag. When little lives are depending on you, you do what it takes to keep them safe by your side.

I know, I know—it isn't polite to invite guests to someone else's holiday party. But when I rescued a litter of bottle babies just two weeks before Christmas, I knew I'd have to ask Andrew if his family would welcome five more to their celebration. Up in the snowy mountains of northern Pennsylvania, his family has a beautiful cabin where they celebrate the holidays, and this would be my first year joining them. They all knew I was a kitten rescuer, but nothing makes an impression quite like showing up on Christmas Eve with gifts in one arm and a kennel full of purring orphans in the other.

When it comes to packing for myself, I'm not high-maintenance. But preparing the five three-and-a-half-week-old kittens we called the spicy kittens (named after hot sauces: Cholula, Frank, Texas Pete, Valentina, and Harissa) for a snowy road trip turned me into a maniac. I tried to anticipate everything those lil' ones might need and packed piles of blankets, extra bottles, emergency medical supplies, and enough formula to fill a swimming pool—you know . . . just in case. Shivering in the cold, we started the engine, defrosted the windshield, and loaded the car with gifts, one small weekend bag, and no fewer than six bags of kitten supplies. To keep the kittens extra cozy, I microwaved two heating disks and filled their large mesh dog kennel with extra plush blankets.

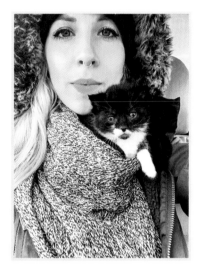

Our drive up took about five hours, meaning we needed to make a pit stop to feed five hungry neonates. We pulled into a rest stop, where I ordered two hot chocolates for us and one hot water for the babies. Parked in the lot, I stirred a combination of powdered formula, bottled water, and hot water to make the kittens a perfectly warm midday meal. Afterward, Cholula nuzzled into my scarf, where she stayed and slept for the remainder of the trip. Bundled up together, we made quite the cozy pair.

We finally made it to the cabin and had a beautiful Christmas. The five babies were the highlight of the visit for everyone. Curled up in their playpen, they were perfectly portable, and there was plenty of time to sneak in feedings between our own hearty meals. Andrew's family was overjoyed to cuddle with the kittens, and many of them had never met a neonate. It was a win-win for everyone: the babies benefited from socializing with many different people, and we all had the joyous opportunity to play with a litter of cuddly, happy kittens on Christmas morning. Watching the snow fall outside, I felt grateful to be warm in my comfy holiday pajamas—and grateful that I could keep my little ones safe and warm, too.

IF I WON THE LOTTERY . . .

"If I ever win the lottery and become a millionaire, I'll spend all my money on saving animals!" is a phrase I hear all too often. In fact, if I had a dollar for every time I heard that, I probably *would* be a millionaire! While it's a thoughtful sentiment, the fact is that you don't have to have a lot of money to save lives.

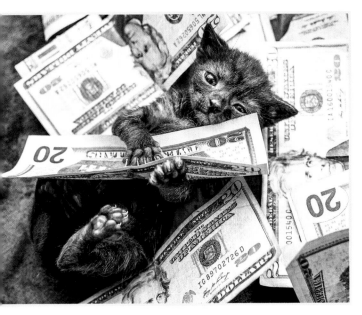

Animal shelters and rescue organizations aren't just kitten suppliers; they're also full-service providers for foster parents. When you work with a local organization, they will provide you with the veterinary services you need, from vaccines to sterilization. Many groups will even provide supplies such as blankets, food, and litter, meaning all you have to do is provide the time, space, and love. Think of yourself as an extension of the shelter; the reason they fund-raise is to be able to save lives, whether in their kennels or in your home. They sponsor your ability to have a revolving door of kittens—how awesome is that? It doesn't have to cost you money to volunteer your support.

Of course, some programs have limited funding, and may not be able to provide you with every supply you need. Fret not—there are lots of creative ways to stock your home with kitten-care tools. Start by tapping into the existing rescue community and seeing if anyone has extra supplies. Rescuers are generous, and many of us have extra bedding, playpens, or even feeding supplies we're happy to share. For new supplies, online wish lists and gift registries are a great way to ask your friends, family, and coworkers to give you a hand. You can even throw yourself a kitten shower, which is like a baby shower for felines! You don't have to do this alone, so don't be afraid to ask for support. Trust me, when your friends find out that you're saving fluffy little lives, they will want to help out! Who doesn't want to come to a party for baby cats?

KITTEN SHOPPING SPREE!

Time to stock up on supplies! Most of my rescue gear is purchased from either a pet supply shop or, if you can believe it, the baby aisle. Diaper bags aren't just for human parents—they're for kitten rescuers, too! Here are some of the common supplies you may want when preparing to save lives:

Keep 'Em Fed

- Kitten formula
- Kitten bottle
- Smoothie shaker or mini-whisk (for eliminating clumps)
- 3 cc or 5 cc syringes (for syringe-feeding neonates)
- Wet canned kitten pâté
- Shallow food dishes

Keep 'Em Clean

- Tissues (for potty time)
- Unscented baby wipes (for easy cleanup)
- A shallow litter box
- Nonclumping, unscented litter
- Unscented baby soap or dish soap (for bathtime)
- Hand sanitizer (for yourself)
- Disinfectant solution

Keep 'Em Healthy

- Small digital food scale
- Flea comb
- Claw trimmer
- Feline probiotics
- Unflavored electrolyte replacer (for dehydrated kittens)
- Dextrose 50% or corn syrup (for combatting low blood sugar)
- 1 cc syringes (for administering medications)

Keep 'Em Cozy

- Soft baby blankets
- Heat source (such as a microwavable heat disk)
- Stuffed animal (with internal heartbeat for extra comfort!)
- Covered playpen
- Portable carrier
- Comfy beds and hideaways

READY, SET, RESCUE!

Now that you're ready to rescue, it's time to get yourself set up to accept kittens. Whether you live in rural Nebraska or downtown Los Angeles, I promise you, kittens need your help. Here's where you can find them.

- Hop on a search engine and type in your city or county plus "animal shelter." Look for information on their website about fostering or volunteering, or give them a call and talk to someone on the phone. If your local shelter doesn't seem to have a website, call your local government and find out who provides animal control services for your area. Some less-populated areas may not have an animal shelter, or may just have a small impoundment facility. While they may not have a foster program, they may let you rescue animals and find them homes, or work with a local rescue group to save animals impounded in your community.

- Do a search online for the name of your city or county plus "animal rescue." You may find that there are several rescue groups working with kittens in your community, so take a look at each of them and see which might be the best fit for you. Find their contact information and let them know you're interested in volunteering.

- Consider looking up your local TNR groups, too. Groups that conduct trap-neuter-return are regularly in need of help with orphans and feral kittens, and they'll be glad to hear from you.

Once you've found the organization you're going to work with, they'll give you guidance about their volunteer orientation process. Remember that just because you get signed up to help doesn't mean you have to say yes to every opportunity—it just means you'll be in the loop so you have the option of lending a hand when it's the right time for you. Getting your foot in the rescue door is your first step into the wonderful world of saving lives. Welcome to the community!

ACT YOUR AGE!

Once you've rescued a kitten, one of the first things to do is to determine the baby's age. It's important to know how to accurately determine the age of a kitten so that you can discern whether she is healthy, what care she may need, and what to expect developmentally. Because each kitten will vary in health and size, physical traits such as weight or appearance are not always a precise indicator of age, so you'll want to examine multiple developmental traits, such as the presence of teeth, in order to precisely determine the kitten's age. For instance, I've rescued many kittens who were the weight of a younger kitten but at the development stage of an older kitten—indicating emaciation. Knowing how to accurately age a kitten will be greatly helpful in developing your game plan for her care. Here are the important developmental and behavioral milestones of a kitten!

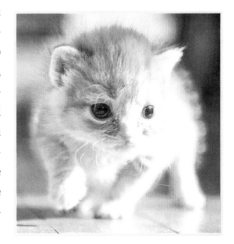

PHYSICAL DEVELOPMENT: Newborn kittens have their eyes closed and their ears folded. They have no teeth, and their gums, nose, and paws may appear bright pink in color. They do not yet have a gag reflex or the ability to thermoregulate. The umbilical cord is attached, and will fall off on its own around four to five days of age (never attempt to remove it manually, as this can cause trauma to the area, which can result in an umbilical hernia or a bacterial infection). Claws are nonretractable.

BEHAVIORAL DEVELOPMENT: Newborns will sleep for the majority of the day. They cannot see, hear, or defend themselves, but they can smell, crawl, and seek warmth and comfort. Starting at two days old, kittens can purr and hiss in response to touch or smell. A healthy newborn will writhe and meow if handled.

AVERAGE TEMPERATURE: 95 to 97 degrees at birth. It's critical to provide a gentle heat source, like a heating disk or heating pad, to keep the kitten warm and stable. The kitten's environment should be kept around 90 degrees during this first week.

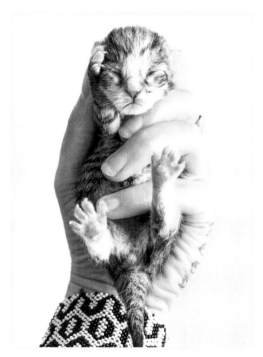

AVERAGE WEIGHT: 80 to 150 grams (premature kittens may weigh less).

CARE INFORMATION: Newborn kittens belong with their mother full-time, as she will provide them with food, cleaning, warmth, and bathroom support. During the first day, a nursing mother may pass immunity to her kitten through colostrum in her milk, which will help the kitten fight illness. Kittens who don't receive the colostrum will be immunocompromised and more vulnerable to disease and infection. If no mother is present, they must be fed kitten formula with a bottle or syringe every two hours (see page 101), stimulated to go to the bathroom (see page 100), and kept at an appropriate temperature.

PHYSICAL DEVELOPMENT: One-week-old kittens have their eyes closed, but no umbilical cord. They still have no teeth, and claws remain nonretractable. Around seven days, the kitten's ear canals will gradually open, and their ears will slightly unfold. Between eight to twelve days, the eyes will slowly begin to open, which can occur over the course of several days. One eye may open more quickly than the other; it's important to let the kitten's eyes open at their own pace. All kittens will be born with blue eyes, which will transition to an adult eye color with age. Although their eyes are opening, their vision will be poor.

BEHAVIORAL DEVELOPMENT: One-week-old kittens, though larger than newborns, are still mostly uncoordinated and sleep for the majority of the day. These kittens may begin to respond to sounds as their ear canals open. At this age they should be able to hold their heads up, move by wiggling their limbs, and be active and vocal if handled.

AVERAGE TEMPERATURE: 97 to 98 degrees. The kitten is still unable to thermoregulate, and it's critical to provide a gentle heat source to keep the kitten warm and stable. The kitten's environment should be kept around 88 degrees at this time.

AVERAGE WEIGHT: 150 to 250 grams. By one week of age, the kitten should have roughly doubled her birth weight.

CARE INFORMATION: One-week-old kittens should be nursed by their mother. Without a mother, they must be fed kitten formula from a bottle every two to three hours, stimulated to go to the bathroom, and kept at an appropriate temperature.

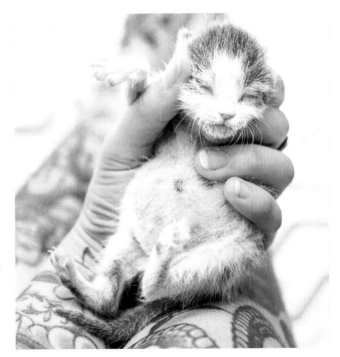

PHYSICAL DEVELOPMENT: At two weeks of age, the kitten's eyes are fully open and baby blue, with enlarged pupils. The kitten's vision will be poor, and she won't be able to see very far. The ear canals will be open and the ears will be small and rounded, like a baby bear cub's. The hearing will be improving, and the kitten may startle awake at the sound of your voice. If you open the kitten's mouth, you will find that there are still no teeth. Claws remain nonretractable.

BEHAVIORAL DEVELOPMENT: Two-week-old kittens slowly become more coordinated and start to attempt their first steps. They will be wobbly on their feet and may fall over while attempting first steps, which is normal. Kittens may exhibit some curiosity about the world around them, but aren't interested in playing and still spend the majority of their time sleeping.

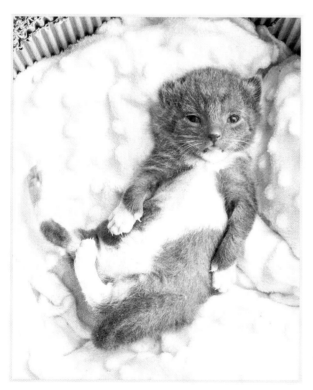

AVERAGE TEMPERATURE: 98 to 99 degrees. Two-week-old kittens still can't regulate their body temperature, and as during the previous weeks, it is critical to provide a gentle heat source to keep the kitten warm and stable. The kitten's environment should be kept around 85 degrees.

AVERAGE WEIGHT: 250 to 350 grams.

CARE INFORMATION: Two-week-old kittens should be nursed by their mother; orphans must be fed kitten formula from a bottle every three to four hours, stimulated to go to the bathroom, and kept at an appropriate temperature. Kittens may begin dewormer at this age (see page 201 for information about deworming).

PHYSICAL DEVELOPMENT: At three weeks of age, kittens have blue eyes and small ears that begin to unfold and point upward, like those of a miniature cat. The kitten's vision and hearing slowly improve, and the tiny teeth at the front of the mouth, called the incisors, begin to emerge through the gums. At this age, kittens slowly begin retracting their claws.

BEHAVIORAL DEVELOPMENT: Three-week-old kittens will be walking, exploring their surroundings, and even beginning to eliminate independently. They may become curious about toys as their visual orienting improves, though they are not yet able to run or chase after moving objects. They will sleep frequently and may begin some small self-grooming behaviors. During this week, coordination improves rapidly.

AVERAGE TEMPERATURE: 99 to 100 degrees. Three-week-old kittens begin to regulate their body temperature but still require a heat source. They will gradually become more active and may stray from the heat source when not sleeping. The kitten's environment should be around 80 degrees.

AVERAGE WEIGHT: 350 to 450 grams.

CARE INFORMATION: Three-week-old kittens who are without a mother must be fed kitten formula from a bottle every four to five hours. At this age, kittens will be transitioning from being stimulated to go to the bathroom to learning how to use a litter box (see page 126 for information about litter training).

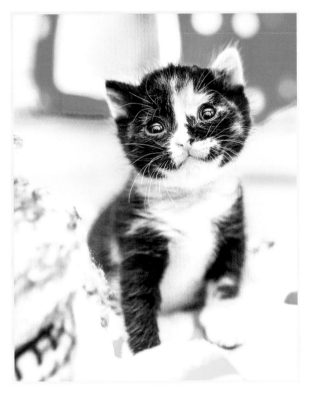

PHYSICAL DEVELOPMENT: At four weeks old, a kitten's vision and hearing improve rapidly. The kitten's canines, the long teeth next to the incisors, start to emerge through the gums, and claws become retractable at this age.

BEHAVIORAL DEVELOPMENT: Four-week-old kittens begin confidently exploring their surroundings and develop more coordination, allowing them to walk, run, and even start to play. With their improved senses, they are notably more responsive, making frequent eye contact with caregivers and reacting to sights and sounds in their environment. As they experience new stimuli, they may exhibit defensive behaviors such as arching their backs. Their grooming skills may still be limited but are improving. Four-week-old kittens will begin engaging in social behaviors with littermates, and can learn tasks through visual cues.

AVERAGE TEMPERATURE: 99 to 101 degrees. Continue providing a heat source, although the kitten will use it only when resting. The kitten's environment should stay comfortably warm, never colder than 70 to 75 degrees.

AVERAGE WEIGHT: 450 to 550 grams.

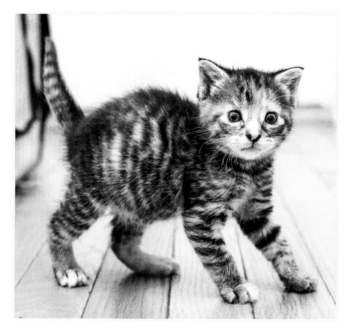

CARE INFORMATION: Motherless four-week-old kittens should be bottle-fed every five hours, including overnight. Although they may show curiosity about solid foods, kittens this age will primarily nurse for sustenance. They will generally be using the litter box on their own, and can begin to be introduced to toys.

PHYSICAL DEVELOPMENT: At five weeks of age, kittens' premolars will start to emerge on the sides of the mouth. Their eyes are blue, ears will be growing and pointed, and claws are retractable.

BEHAVIORAL DEVELOPMENT: Five-week-old kittens run and play confidently. Their social skills develop, and they begin to interact more with humans and other animals. Their grooming skills improve, and by this age, they will have perfected their use of the litter box. At this age kittens are honing their hunting skills and will be practicing taking down prey (toys).

AVERAGE TEMPERATURE: 100 to 101 degrees. A heating source is no longer required as long as the environment is a comfortable temperature of 70 to 75 degrees.

AVERAGE WEIGHT: 550 to 650 grams.

CARE INFORMATION: Five-week-old kittens, if healthy, may begin the weaning process. Kittens should receive ample wet kitten food every five to six hours, in addition to access to their mother's milk or, if orphaned, a bottle. If weaned, food and water should be provided at all times. Always provide supplemental bottle-feeding as needed to ensure that the kitten is maintaining a healthy weight and body condition during weaning. Provide a shallow litter box at all times.

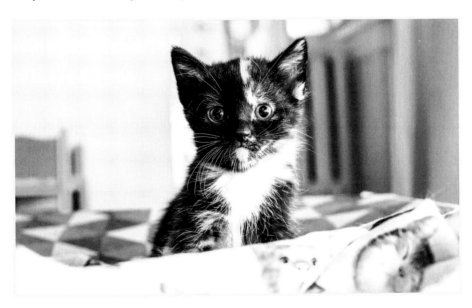

PHYSICAL DEVELOPMENT: At six weeks of age, a kitten's deciduous teeth will be fully descended. The eyes are still blue, and vision and hearing are fully developed.

BEHAVIORAL DEVELOPMENT: Six-week-old kittens socialize confidently with peers, play-fighting, pouncing, hiding, and defending themselves against threatening stimuli. They are curious about their surroundings and eager to explore. At this age they are perfecting their grooming skills, and becoming coordinated enough to jump off furniture and land on their feet.

AVERAGE TEMPERATURE: 100 to 101 degrees. A heating source is no longer required as long as the environment is a comfortable temperature of 70 to 75 degrees.

AVERAGE WEIGHT: 650 to 750 grams.

CARE INFORMATION: Kittens should receive ample wet kitten food if weaned. Provide supplemental feeding if needed to ensure that the kitten is maintaining a healthy weight and body condition. The kitten should have access to water, food, and a shallow litter box at all times. At six weeks, kittens should receive their first FVRCP vaccine to protect them against viruses (see page 180 for more about vaccination schedules).

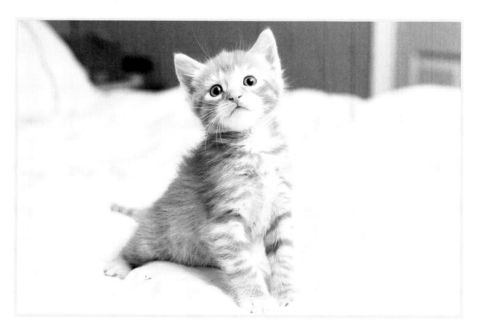

PHYSICAL DEVELOPMENT: All baby teeth are present at seven weeks of age. At this age, the kittens' eyes change from baby blue to their adult eye color. (Kittens with green, gold, or copper eyes are likely seven weeks or older.) Male kittens' testicles may begin to descend around seven weeks.

BEHAVIORAL DEVELOPMENT: Seven-week-old kittens experience a spike in energy. They sleep less and spend more time playing, running, climbing cat trees, and confidently jumping off furniture. Their sleep pattern becomes much more adult-like, and their hunting skills are mature.

AVERAGE TEMPERATURE: 100 to 101 degrees. A heating source is no longer required as long as the environment is a comfortable temperature of 70 to 75 degrees.

AVERAGE WEIGHT: 750 to 850 grams.

CARE INFORMATION: Kittens should receive ample wet kitten food, and may have dry kitten food as a supplement. Provide access to water, food, and a shallow litter box at all times.

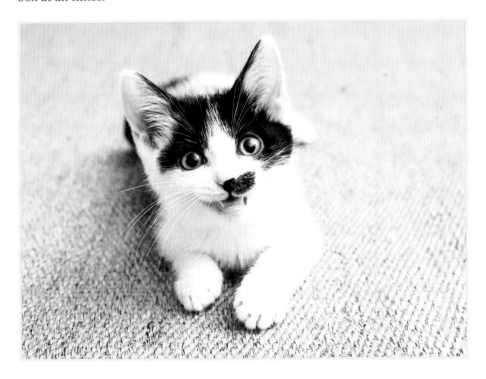

PHYSICAL DEVELOPMENT: All baby teeth are present at eight weeks of age. The eyes will have completely transitioned to their adult color of green, gold, copper, or blue. The ears will be proportional to the kitten's body.

BEHAVIORAL DEVELOPMENT: Eight-week-old kittens are energetic and independent. Their agility and coordination are nearly fully developed. They will be highly interested in social play with littermates.

AVERAGE TEMPERATURE: 100 to 101 degrees. A heating source is no longer required as long as the environment is a comfortable temperature of 70 to 75 degrees.

AVERAGE WEIGHT: 850 to 950 grams.

CARE INFORMATION: Kittens should receive wet kitten food three to four times per day, and may have access to dry kitten food as a supplement. Provide access to water and a shallow litter box at all times. If two weeks have passed since their first FVRCP vaccine, kittens may receive a booster at this time. At this age, if at least two pounds and healthy, they may be spayed/neutered, FIV/FeLV-tested, microchipped, and adopted into loving forever homes.

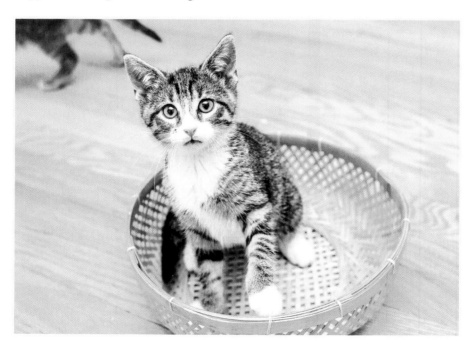

One of the great joys of raising young kittens is watching their behavioral and physical development during their first weeks of life. You might not realize it yet, but at each stage of growth, biology dictates behavior! If you're wondering why kittens develop at the rate they do, let's dive a little deeper into the development of each body part, and discuss how the changing body influences the kittens to engage with the world around them in new and exciting ways.

THE TRUTH IS IN THE TOOTH

Kittens are born toothless, with nothing but a cute lil' set of pink gums for the first three weeks of life. After this period the kitten's baby teeth, also called deciduous teeth, will start to descend in sets: first the incisors at three weeks, then the canines at four weeks, and finally the premolars at five weeks. By six weeks of age, kittens will have a set of twenty-six baby teeth. While it can be challenging to tell a kitten's age based on her weight or appearance, tooth development is a more reliable way to make a determination. That's why when it comes to aging kittens, I always recommend peeking inside the mouth . . . because the truth is in the tooth!

Kittens' teeth each serve specific purposes, and I find it fascinating that their behavioral development so closely echoes their baby-tooth development. For instance, the adorably tiny incisors at the front of the mouth are totally useless for hunting, but they're great for grooming—and around three weeks of age is when I start to notice self-cleaning behaviors. Canines aren't great for shredding meat, but they're perfect for hunting, and four weeks is right around the time that I see kittens start to practice predation. Premolars act as shears that are perfect for chewing on meat, and they tend to come in right around the time that meat becomes both appetizing and healthy for kittens to consume—at five weeks of age. The teeth are therefore a reflection of the kitten's preparedness for the world.

Between three and a half and seven months of age, the kitten's adult teeth will begin to push against the twenty-six deciduous teeth, causing them to absorb their roots and pushing the crowns of the teeth from the mouth. The baby teeth are replaced by a full set of thirty permanent teeth. As the baby teeth fall out, kittens will typically swallow them, or you may even find a tooth that has fallen out in bedding. During this time, it's normal to see things like two canine teeth right next to one another for a period of about a week—so don't panic if your kitten temporarily resembles a fluffy shark! However, if two teeth occupy the same space for more than a week, you'll want to make an appointment with a veterinarian to discuss the retained tooth and potentially have it extracted.

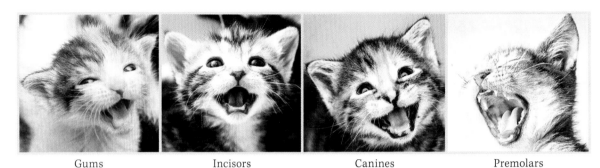

| Gums | Incisors | Canines | Premolars |

Age	Tooth Development
0–2 weeks	No visible teeth
2–3 weeks	Incisors beginning to emerge, forming tiny bumpy ridges at the front of the gums
3 weeks	Incisors present
4 weeks	Incisors and canines present
5–14 weeks	Deciduous incisors, canines, and premolars present
14–16 weeks	Twelve adult incisors emerge, six on the top and six on the bottom, beginning with the center set
16–20 weeks	Adult incisors present; adult canines emerging
20–24 weeks	Adult incisors and canines present; adult premolars emerging
24–28 weeks	Adult incisors, canines, and premolars present; molars emerging
28 weeks (7 months)	Full set of permanent teeth present

Born with their eyelids sealed shut, kittens are blind throughout the first week of life. At between eight and twelve days of life, the eyelids will slowly separate, giving kittens their first peek into a blurry world. This doesn't happen all at once—instead, the eyes tend to slowly peel open over the course of several hours or days, starting at the tear ducts and opening outward. They may look a little silly during this process, like their globes are microscopic or like they're winking at you, but soon enough their eyes will be fully visible . . . and absolutely adorable!

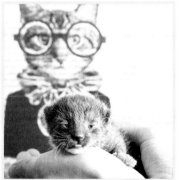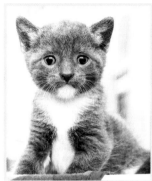

Just because their eyes are open doesn't mean their ocular development is complete—in fact, it's only just beginning! During the first seven weeks of life the kitten's eyes will continue to develop, both in function and in appearance. You'll notice that young kittens don't have particularly good eyesight, and will not respond to visual stimuli during the first weeks of life. This is due in part to corneal edema that wanes over the first weeks of life, and in part due to the immaturity of the retina, which makes it a challenge for them to see clearly. Neonatal kittens tend to have large pupils, resulting in eyes that look cartoonishly dilated and innocent, with hardly visible irises.

Around four weeks of age you'll notice the eyes beginning to change. As the retina matures, the pupillary light reflex begins to improve, allowing the pupil to constrict relative to the brightness of the room. At this point you'll be able to see more of the blue-colored iris as the pupil takes on the iconic vertical slit of the feline eye. I adore this age because it's when kittens first start to visually connect with me—they'll make direct eye contact, visually follow my movements, and even react to toys and objects in their environment. I can't help but smile when I realize that for the first time, I'm not just looking at the baby; the baby is also looking back at me!

From there, things only get better. By five weeks of age, kittens are able to learn tasks through visual cues, such as watching their playmates play, eat, or groom. As their vision improves, so does their ability to navigate the world around them, and they begin understanding how to avoid obstacles . . . and how to jump, climb, and squeeze their way around and over objects in order to get to their desired destination. Coinciding serendipitously with the maturation of their motor skills, vision reaches adult standards around six weeks of age, at which point the kitten engages with the surrounding environment much like a miniature cat. Let the fun begin!

SPOTLIGHT: BABY BLUES

All kittens are born with baby blue eyes, a sweet feature that surprises many first-time caregivers. This coloration is not due to actual pigmentation, but rather a lack thereof. What we are seeing when we see a kitten's baby blues is actually refracted light and an immature iris. As the eyes mature, melanin production increases and we begin to see specks of the true adult eye color. By seven weeks of age, the kitten's eyes will have transitioned to a beautiful hue of green, gold, copper, or, in some cases, a permanent shade of blue.

LISTEN UP, LITTLE ONE!

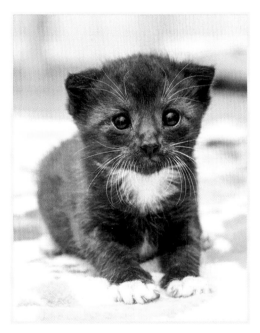

It's not that newborn kittens don't *want* to listen to you telling them how adorable they are—it's just that they can't actually hear you! Like the eyes, the ears are not fully mature when a kitten is born. The external ear canal stays closed throughout the first week of life, and begins to open up between one and two weeks of age. This protects the ears from dirt and residue, allows the auditory system to safely develop, and prevents hearing damage from changes in pressure. While the ear canal is open at two weeks, their hearing continues to improve over the next several weeks. As the inner ear develops, so does its outer shape—helping the kitten's silhouette blossom from a rounded lil' bear cub to a pointy-eared micro-cat.

Kittens may be deaf and blind at birth, but their sense of smell is already intact. Until the eyes and ears are open, kittens navigate their world primarily through tactile, thermal, and olfactory senses—with the nose playing a major role in their ability to locate their mother (or bottle). By three weeks of age, the olfactory system is completely developed, allowing them to take in information through the nose. Kittens will display a natural rooting reflex wherein they press the nose and mouth toward the scent or feel of their food source, such as the mother's belly or the orphan caregiver's palm. When all other senses leave the kitten in the dark, the nose always knows!

CLAWS OUT

Ouch! If you've noticed that kittens are pricklier than a cactus, that's because their claws are nonretractable for the first month of life! This aids in kneading the mother

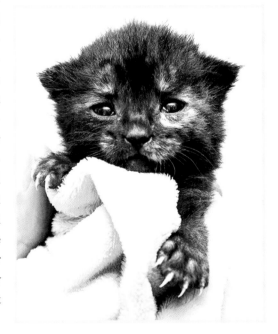

to stimulate milk production, and may be useful for reflexes such as clinging. Their small white nails are visually present at all times until about four weeks of age, at which point kittens gain the physical ability to retract the claws into the paw. Claws are an essential part of the feline body and are necessary for stretching, balancing, climbing, and expressing other natural behaviors, so please never declaw! Declawing is the cruel mutilation of an essential body part. Instead, train kittens to engage in appropriate clawing behaviors and to get used to having their claws trimmed. Around the time that claws are able to retract at four weeks, you can start gently clipping the pointy white tips of the claws to help the kittens get used to a trim.

If you're trying to determine the sex of a kitten, the first step is to gently lift the kitten's tail and take a peek at what's going on under the hood. Never be forceful with a kitten's tail, which is an extension of his or her spine! Hold the kitten in one hand and lift the tail with the other.

A **male** kitten's genitals will look like a circular mound or bulge of fur (the scrotal sac) with a small fleshy circle at the center (the penis). The genitals of a male cat are a greater distance from the anus than the genitals of a female cat, and you will therefore see quite a bit more fur separating the two. Note that kittens' testicles do not descend until around two months of age; before this point the scrotum is empty.

A **female** kitten's genitals will look like a vertical line or teardrop (the vulva). Unlike their male counterparts', a female's genitals will appear flat and will be close in proximity to the anus.

When in doubt, ask yourself: *Does this look like a circle or a line?*

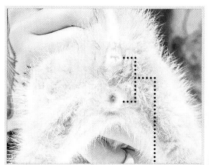 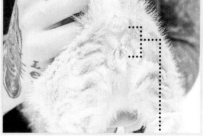

Male: Longer distance   Female: Shorter distance

YOU'VE GOT THIS!

Preparing for kittens might feel overwhelming, but don't worry—you can do this! Sometimes the best way to get comfortable with kitten rescue is to work backward, starting with older kittens and working your way toward saving the younger and more delicate babies. In the next two chapters, I'll tell you what you need to know about working with kittens in the first and second months of life, from the tiniest neonate to the big kids who are getting ready for adoption day. Soon enough, you'll be comfortable helping kittens of all different ages!

CHAPTER FOUR

FIGHT FOR THE LITTLE GUYS

NEONATAL KITTENS

They're miniature, they're squirmy, and they're the most fragile of them all: neonatal kittens are undeniably my favorite population to work with, partly because I love a challenge and partly because I love a transformation. To hold an entire life in your palm, knowing that life is entirely dependent on you for survival, is a call to action. When we answer the call,

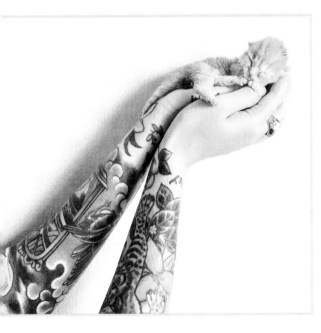

we witness a profound metamorphosis that changes not only the kittens' lives but also our own. When they look up at us with bright eyes and ears wiggling, every drop we feed is a chance for them to live—not just for that moment, but for an entire lifetime. Like a gardener who sows a seed and tends it with care, we can watch every step of the way as they bloom. We discover that we are capable of incredible things, and our hard work is rewarded with the kitten's vitality, affection, and downright cuteness.

I wasn't prepared for the first newborn kitten I raised.

On a cold and rainy night in South Philly, my friend Jeanne called to ask for help with a little black kitten she'd found in the alley outside her row house. After twelve hours of watching and waiting for a mother cat, it seemed that he was alone for good and would need specialized help. I'd rescued a few kittens by then and felt certain I'd be able to assist, but the truth is, I had no idea what I was walking into when I headed over that evening. When she opened the door, I gasped. I had never seen a cat so small! I felt a rush of anxiety pour through my body. He was barely the size of my palm and looked like a little black mouse curled in a fetal position. His eyes were closed, his umbilical cord was attached, and his little body felt cold in my hands. To be honest, I didn't think he would survive the night.

But the little guy had a strong will to live. We got him through that first night using a syringe and some kitten formula, a heating pad made out of some microwaved dry rice in a sock, and a healthy dose of luck. As the sun rose on my second day with him, so did my hope that I might be able to keep him alive. Jeanne and I scrounged together enough cash to afford an exam with a vet, and while they tried to help, it seemed that even cat specialists didn't have expertise in orphaned kitten care. The learning curve was steep. I relied on information I gathered from the vet, a mishmash

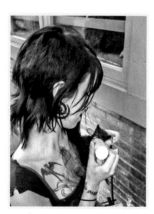

Bottle-feeding my very first neonate. Let's just say I've since improved both my bottle-feeding skills and my hairstyle!

of questionable and often contradictory resources I found online, my gut instinct, and a fierce determination to help him through his first weeks of life. Incredibly, he continued to grow and grow, and Jeanne and I lovingly referred to him as Wolfman because of the downy black wisps of kitten fur that radiated around his little face.

During his first weeks, Wolfman spent most of his time hidden in my shirt, only waking up so I could secretly bottle-feed him in a bathroom stall at the public school where I worked as a counselor for children with special needs. I became a total helicopter parent, obsessing over every aspect of his well-being, constantly anxious about whether I was doing everything I could for him. When he didn't poop for two days, I took the day off work and canceled my plans until I was sure he was passing stool. When my alarm clock went off for his middle-of-the-night feedings, I'd shoot right out of bed, anxious to fill his belly. With all the time he spent curled in my hand, it turned out *I* was the one wrapped around *his* little finger!

With a little luck and a lot of hard work, he made it to adoption age, and it was time to find him a forever home. My friend Ginny knew she wanted to adopt him, and I couldn't think of a better mom for my little Wolfman. We'd been friends since fifth grade, and she and her mother had always been the biggest cat ladies I knew as a kid. After the adoption, Ginny changed his name to Zeke, and all these years later, he is still living the good life in her Virginia home.

YOU MUST BE NEW HERE

I was clueless when I saved my first baby, but you don't have to be. The delicate art of neonatal kitten care can be learned through research, mentorship, and personal experience, and you'll soon be astonished at your ability to help a budding life begin to bloom! Once you know the basic building blocks of a healthy baby, you'll be able to assess each situation and take appropriate action.

When you're meeting a kitten who is new to the world, the first step is to assess her condition so you know what course of action to take. It can certainly feel overwhelming when you're saving your first baby and you're not sure what's normal and what isn't. While a veterinarian can (and should) do a more thorough examination than you can, we can immediately learn a lot about a kitten's health based on some basic observations. These observations should be made and documented the moment you bring the kitten home, but also throughout the kitten's first weeks of life. The following is a list of things to consider when observing the kitten:

🐱 **Temperament** should be active and alert when awake. Even a one-week-old kitten with her eyes shut should be responsive when handled. The kitten should be able to lift her head, vocalize, and make age-appropriate movements of her limbs. In cases of extreme lethargy, a vet should be consulted without delay.

Temperature should be comfortably warm. *Never feed a hypothermic kitten*; hypothermia decreases the ability to suckle and slows gut motility, and feeding a cold kitten can result in aspiration, bloating, or even death. If he's cold to the touch, warm him gradually over the course of at least thirty to sixty minutes. If the body is overheated, gradually cool by placing him in an air-conditioned space or by an ice pack wrapped in a cloth until his temperature returns to normal.

Fur and skin should be smooth and clean. Look for any wounds, abscesses, or fur loss. Look for evidence of external parasites, such as dirt-like residue from fleas. Always treat fleas within twenty-four hours of arrival to avoid infestation or anemia, and seek veterinary advice about skin conditions.

If the **umbilical cord** is still attached, do not pull it. Never touch a fresh umbilical cord with dirty hands. If it's still wet, clean the cord with iodine, tie it off close to the skin with a piece of unflavored dental floss, and cut it with sterile shears. If it's dry, simply allow the stump to fall off naturally.

Mouth should be closed unless meowing or yawning. Open-mouth breathing is a sign of overheating or serious distress. Take the kitten to the vet if she's breathing through the mouth.

Gums should be pink and wet. White or bluish gums could indicate lack of oxygenation or anemia. Pale gums could indicate hypoglycemia. A drop of corn syrup or oral dextrose can be given to temporarily boost the blood sugar of a hypoglycemic kitten in an emergency situation, but it's critical to follow up with a visit to a veterinarian. (See pages 215–216.)

Eyes should be bright and clear of any discharge. (See pages 168–169.)

Ears should be clean. Check for signs of ear mites, which may cause dirt-like residue. (See pages 200–201.)

Nose should be clear of any discharge or sneezing. If discharge is present, you'll want to consult a veterinarian. (See pages 167–168.)

Urine should be pale yellow. If it's dark, your kitten may be dehydrated and will benefit from careful hydration support. (See pages 213–215.)

Feces should be well formed. If diarrhea is present, you'll want to address the issue with haste. (See page 206.)

SOME LIKE IT HOT (JUST NOT TOO HOT)

Neonatal kittens cannot thermoregulate, and therefore rely on their mother's bodies to keep them warm. When orphaned, young kittens quickly become hypothermic. It is critical to provide kittens with a heat source until at least four weeks of age.

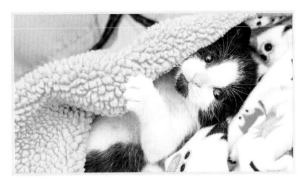

Heat Source	Pros	Cons
Electric heating pad	Long-lasting heat	Cannot use while in transit, automatic timer may turn off, cannot move kittens easily
Microwavable heating disk	Portable, durable, can retain heat between feedings	Must reheat every four to six hours; can scald if overheated
Single-use hand warmers	Easy heat source for on-the-go needs	Not a sustainable approach for ongoing heat
Rice mom (uncooked rice in a sock, microwaved)	Cheap, portable, made of resources available at home	Can lose heat more quickly than other heat sources
Incubator	Consistent, precise regulation of temperature and humidity	Expensive and bulky medical device

At birth, kittens will have a low body temperature of around 95 degrees, which will increase over the first month of life until it reaches a standard cat temperature of roughly 101 degrees. During the first four weeks, it's critical to provide a warm environment.

Kitten's Age	Average Body Temperature	Target Temperature for Environment
0–2 weeks	95°–99°F (35°–37.2°C)	85°–90°F (29.4°–32.2°C)
2–4 weeks	97°–100°F (36.1°–37.8°C)	80°–85°F (26.7°–29.4°C)
4+ weeks	99°–101°F (37.2°–38.3°C)	≈75°F (23.9°C)

It was unseasonably cold in Washington, DC. Spring was coming, but not quickly enough—and after several weeks of warm weather, we had been hit with a sudden cold front that dumped a foot of snow on the ground. It was on this frozen day that a community cat in my neighborhood went into labor prematurely and, seeking shelter, slipped through a local artist's studio door, which had been left ajar. Under the refuge of a large oil painting, she gave birth to two underweight kittens . . . and then exited the building, never to return.

By the time I received the call about the two kittens, they were four hours old and nearly dead. I rushed down the street with a heating pad and a rescue kit, and entered the studio to find the artist in a state of panic. The studio wasn't much warmer than the street, and the two newborns were frozen stiff like little Popsicles. Still wet from birth, they were covered in a chilled, bloody residue. They made no sound or movement, other than shallow breaths from the small tuxedo kitten. The black kitten appeared to have no life in her body.

As I reached for the kittens, the artist asked, "Are you sure it's okay to touch them? I wasn't sure, so we didn't."

"Yes—you have to touch them in order to help them," I said, lifting their lifeless bodies to my mouth, breathing hot air into their damp fur. Externally, I was composed, but internally, my heart was flooded with sadness, knowing they'd been left there to freeze without any assistance or warmth. Situations like these are why it feels so important to me to educate people about kitten welfare. People just don't know what to do.

I placed them side by side on a heating pad. They were in a very bad state: clearly born prematurely, left with no heat source for hours, never having had a lick of food from their mother. Using a cloth, I got to work cleaning the afterbirth from their fur and clearing the residue from their airways. I brushed their bodies vigorously with a soft-bristle toothbrush, trying to get their blood flowing. After a few minutes, the little black one began to breathe. The artist gasped. The kitten was still alive after all, but barely.

A cold kitten is a dead kitten; neonates cannot survive without a heat source. Once it was clear that the kittens were still clinging to life, I brought them back to the nursery, naming the black kitten Mink and the tuxedo kitten Badger. They were underdeveloped and so, so tiny—it doesn't get tinier than a preemie. Despite everything we tried for Mink, she sadly passed on her second day, leaving baby Badger all alone to fight for his life.

Badger spent his first three weeks of life alone in an incubator, nesting like a little baby bird who wasn't yet ready to hatch. My heart broke for him as he wiggled around, navigating the world with closed eyes and no mother or sister to cling to. He had a stuffed puppy and a stuffed moose, which he'd rest his little white chin on during his long naps in between feedings. Every few hours I'd lift his tiny body, weigh him, feed him, help him go to the bathroom, clean him up, and give him approximately one million kisses before placing him back in his warm isolation unit.

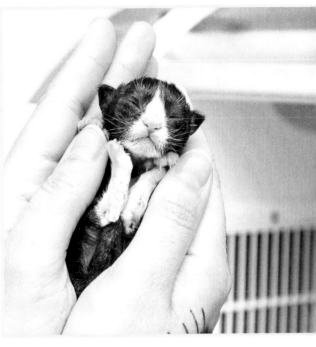

As a preemie, Badger's body developed roughly seven days behind schedule throughout the duration of his upbringing. His umbilical cord clung on until he was twelve days old, his eyes opened at sixteen days old, and his motor skills were delayed. It felt like he would be a little guy forever! As his body grew, it became clear that the cards were stacked against him. He had a belly full of parasites, skin that flaked off in chunks, and a congenital defect called megaesophagus that caused him

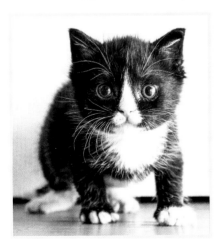

to regurgitate his food. He was constantly gassy, and his bloated belly gave him a pudgy pear-shaped look. With all his woes, I jokingly referred to his condition as "neonatal hot mess syndrome." He was a mess, but he was my favorite mess; in all our time together, he had become my little sidekick.

Some would lose hope for a kitten with so many troubles, but I'm not one to give up on a baby who clearly wants to live. For as many troubles as he had, Badger would gulp down meals like a competitive eater, seek human interaction, and melt in your hands if you gave him a gentle scalp massage. This was a kitten who desired to someday be a cat, but getting him there would be such a delicate process. Badger's treatment involved antibiotics, deworming medications, and daily butt baths to deal with his poopsplosions. As he weaned onto solid foods, he had to use a special feeding station to help him eat at an upright angle and prevent regurgitation. It was a bumpy road, but over time, he started to get the hang of life, and even started thriving!

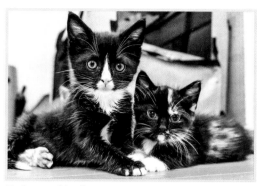
Badger and his bestie, Leeni.

As Badger's health improved, I decided to introduce him to a litter of five kittens I was also fostering at the time—kittens who had been raised by a mother cat, and had thus grown up to be robust, social, normal kittens. Here I was, feeling like the mother of a homeschooled, dorky, stinky little boy who had no social skills, bringing him to his first day at a prep school with the privileged little milk-feds. I kissed him on his head, placed him in the room with the others, and held my breath, thinking: *Please, please, please accept my awkward son!*

It took a few days, but he slowly started to fit in. Next thing I knew, he was figuring out how to cuddle. After that, he was learning how to play. He took a liking to Leeni, a swirly tortie who looked like a beautiful little peanut butter brownie, and over time, Leeni took a liking to him, too. My heart exploded with joy; it was like watching an '80s rom-com unfolding before my eyes. The nerdy outcast was winning over the cool girl, and it was *the best*. As time passed and their friendship flourished, his health conditions withered away. Suddenly he was no longer a weird little pear—he was a handsome, normal(ish) boy with a best friend.

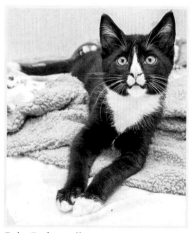
Baby Badger, all grown up.

Badger and Leeni found an adoptive home together, and as I placed them in their carrier to say good-bye, I kissed him one last time and tears filled my eyes. I remembered Badger and his sweet sister, Mink, huddled together, so cold on their first day of life, and how impossible it felt that either of them would survive. I wept for his sister, and for all that Badger endured in order to become the beautiful young cat who sat before me. "I'm so proud of him," I said, and zipped him up with a lump in my throat. Badger comfortably curled up next to his new sister, Leeni, and he looked at me through the mesh with big, soft, loving eyes. He now had a best friend and a loving home, and from that day forward he would always be warm.

FIVE WAYS TO COMFORT AN ORPHAN

Mother cats don't just provide food for their babies; they also provide love and comfort. When caring for orphans, we want to make sure we're providing them with all the comforts of mom so that they can have a cozy, relaxing, stress-free experience. Here are five ideas for comforting an orphaned kitten:

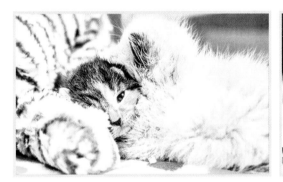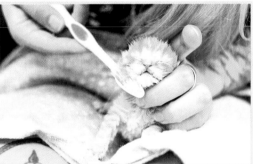

🐱 **Warmth:** A heat source is essential for body temperature regulation, but it's also a nice source of motherly comfort for a kitten. In addition to keeping her nest heated, make sure that her formula is a comfortable temperature so that she can rest contentedly after filling up on a warm bottle.

🐱 **Heartbeat:** The gentle vibration and comforting sound of a mother's heartbeat can lull kittens to sleep. Orphans will benefit from having an audio heartbeat simulator placed near their space or inside a plush toy, or you can even hold the kitten against your own chest for a soothing sound.

🐱 **Plush blankets:** Cat blankets are okay, but human babies get all the best stuff! Consider buying a few nice plush micro-fleece baby blankets for the kittens to curl up in. They're especially fond of blankets with some texture to them, which resemble their mother's soft fur.

- 🐱 **Recycled fur scraps:** Anyone who loves animals knows that fur coats are the product of immense cruelty. But rather than toss your grandma's old mink stole, why not repurpose it and allow it to actually *help* animals? Kittens love curling up on a recycled fur scrap. Take some scissors to that mean old coat and transform it into a bunch of cozy kitten beds!

- 🐱 **Toothbrush:** A toothbrush is a similar size and texture to a mother's tongue, and kittens will love feeling the toothbrush against their fur every day. Gently brush their backs, their heads, and even the sides of their faces to give them the comforting sensation of being lovingly groomed.

WORTH THE WEIGHT

Weight gain is an important indicator of health, so it's essential for caregivers to monitor the weight of kittens daily. Weight loss can be an early indicator that something is going wrong. Monitoring allows us not only to celebrate their growth and progress but also to catch small problems and address them before they become more serious. I can't overemphasize the importance of this step. It takes only a few minutes, and those few minutes are worth it!

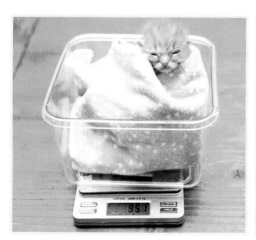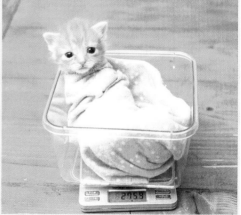

You may choose to monitor the pre- and post-feeding weights at every feeding, weigh twice a day, or just get a daily weight summary every morning, but it's important to do some form of daily weight monitoring. For me, the younger or more vulnerable the kittens are, the more often I'm checking in on their weight throughout the day. Whatever you choose, be sure that you're writing the weights down and tracking their progress (see page 303 for a Kitten Growth and Monitoring chart that you can photocopy for future use).

Remember that all kittens are different, and the weight and feeding chart below is just a guide, not a rule book. That said, you should be seeing an incremental gain of roughly 10 grams per day or more in a healthy kitten. Here's what you need to know about how to weigh a kitten "purrito":

You'll need

- A small digital food scale
- A small baby blanket or washcloth
- A bowl
- A notepad and pen
- A kitten

Kittens are squirmy and won't do well sitting directly on top of a small digital scale, but using this technique, weighing kittens is as cute as it is easy. Set the scale to weigh in grams. Place the cloth inside the bowl, put it on top of the digital scale, and tare the scale so that it says 0. Remove the cloth and wrap it around the kitten to form a loose purrito. This will lightly restrict movement while you weigh the kitten. Place the purrito into the bowl, note the weight in grams, and write it in your notepad along with the date, time, and the kitten's name.

KITTEN WEIGHT AND FEEDING CHART			
Age	Weight	Amount per Feeding	Schedule
0–1 weeks	75–150* grams	2–6 ml	Every 2 hours
1–2 weeks	150–250 grams	6–10 ml	Every 2–3 hours
2–3 weeks	250–350 grams	10–14 ml	Every 3–4 hours
3–4 weeks	350–450 grams	14–18 ml	Every 4–5 hours
4–5 weeks	450–550 grams	18–22 ml	Every 5–6 hours
5–8 weeks	550–850 grams	(weaning: offer ample wet food)	Every 6 hours

*Premature or underweight kittens may weigh less.

What goes in must come out, and you'll be amazed at how quickly food moves through the tiny body of a neonatal kitten. For the first three weeks of life, kittens can't pee and poop on their own—they need a little bathroom assistance. Mama cats stimulate their young to go to the bathroom by regularly licking their bottoms, keeping them comfortable and clean. If you're raising an orphan, you'll need to mimic this behavior (. . . no, not by licking them!) by gently rubbing them with a soft, absorbent tissue every few hours.

Before each feeding, you'll want to empty them out so that they're comfy and ready to accept a meal. Use a soft disposable cloth such as a tissue or toilet paper, avoiding harsh products like heavy paper towels, which could irritate the kitten's

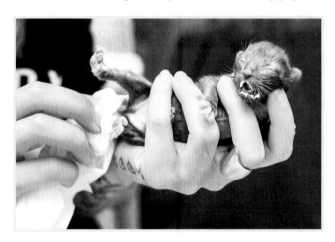

skin. Hold the kitten steady with one hand, and gently rub the genital region in a circular motion with your soft tissue. The tissue will become saturated as the kitten begins to pee. Continue to stimulate the kitten until she is no longer peeing. Depending on the kitten's age, this may take anywhere from ten to thirty seconds. If the kitten needs to poop, you may feel her abdomen flexing as she works to push. Stimulating helps encourage her to use her muscles to pass waste, so continue rubbing until the kitten has finished her business.

Monitor the urine and stool for any concerning symptoms. Pee should be clear or light yellow in color and should occur at every feeding. Bottle-baby poop should be well formed and mustard yellow in color, and can occur anywhere from one to five times a day, depending on the kitten. If you're concerned about the frequency or consistency of the kitten's poop, learn more about poop problems on page 210 and consult a veterinarian to get help.

Don't forget to clean the kitten up after potty time! Mama cats meticulously clean their babies, and you should do the same. Even if the kitten's skin feels dry after peeing or pooping, you still want to wipe her butt down with a wet cloth or a baby wipe afterward to keep her clean. Kittens have sensitive skin and are susceptible to urine scald, a form of moist dermatitis caused by urine residue that burns and irritates the skin. You can help kittens stay comfortable by gently wiping them down after stimulating. If the kitten does get urine or fecal scald, keep the area clean at all times and apply a light zinc-free topical ointment to help her heal.

Once the kittens are three to four weeks old, you'll notice that they'll start wanting to go on their own, which means it's time for a litter box! Learn all about litter box training on page 126.

BOTTLES UP!

If a kitten is orphaned or unable to get enough nutrition through nursing, you'll need to bottle-feed. Bottle-feeding is an acquired skill, and it's totally normal to feel a little awkward the first time you do it. Be patient and don't give up—soon enough, you'll be a pro! Here's what you need to know about helping kittens nurse on a bottle.

Preparing to Feed

ASSESS THE KITTEN.

- If a kitten is cold, it is unsafe to feed until you have stabilized her temperature. This should be an issue only during the first feeding, as orphans are often hypothermic when rescued but will be kept warm once in your care. If a kitten is hypothermic, gradually warm her for at least thirty to sixty minutes with a gentle heat source, and do not feed until she is warm to the touch and moving freely.

- If a kitten is not able to swallow, it is not safe to feed her. For instance, if a kitten is too lethargic to lift her head, you should not flood the mouth with food and should instead seek veterinary support. If a kitten has a cleft palate, it may be riskier to feed her, and caregivers should be especially cautious. Ensure that the kitten is able to swallow by placing a drop of formula on her tongue and feeling the throat with one finger. If the kitten appears stable and is swallowing, proceed. Kittens who are unable to swallow should see a veterinarian immediately.

GATHER YOUR SUPPLIES.

🐱 You can purchase a kitten bottle at any pet supply store or feed store, or online. Be aware that many bottle nipples don't come precut; you will need to cut a hole in it yourself using sharp scissors. The hole should be big enough that if you hold the bottle upside down, formula will slowly drop out of the nipple— but not so big that formula flows out freely.

🐱 Purchase kitten formula. Kittens have special nutritional requirements and require a meal that is formulated for their needs. Never feed a kitten cow's milk, other dairy products, dairy alternatives, or human baby formula, as this can be dangerous or even fatal to the kitten. Instead, purchase kitten formula in powdered or liquid form. Once it's opened, keep the formula refrigerated and follow the labeling for storage, use, and expiration.

PREPARE THEIR MEAL.

🐱 Make fresh formula every one to two feedings, as old formula can spoil or develop unhealthy bacterial content.

🐱 Use a smoothie shaker or a miniature whisk to completely eliminate clumps, which can clog the bottle or lodge in the kitten's throat.

🐱 Formula should be a comfortable temperature. Fresh formula can be made with warm water; refrigerated leftovers can be microwaved for eight to fifteen seconds (microwaves vary, so be cautious!) or placed in a mug of hot water for thirty seconds to gently warm. Always shake the bottle thoroughly before feeding, and test the temperature on your wrist. If it is too hot or too cold for you, it is not the right temperature for the kitten.

Feeding

ASSUME THE POSITION.

🐱 Lay the kitten in a natural, belly-down position—never on her back. Think of how a kitten would nurse from her mother: with her belly facing the floor, lying down or seated. When bottle-feeding, it's normal for her to eagerly sit up or even try to stand, but it's crucial that you keep her in a forward-facing position. If a kitten is fed belly-up, it's not just unnatural; it's dangerous and can cause aspiration.

🐱 Hold the kitten's head stable with your nondominant hand. The index finger and thumb can be used to gently keep the head in place, while the middle finger can lie lightly across the throat to feel if the kitten is swallowing.

🐱 Gently slide the nipple into the kitten's mouth and invert the bottle so that the liquid line completely covers the opening of the bottle. This should start the downward flow of formula into the kitten's mouth. Be very careful not to squeeze formula into the kitten's mouth, as this can cause aspiration. If you are feeding a very young kitten and having a difficult time controlling the flow, consider syringe-feeding.

LOOK FOR THE LATCH.

🐱 The goal is to have the kitten roll her tongue into a U shape and begin to swallow. This is called latching and is a sign that she's fully engaged and eating well. Kittens who are latched will suckle at their own pace, with their tongue rolled, and may wiggle their ears as they chow down. Latching is the goal, so if you've gotten that far, pat yourself on the back!

🐱 If the kitten latches, that's great, but it's okay if it takes a while for her to get the hang of things! Bottle-feeding is an art form that improves with time, so be patient and don't give up.

FILL 'EM UP!

🐱 In general, kittens will tell you when they're done eating by unlatching and turning their head away from the bottle once they're full. However, you'll want to check out the Weight and Feeding Chart on page 99 to determine the proper amount and frequency of feeding so you know if the kitten is undereating or overeating. Remember that every kitten is different, and this chart is a guideline, not a rule book! Some kittens prefer to eat smaller meals more frequently, or may eat a large amount at one feeding and less at the next.

🐱 Some kittens may benefit from being offered seconds. If I'm not positive a kitten has had a big enough meal, I'll revisit her once I've made the rest of my rounds, and offer her another try.

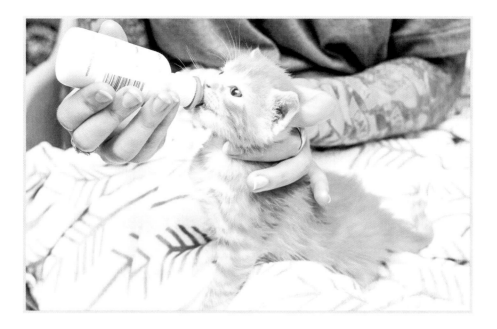

Feeding Tricky Bottle Babies

BE PATIENT AND PRESENT.

🐱 Got a kitten who just doesn't get it? That's pretty normal, especially when one or both of you are still new to bottle-feeding! The keys are patience and presence. You must remain calm and present during the process and guide her along the way. If you're feeling frustrated, "reset" yourself and the kitten by taking sixty seconds to put her down, stretch, take a breath, and try again.

🐱 Be sure you're really holding the head and body stable. Kittens don't necessarily understand what you're trying to do when you bottle-feed them, so the first few times, you may need to hold the head firmly (but gently) in place until they learn what you're doing.

CHECK FOR USER ERROR.

🐱 The kitten might not be eating because she *can't* eat due to a blockage or a poorly cut nipple. If you're using a nipple that you manually cut, make sure the hole hasn't been cut too big or too small. Check for clumps in the formula that may be blocking the hole.

🐱 Ensure that the formula is adequately warm; many kittens will not accept a cold or lukewarm bottle.

SWADDLE 'EM.

🐱 You can gently purrito the kitten if need be with a small receiving blanket to contain wandering limbs and keep the kitten focused on her goal; just make sure she is still in a proper belly-down position.

SIMULATE TRUE NURSING.

🐱 When a kitten nurses from his mama, his face is in her fur, and she may comfort him by licking. You can comfort an orphan by feeding him on a heat pad next to a stuffed animal, gently covering his eyes to help him feel contained, and rubbing his face with a cloth or toothbrush to simulate a mother's tongue. Kittens' suckle reflex is strongest when they first wake up, so try feeding a fussy eater as soon as he wakes.

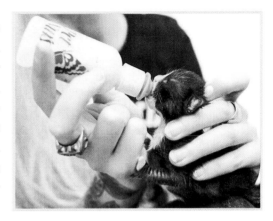

After Mealtime

NO MILK MUSTACHES.

🐱 Milk mustaches are cute, but not if they're left to dry. After feeding, always clean the kitten's face by wiping away any formula with a warm, wet cloth or baby wipe. Formula left behind can cause the kitten to get a crusty face or moist dermatitis that causes the fur to fall out, so keep her nice and clean.

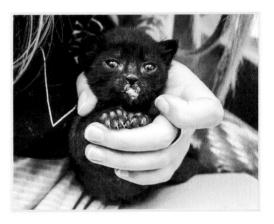

LAST CALL FOR POTTY TIME!

🐱 Even if you've helped the kitten go to the bathroom before the feeding, some kittens may have to go again after the feeding. I like to stimulate them one last time after they eat so that they can be comfortable during their next nap. Don't forget to wipe them up after!

STORE YOUR FORMULA SAFELY.

🐱 If there's still formula left over, put the bottle back into the refrigerator until the next feeding. If you've used the same batch of formula for more than a few feedings, it's a good idea to dump it out and start fresh.

SLOW AND STEADY SYRINGE-FEEDING

Bottle-feeding is the standard method for feeding orphaned kittens, but if you're having difficulty feeding a small newborn kitten, you may want to consider switching from a bottle to a syringe. A syringe can be greatly beneficial for kittens under two weeks of age. Syringes make it easier to measure in small increments, so you can feel confident that the kitten has eaten a full meal. However, it does come with some risks, as very young kittens don't have a gag reflex and can easily aspirate if fed too quickly.

For small babies, I recommend a 3 cc or 5 cc oral syringe (without a needle, of course!). You can find these online for less than ten cents apiece. In a pinch, ask your local veterinarian or animal shelter for a few syringes; they will definitely have some on hand. Ideally, you will use a syringe in combination with a nipple attachment to help the kitten get a good latch. Be sure to pick up at least a dozen syringes, as you don't want to use them for more than a few feedings, even if you're sanitizing them. Used syringes can operate less smoothly, and it's dangerous to syringe-feed if you can't control the flow.

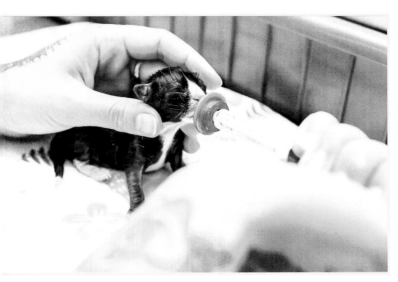

Prepare the formula according to the manufacturer's instructions, making sure that it is fresh, clump-free, and comfortably warm. Pull the formula into the syringe. Just like with bottle-feeding, you should always lay the kitten in a natural, belly-down position—never on her back. Gently slide the syringe into the kitten's mouth and slowly drip formula onto her tongue. The kitten should begin to swallow. Hold the kitten's head and lightly feel her throat to ensure she is swallowing. If the kitten latches on and is suckling, that's great! Very slowly continue to drip formula into her mouth, as slowly as necessary in order for her to swallow each drop. Exercise extreme caution while syringe-feeding to avoid aspiration.

ASPIRE NOT TO ASPIRATE

If you've ever swallowed "down the wrong pipe," then you already know what aspiration is. At the back of the throat, there are two pipes: the esophagus, which leads to the stomach, and the trachea, which leads to the lungs. Most of the time, the trachea is open so that air can easily pass through to the lungs, but when we swallow, a series of muscles constricts and the trachea is closed to allow food to enter the pathway to the stomach. In order for the body to choose the right pipe, the brain and the body have to work together to close the trachea through swallowing.

Neonatal kittens are at special risk of inhaling food into the trachea, especially if they are being bottle-fed. This can occur if the bottle is squeezed and fluid is forced into the kitten's body, if the kitten's feeding posture is incorrect, or if the kitten is struggling to swallow due to a congenital issue such as a cleft palate or megaesophagus. By feeding slowly in a natural upright position and monitoring to ensure the kitten is swallowing, we can reduce the risk of aspiration and keep the food going where it needs to go.

If a kitten does aspirate, you may notice that formula is sneezed out of the nostrils or coughed up. If this occurs, stop feeding immediately and assist the kitten in coughing up the formula. In some cases, aspiration will not be evident right away, but the kitten may develop lethargy, inappetence (loss of appetite), or respiratory distress. Consult a vet immediately if these symptoms of aspiration pneumonia arise, and discuss the option of

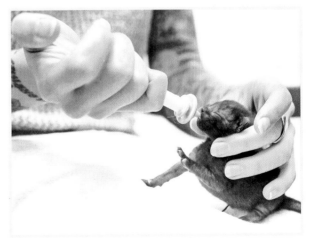

an antibiotic or nebulizer. Of course, the best way to fight aspiration pneumonia is to prevent it from occurring to begin with, so stay present when feeding and ensure that the kitten is actively engaged in swallowing during mealtime.

OH, MAMA

If you're not quite ready for the responsibility of bottle-feeding and potty time, but you still want to help baby kittens, why not foster a litter that comes with their very own kitten-care expert: a mama cat! Lactating moms and their babies are in regular need of foster families, and it's a unique and fun experience to care for a family unit. Mama cats can be incredible caregivers, giving their babies almost everything they need, including warmth, breast-feeding, grooming, and bathroom stimulation. I'm always amazed how perfectly pudgy and sparkling clean their babies tend to look. Mamas even clean up and ingest their babies' waste. Now, that's motherly love!

Before you foster a family, make sure you know what to expect and how to prepare. Mama cats require a little more room to roam than baby kittens do and can get antsy when kept in tight quarters for extended hours. If you can, it's a good idea to dedicate a room to the family. Set up a comfortable nesting area in one corner of the room using a kennel or playpen lined with a soft blanket. Until the babies are about four weeks old, the mama cat will likely spend nearly all her time in this space, nursing and cleaning her babies.

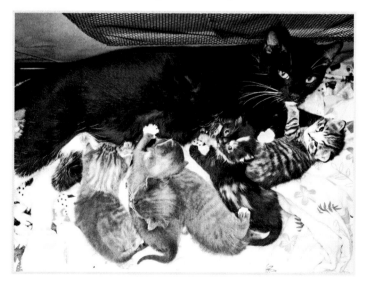

Outside of the nesting area, provide the mama cat with a litter box, fresh water, and ample amounts of kitten food for her to eat. You may notice that the mama is *hungry*, and that's normal! It's important to feed mama cats large amounts of kitten food, as their bodies need the higher fat and protein content while they are nursing their young. In addition to feeding the mama cat, you'll want to keep an eye on her belly to ensure she's having a comfortable lactation experience. If you notice that she has any swelling, redness, or pain from nursing, make sure she sees a vet right away.

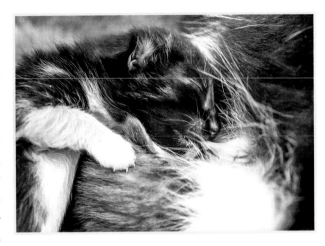

As the babies grow and become more independent, the mama will start seeking distance from them for several hours of the day. It's nice to give her a place she can get away for a bit, like a perch or a raised bed, so she can have a little bit of "me time"! Mama cats typically appreciate the opportunity to gradually get back to life as usual after several weeks of baby care, and by the time the kittens are old enough for adoption at eight weeks, they'll be more than ready to say good-bye.

Most important, don't assume that every cat knows how to be a good mama. Every day, you'll still want to weigh the babies, examine them, and ensure that they are in good health and growing appropriately. In some cases, mama cats aren't able to provide adequate care to their young, and in other cases, babies may have health conditions that a mama cat can't tackle alone. Monitoring the kittens will be important so that if any of them begin to struggle, you can intervene by providing supplemental bottle-feeding and additional care.

THE NAMING OF KITTENS

What's in a name? It's a single word, but it's packed full of meaning. Just like the title of a favorite book or movie, names can give us a first impression of something much more complex. To name a cat is to uniquely convey his individuality. While it may seem silly to put thought into giving a name to a kitten who can't possibly comprehend the *meaning* of the word, I believe naming kittens is more about developing a bond with each animal—making her more than a number. Choosing a kitten's name links her to us as a valuable being with a singular identity. Names can be descriptive or random, refined or downright silly. If you ask me, names do two things for kittens: they dignify, and they signify.

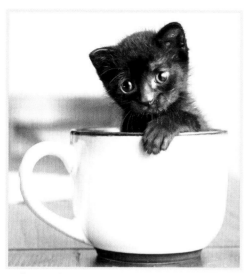
Tetley was brought to the shelter in a tea box.

I've named hundreds of kittens over the years, but it's still one of my very favorite things to do. Depending on the individual kitten, I've given them names that are sweet and simple, like Primrose and Estelle, or totally bizarre, like Jumbo Slice and Texas Pete. I often find myself naming kittens after their origin story, such as Tetley (who arrived in a tea box), Hankie (who arrived in a tissue box), and Beanie (who arrived in a coffee bean box!). Themed names are great for litters of kittens; I may decide to name a whole crew after different pastas or different types of bears. I try to have fun with the names, choosing something suitable and completely unique . . . which isn't always easy after naming as many as I have!

Every time I hear a word I think would make a great name, I write it down. Open my notepad, and you'll find a massive stockpile of names waiting to find their home in a baby cat. Of course, while building this archive has been fun, naming a kitten is always more involved than pointing to a word on a list. I typically need to get to know the kitten for a day or two before I can choose a name that fits just right.

Try creating your own list of potential names! Here are some ideas to get you started:

- Tasty foods or desserts
- Characters from books, movies, or TV shows
- Terms of endearment
- Favorite toys from your childhood
- Historical figures, celebrities, or personal heroes
- Words relating to the kitten's background story

Get creative! You can consider the kitten's personality traits and physical attributes, or choose something totally random. What'd you eat for breakfast? . . . I bet it'd make a cute name for a kitten!

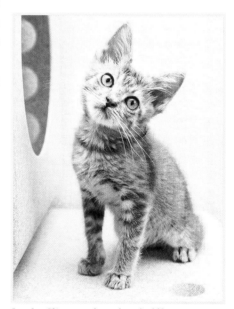
Jumbo Slice was less than half his target weight when rescued, so I named him after a gluttonous meal to encourage weight gain!

It was almost midnight, and I was on a long drive home from Philadelphia. Passing through the tollbooths by the Baltimore tunnel, I noticed a message on my phone: "Urgent! A kitten needs your help!" A friend of a friend of a friend had found a newborn kitten outside ten hours earlier, brought him inside and put him in a box, then fell asleep for the night. By the time this information made it to

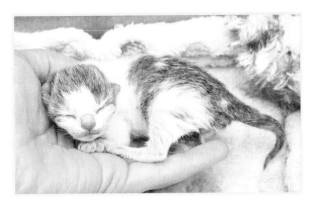

my friend, there was total panic about whether the kitten would survive, having had no food or care during these critical early hours of life. Even though I could barely keep my eyes open, I couldn't say no. I started coordinating with the friends of friends to get the kitten to my house by the time I arrived around one in the morning.

The kitten arrived wrapped in a gym shirt. I unwrapped the cloth and there he was: undeniably a newborn. He had an umbilical cord, a pink nose, and was no larger than a mouse. I named him Tidbit because of his tiny stature, and that night I stayed up monitoring him obsessively—weighing him, keeping him warm, and waking up every two hours to slowly syringe-feed tiny drops of formula into his mouth. After each feeding he'd curl up between his heating pad and a stuffed animal, and his vulnerability broke my heart. When a little bean like Tidbit is depending on you to survive, you're honestly more than happy to wake up to an alarm for feeding time, no matter how tired you are.

The first week of life is always the scariest, so when he made it to one week, it felt like an accomplishment worth celebrating. I made him a tiny hat and a celebratory

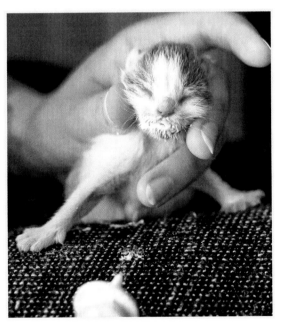

Tidbit ate every two hours via syringe.

banner out of construction paper, pulled out a camera, and snapped Tidbit's one-week birthday photo. A few days later, his eyes began to slowly peek open, and by day fourteen, they were open to the world. I snapped a two-week birthday photo of his new lil' face, with a sweet and sleepy expression that seemed to say, "I just woke up, what'd I miss?" After his two-week birthday photo, I began the tradition of documenting his weekly birthdays.

There's something about the solo orphan babies that tugs at my heartstrings. I hate to leave them alone. For this reason, I bond very closely with the singletons because of how much time I spend interacting with them. With no one to lick him and teach him to groom, I brushed him with a toothbrush every day until he started to learn to clean himself. While I worked at my computer, Tidbit made himself cozy on my shoulder, batting at my long hair. While I showered, Tidbit sat on the bath mat, staring at

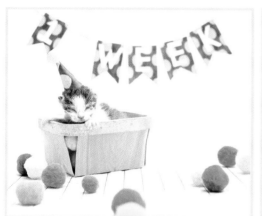 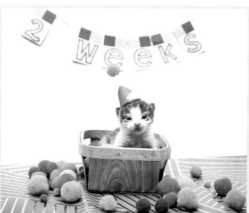

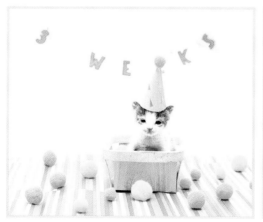 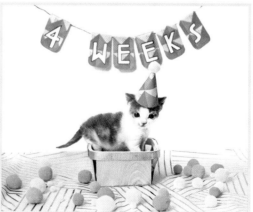

me with his head cocked in confusion. Tidbit even came along for a work trip to New York City, taking meetings with me, attending one of my lectures, and even joining me for a radio interview. For eight adorable weeks, Tidbit was my lil' sidekick.

Meanwhile, the weekly photos continued, and before I knew it, he was outgrowing his photo props. When you spend every moment with a baby, his growth seems incremental, but the photos show just how quickly change happens for kittens. They track his unlikely transformation from a helpless little bean (Tidbit) to a confident young cat celebrating his adoption day (Big Tiddy!). To me, these images serve as evidence that we can impact the fate of an animal in the blink of an eye and change his life forever. Just a matter of weeks takes kittens from vulnerability to strength, from hopelessness to hope. The key is having someone who cares enough to share some time, food, and love . . . and maybe to snap a few cute photos along the way.

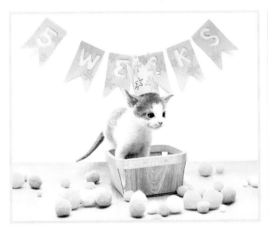 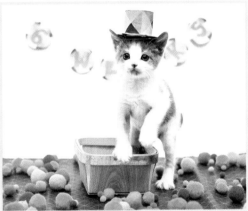

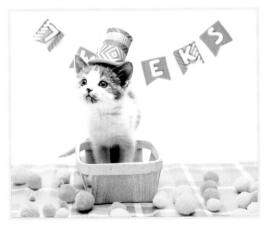 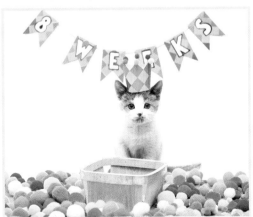

GROW, BABY, GROW

Sometimes Andrew and I jokingly refer to our home as the "baby farm," because this is where baby cats come to grow. While caring for a neonate might sound complex, it's really all about establishing a simple routine and sticking to it until the kitten grows old enough to perform these functions independently. As kittens age, their care routine becomes increasingly easy as they gain more mass, more strength, and more skills. In the next chapter, we'll talk about what happens as kittens become more independent, getting bigger and stronger as they prepare for adoption.

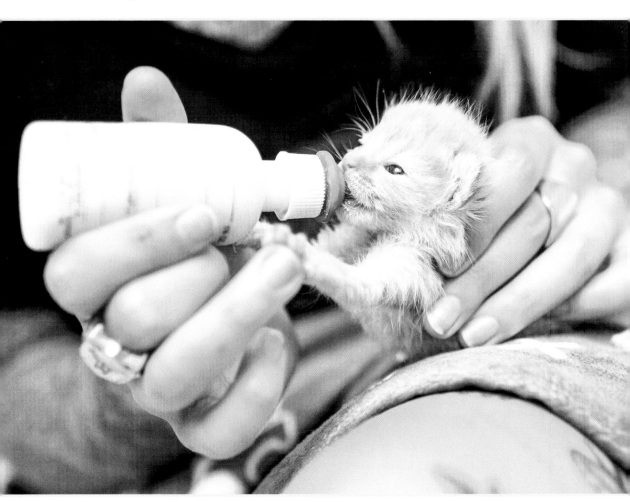

CHAPTER FIVE

FROM TINY TO MIGHTY

I'M A BIG KID NOW

As kittens reach one month of age, everything starts to change. Their vision is sharpening, their coordination is improving, and they're becoming much more curious about the world around them. During this exciting period of change, kittens are testing the waters of being a big kid—and it's up to us to be their life vest as they do! There's nothing more fun (or funnier) than watching kittens try out their first toy, practice their first pounce, or take their first bite of meat, and seeing them discover the fierce feline inside of them. Let's learn about what happens as tiny kittens transform into big kids!

TEENY WEANIES

Cats' bodies may be designed for hunting, but these carnivorous critters aren't born ready to chew on a chunk of meat. During the first weeks of life, kittens subsist entirely on a liquid diet, either by nursing from their mother or, if orphaned, drinking formula from a bottle.

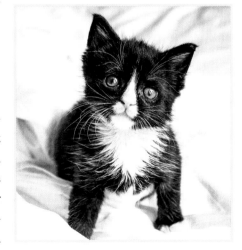

As their teeth begin to fill in and their bodies begin to develop, they start the process of *weaning*, or transitioning from a liquid diet to a solid diet.

Weaning can be a fun and messy endeavor. Just like a toddler covered in spaghetti sauce, kittens are often adorably ungraceful when learning how to consume solid foods. I've always enjoyed the weaning process because watching kittens consume meat for the first time is like watching a light turn on in their tiny carnivorous minds. There's something hilarious and endearing about watching an innocent one-pound furball discover her true nature as a predator. They typically start exhibiting their first hunting behaviors around this age, like pouncing and attacking toys, and they may even let out a tiny growl. What petite, fearsome beasts!

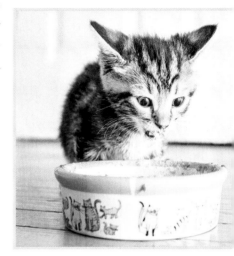

Weaning Supplies

- Kitten formula
- Wet kitten food (make sure it says "kitten"!)
- Shallow food dish
- Small scale (for monitoring weight)
- Puppy pads and baby wipes (for easy cleanup!)

WHEN TO WEAN

In order to give kittens a successful weaning experience, it is critically important to get the timing right. Weaning is one of the most vulnerable periods of a kitten's life; she is being introduced to new nutrients and a new method of eating, leaving lots of opportunity for something to go awry. Weaning is therefore most successful when a kitten is biologically prepared to handle both safely consuming and digesting the new nutrients that are being introduced.

The digestive system changes greatly during the weaning process. The intestinal villi develop rapidly, increasing the intestines' internal surface area and allowing the kitten to properly absorb the new nutrients. This process is critical for ensuring that the kitten can safely absorb the vital proteins and sugars through the gut. The digestive enzymes also begin to shift at the time of weaning; the lactase, which breaks down milk sugars, changes to sucrase, which breaks down the sugars present in meat. Even though you can't see the gut, it's changing and developing rapidly inside the growing kitten, preparing him for his future.

Kittens weaned prematurely are at risk of weight loss, diarrhea, vomiting, dehydration, and malabsorption. Their bodies may not be able to properly digest or absorb nutrients from meat. They also may not be able to safely or effectively eat the food, and can choke or undereat, consuming an insufficient quantity to meet their caloric needs. Premature weaning is a common risk factor for serious illness in kittens, so it's best to wait until five weeks to wean. Of course, weaning too late can be an issue, too—in addition to not gaining the right nutrients, kittens weaned too late risk shredding the nipple of a bottle with their sharp teeth!

The first baby teeth will be descending at three and four weeks of age, but don't be fooled—these teeth are not designed for eating meat. Incisors are useful for grooming and nibbling at the fur, and canines are useful for learning to hunt prey; but it isn't until the premolars descend at five weeks that the kitten is ready to start shredding solids. At this age, kittens' bodies are coordinated enough to begin seeking, finding, chewing, and swallowing food independently.

Ultimately, however, the age of weaning often depends on the kitten's real-life circumstances. Many shelters and rescue organizations routinely begin introducing kittens to solid foods as early as three and a half to four weeks old due to the difficulty of finding foster homes for kittens who are unweaned. This isn't what I'd recommend in a perfect world, but my perspective is that we have to make pragmatic decisions with the specific conditions in mind, doing right by each individual within his or her own context. If a kitten is four weeks old and is at risk of euthanasia if unweaned, it's obviously preferable to give the kitten a chance to live by introducing him to a solid diet. That said, kittens are more robust and healthful when given an extra week to nurse or at least supplemental bottle-feeding; 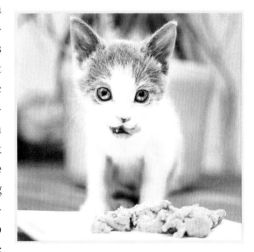 whenever possible, it's better to adjust the caregiver duties to meet the needs of the kitten than to adjust the care of the kitten to meet the needs of the caregiver. When kittens are given age-appropriate care, it's a better experience for everyone involved. My hope is that one day there will be fewer kittens in need of homes, and that those who are in need will be able to be cared for on a timeline that gives them the best experience possible.

GIVING MOM A BREAK

If you're caring for a mother and her babies, you'll find that weaning often happens quite naturally. As the kittens become more mobile and inquisitive, they may start being curious about their mama's food and trying to take a few nibbles. Whether they do or don't show interest in her food, you'll want to start hand-feeding wet food to them around five weeks of age. The goal should be to help them become independent eaters by six weeks of age so that you can slowly begin to give mama a break.

Once the kittens are eating on their own, it's a good idea to start giving mom a little space. As kittens' sharp teeth grow in, mom cats are often pretty ready to get

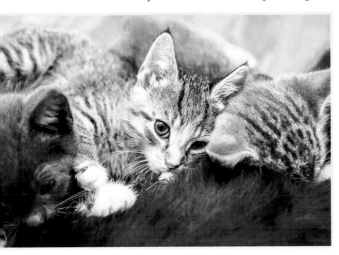

them off her teats! While she may allow them to supplementally nurse, you want them to be primarily subsisting on wet food by six weeks. How you give her a break will depend on the situation. If the family has full run of a room, it should be relatively easy for the mom to create distance for herself, and if she can, she will! It can be helpful to give her a perch or platform where she can get some solo time. However, if the family is being kept in close quarters such as a kennel or playpen, it's a good

idea to physically separate the babies and mama during part of the day to encourage independent eating. Part-time parenting for a one-week period gives both the kittens and the mother a slow, comfortable transition. Four to seven days after nursing ceases, the mother's milk will begin to dry up and she'll be back to her independent ways. You can then move mom to a separate room, to her adoptive home, or TNR if she's a community cat, and prepare the kittens for adoption.

Whenever possible, avoid pulling the babies off the mama too early or too quickly. In addition to being dangerous for the kittens, premature weaning can also have a negative impact on the mother. Abruptly ceasing nursing can cause milk to accumulate in the mammary glands, leading to pain or even an infection called mastitis. If the mother develops signs of swelling or discomfort, you'll want to talk to a vet about antibiotics, and apply warm compresses if the cat is friendly and safe to work with. However, it's best to avoid this situation altogether by allowing the weaning process to occur at a comfortable pace for all!

DON'T HURRY—TRY SLURRY

One way to start introducing meat to kittens, especially those who are orphaned, is to create a transitional food called slurry. Slurry is a combination of the food they are used to consuming (kitten formula) and the food they are moving on to (wet food). The great thing about slurry is that you can create different concentrations so that the kitten can become gradually more acquainted with the new food, both texturally and digestively. You can introduce slurry around five weeks of age.

Purchase wet kitten food and mix it with your kitten formula. You can start by making a soupy texture that can be lapped up, and over time increase the concentration of meat as they learn to chew. Many kittens will not automatically understand slurry, so be ready to offer it to them via a finger (or a tongue depressor if you don't want to use your hand). You can place a little bit into the mouth and observe to ensure they are swallowing, then repeat the process so they get used to the idea of solid foods. Over time, you can lower your finger into the dish to show them that they can lap it up independently.

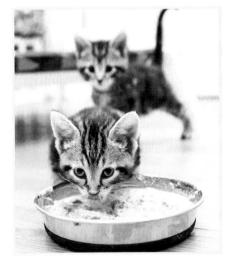

Never assume that a kitten can eat on her own until she has a track record of successfully doing so. By sitting with the kittens and actively supporting the feeding process, you can physically introduce them to the food until they're able to do it on their own. To make sure they're getting a full tummy, I recommend continuing supplemental bottle-feeding after each slurry trial until they're eating a full meal on their own.

Once the kittens are confidently eating slurry, you can transition them completely to their diet of wet kitten food. Of course, there are some kittens who may automatically understand wet food without the transitional slurry, and that's okay, too—it's all about getting to know the individual and supporting his unique needs. Either way, most kittens will be totally transitioned onto wet food by six weeks of age, which means life will be getting a whole lot easier for you. Woo-hoo!

WEANIN' AIN'T EASY

It was a crisp February evening in Philadelphia, and while kitten season hadn't started yet, this crew of two-week-old tabbies clearly hadn't gotten the memo. When I picked up my new quintuplets, they had just opened their eyes, and were ravenous bottle babies. Every few hours Velouria, Margot, Barnaby, Winston, and Phillip would take turns chugging a warm bottle and then fall sound asleep with fat, happy bellies. Andrew and I took turns on the night shift, waking up several times throughout the night to feed the feasters.

Bottle-feeding five kittens is a wild ride. At first, the kittens were peaceful and gentle sucklers . . . but as they got older and more aware of their surroundings, they became more competitive. By the time they were reaching five weeks of age, it was an absolute riot as they all clamored over the bottle, squealing and begging to be next in line. Waking up at 3 a.m. to satiate five eager gluttons is an amusing experience, but I'd be lying through my teeth if I said that you don't look forward to the day they learn to eat on their own.

There's no way around it: weaning is messy. When you first show kittens a bowl of food, they're honestly not sure if they're supposed to be eating . . . or finger-painting! Velouria seemed to pick up on it relatively quickly, shoving her tiny face into the bowl and slurpin' slurry. Winston and Phillip did their best to figure it out, too, dunking their faces into the dish and looking back up at me with little meat mustaches. But Barnaby and Margot had a harder time of it. Barnaby basically submerged his entire snout in the slurry, resulting in

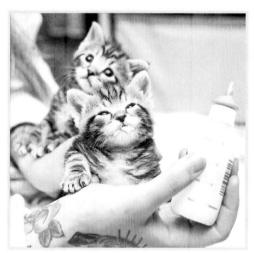

Phillip and Winston get a midnight meal.

more than just a mustache . . . It was honestly more like a massive meat beard. And Margot—bless her heart—she didn't know *what* was going on. She stood with her paws fully saturated in slop, as if she might absorb some nutrients through her paws by osmosis.

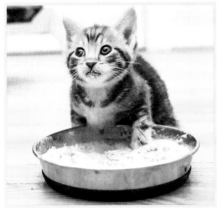
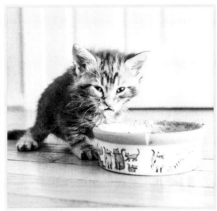

Margot doesn't quite get it . . .   Barnaby is a mess!

While the brown tabbies all picked it up quickly, I continued supplemental bottle-feeding Margot and Barnaby for about a week until I was convinced they'd finally figured it out. Weaning is just like growing up: it's a little awkward, it's a little sloppy, and everyone has to do it at his or her own pace. A little patience and humor go a long way when fostering fledgling felines!

MEAT THEM WHERE THEY ARE

Remember when you were a little kid and your caregiver would say, "If you don't finish your veggies, you can't have dessert"? Take that idea and throw it out the window when it comes to weaning kittens. If a kitten doesn't want her meat, the last thing you want to do is shrug and tell her it's too bad. Give her something else! If she doesn't want wet food, try slurry. If she doesn't want slurry, offer her formula. Some kittens may even reject wet food altogether, but may love crunchy food. Try different things until you find what works. There's no such thing as "tough love" when it comes to kitten weaning. We have to meet them where they are. The important thing about the weaning process is not to rush.

I highly suggest that you continue to have the kittens nurse at the end of the meal for the first several days of the weaning process. By providing supplemental bottle-feeding (or nursing with mom), you ensure that the kitten is truly getting a full meal and meeting all her caloric and nutritional needs. This is a more natural and gradual approach than switching abruptly, and reduces the risk of weight loss during this critical period. The kittens will be grateful for a few last chances to nurse!

Most important, make sure you're monitoring the kittens throughout the weaning process, and paying attention if their health starts to decline. Weigh your kittens twice a day while they are transitioning onto solid food, and ensure that their weight is going up—not down. Take a look at their stool, and notice if it's loose or pale in color. Notice their energy level: Are they playful and active, or are they listless and lethargic? If you've started weaning a kitten and his health is declining, it's a good idea to scale back and let him nurse (or bottle-feed) until he is a little older. Slow and steady wins the race!

TINY CARNIVORES

Cats are obligate carnivores, and like with all felids, eating meat is a biological necessity for them. They have evolved to be perfectly designed for consuming the bodies of other animals, and to thrive on an all-meat diet. For instance, cats have carnassial teeth, which are paired upper and lower teeth that pass by each other sharply in a manner that allows them to shear flesh and tendons. They have short-

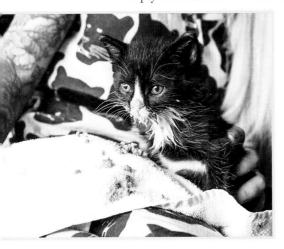

ened intestines that allow them to pass food through the gastrointestinal tract quickly, absorbing the nutrients and completing the digestive cycle in a matter of hours. Unlike plant-eating species, cats are unable to self-produce certain vitamins and amino acids, and must instead obtain them by eating others. Whether hunting in the wild or circling our feet in the kitchen, cats have always thrived on a diet of meat.

If it seems like the kittens are eating like ravenous little piggies, it's because they are! "Kittens require more energy from their food as they grow—up to twice as much food per pound of body weight as adult cats," says cat expert In-grid King, author of the award-winning blog The Conscious Cat. In addition to eating a larger quantity, kittens also need to eat more frequently, and with a greater amount of protein and fat. Choosing a diet that is rich in protein and fat and offer-ing it generously during the first six months of life will help to develop the building blocks of a healthy body. Once they reach six months old, most kittens can be transitioned onto their adult diet and feeding schedule.

When choosing a kitten food, one important consideration should be hydration. Wet canned food is always preferable to dry food, as a higher moisture content is present. Because cats lack a strong thirst drive, obtaining plenty of water through the food is critical. This is especially true for kittens, who may still be learning to consume water, and may have more opportunities to lose hydration if sick. But that's not the only reason wet food is preferable. King continues, "Cats lack the specific enzyme that processes plant-based proteins metabolically, and as a result, they need few to no carbohydrates in their diet." With dry food tending to be sub-stantially higher in carbohydrates, it is not an optimal diet for a kitten, and should be used sparingly or as a supplemental snack.

The commercial pet food industry has several wet diets marketed specifically for kittens, which is a great place to start when shopping. Not all kitten foods are created equal, though, so if you're looking for the highest-quality food for your kit-ten, I recommend getting a moist canned food that contains high protein and fat content. It can be a challenge to find kitten food at some grocery chains and big-box stores, but online retailers and pet supply shops tend to carry a wide variety of options.

Some kitten rescuers swear by raw diets for kittens, and while it can be done with great success, I will caution that it is a potentially risky decision if done incor-rectly. While raw diets are high in nutrients and water, they also quickly develop bacteria that can harm a sensitive young tummy. If you plan to feed a raw diet, choose a balanced commercial raw diet and be very mindful of storing and prepar-ing it properly.

At the end of the day, the deciding factor may end up being . . . the kitten! Inter-estingly, many kittens have picky palates and may reject one food but love another, so don't be afraid to try a few brands or flavors until you find the one they love. I keep three different kinds on hand in my home nursery, and find that when it comes to palate preference, kittens are every bit as choosy as people are—but once they find something they like, they tend to stick with it. Bon appétit, little ones!

Kittens' bodies contain a higher water content than their adult counterparts, and hydration is therefore central to their health and well-being. Water aids in digestion and bowel function, maintains the kidneys and other organs, energizes the muscles, protects the bones, and keeps kittens feeling refreshed and healthy. Water is life!

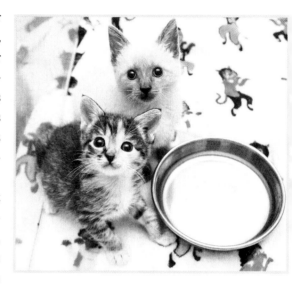

Neonates receive their water content completely through breast milk (or formula). However, as they begin to wean, kittens will need to obtain their moisture content elsewhere. Once kittens are weaning and tapering off their liquid diet, you can begin to introduce them to a shallow bowl of fresh water. Most kittens will not naturally understand water until they understand eating from a dish, so don't fret if it takes them several days to figure it out. As they discover water for the first time, it's normal for them to dip their faces into it awkwardly, almost pecking at it like a bird eating seed. This is how they learn! Just make sure it's a shallow dish and that they're old enough (and big enough) not to fall in. Once the kittens are at the weaning phase, they should have access to clean, fresh water at all times.

It's common for kittens to become dehydrated (see page 213 to learn about kittens and dehydration), and because it's one of the biggest dangers they face, you'll want to think about ways to increase their moisture content. It doesn't hurt to stir a splash of water into their wet food to help boost their hydration, especially if you're concerned that they aren't consuming enough water. Of course, providing wet food is highly preferable to dry food, as it is 70 to 80 percent water, versus dry food, which typically is about 10 percent water. Wet food is therefore a great way for kittens and cats to consume water without even realizing it!

Cats tend to be spectacularly clean, making them a wonderful low-maintenance animal when it comes to grooming. However, kittens aren't always spick-and-span (especially during the weaning process!), so they need to learn self-grooming behaviors in order to develop a healthy cleanup routine. Getting kittens accustomed to being meticulously clean is important for both their physical health and their grooming awareness. Here are a few pieces of advice to help kittens learn how to primp:

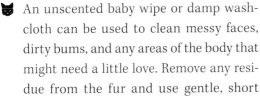

- An unscented baby wipe or damp washcloth can be used to clean messy faces, dirty bums, and any areas of the body that might need a little love. Remove any residue from the fur and use gentle, short strokes to mimic a mother's tongue. Just make sure the kitten is warm and dry after you wipe her down.

- A soft-bristle toothbrush is a great way to comb through the kitten's fur and encourage licking. By regularly brushing the kitten, you'll teach him that it feels good to get his fur feeling sleek and spotless.

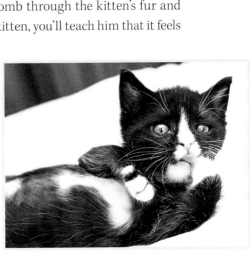

- Groom after mealtime. This gets kittens into the rhythm of a cat's natural routine: hunting, eating, then grooming. By spending some time on cleanup after each meal, you'll get them into the swing of a healthy grooming ritual for the rest of their lives.

- Help the kitten maintain claw health by providing a scratching post, and by introducing claw trimming at one month of age.

As kittens reach three to four weeks of age, they begin looking for somewhere to go to the bathroom, making this a great time to introduce the litter box. Luckily for caregivers, the litter box comes instinctively to most kittens, and by a month of age the majority of them will be using it with ease. I've always felt that the term "litter training" is a bit of a misnomer when it comes to kittens; it's less about training and more about simply providing the right set of circumstances for them to succeed. By giving them a consistent and proper experience from day one, we can set kittens up for a lifetime of good litter box habits.

Cats are marvelously clean animals, and they tend to seek out places where they can discreetly do their business and then cover it up. These instinctively polite poopers don't want to leave behind a strong scent, which is why outdoor cats tend to choose loose soil for a toilet rather than pavement. The fine grain of the litter provides a similarly attractive place for kittens to pee, and the goal of litter training is to make the litter box the simplest and most obvious place for them to bury their waste. It's important to simultaneously decrease alternative areas, such as piles of laundry or bedding, which can seem to a young kitten like a similarly suitable place to cover up their waste. Keep bedding smooth and avoid these unwanted potential potties, especially while kittens are learning to use a litter box, *or* whenever they are entering a new and unfamiliar space. You want to make the litter box the only desirable option for bathroom time!

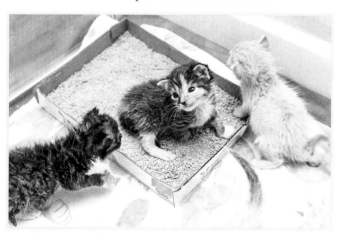

A shallow, disposable box or tray is a great way to introduce kittens to litter training!

What makes a good kitten litter box? While many adult cat litter boxes have tons of bells and whistles like steps, covers, or even self-cleaning capabilities, none of that is appropriate for a young kitten. Kittens need a box that is low to the ground, with a shallow lip that is easy for them to walk over. One great option for the truly teeny guys is to use a cardboard tray (such as the kind that holds wet cat food) or a disposable baking pan, both of which are small and can be tossed out once used. Most kittens will prefer to use the bathroom in a corner, and boxes should be placed within close proximity to the kitten. If the kitten has access to more than one room, ensure that there is at least one box in a corner of every room the kitten has access to until she has fully acclimated.

Kittens are curious animals who explore their worlds just like human babies do: with their mouths! While it's obvious to us that a litter box is no place for a snack, kittens are still figuring out what it's all about and may do a taste test to see if the litter is worth munching on. To avoid any unfortunate circumstances, use a kitten-safe litter that won't harm the kitten if ingested. Clumping litters and highly fragrant litters should be avoided; a more suitable alternative is a scent-free, nonclumping clay litter, paper litter, or corn litter. Once the kitten has established several weeks of appropriate litter box usage, you can switch to any litter of your choice.

Of course, the most important way to teach a kitten good litter box habits is to start by having good litter box habits yourself. There's an unfortunate stereotype that homes with cats are stinky—but that's just not true. The litter box is only stinky if you don't clean it! It's important not to look at scooping as a chore, and to think of it as a simple routine instead. If you walked past a dirty toilet in your home, would you just shrug your shoulders and leave it for tomorrow? No way! You'd flush it. The litter box is no different. You should scoop it every time you notice that it is dirty. Kittens don't like a gross litter box any more than you like a dirty porta-potty, so keep their box clean for your sake and theirs. You'll reduce the likelihood that they will go outside of the box, and you and the kitten will both be happy to have a fresh home. Cats aren't smelly animals . . . but people who don't clean the litter box sure are!

When a kitten first uses the box, it's great to provide positive reinforcement such as a happy and congratulatory tone or gentle head scratches to say, "Good job!" But if the kitten doesn't get it at first, you don't want to punish her for going outside of the box. Despite popular belief, rubbing a kitten's nose in her waste teaches her nothing except to fear you. Instead, have patience and try to troubleshoot the issue. Is the kitten unable to easily find or access the box? Is the specific litter bothering her? Try a few different brands, boxes, and placements.

When kittens are learning to use the box for the very first time, it can be helpful to place their waste into the box to signal to them that that's where it belongs. If the kitten poops outside the box, move the waste into the box where she can see it.

If the kitten is only a few weeks old, you can even stimulate her directly into the box to help her associate it with the scent of her urine. Until kittens have learned

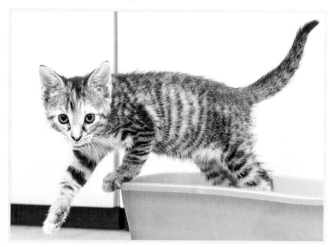

good litter box habits, it's important to keep them in a small area so they can quickly find the box and so that they don't begin eliminating in any unwanted areas—after all, it's a lot harder to break a bad habit than to avoid having it start at all. Keep the kitten's world small until she has conquered it—then she'll be ready to go forth into the home with polite potty skills!

LITTER BOX DOS AND DON'TS

Do	Don't
Use a shallow, uncovered box that is easy for the kitten to walk into.	Use a covered box or a box that is too tall to be easily entered.
Use a kitten-safe litter that is nonclumping and fragrance free.	Use a highly fragrant or clumping litter, which is dangerous to kittens if ingested.
Clean the litter box at least once a day, if not more frequently.	Allow the box to become saturated with urine or filled with feces.
Eliminate other potty options by keeping the kitten's surrounding environment clean, smooth, and free of piled bedding.	Keep around piles of loose bedding or laundry, which can appear like a good place to use the bathroom and cover it up.
Make it easy for the kitten to find the box; put out at least one litter box in every room that the kitten has access to while learning.	Make the kitten go on a hunt for the potty by having only one litter box for a four-bedroom house.
Put the box in a corner.	Put the box in the center of a room.
Praise the kitten when she uses the box!	Punish the kitten for not using the box.

Keep your feet off the dinner table.

Look both ways before you cross the street.

Say "please" and "thank you."

As children, we are taught all sorts of behaviors that are meant to keep us healthy, safe, and in good social standing. When raising kittens, we similarly take on the role of the adult figure who guides the appropriate behavioral development of the adolescents, ensuring that they will someday flourish as sociable and well-mannered members of cat society. By working with them from a very young age, we're able to influence how they interact with their surrounding environment, humans, and other animals, and we help them become the very best cats they can be.

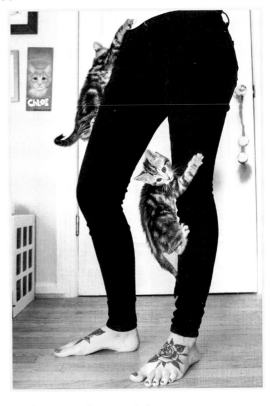

But it isn't as easy as telling them what to do. Kittens may not understand spoken words, but they respond very well to routines and interactions that suit their needs and ours. To help kittens develop healthy behaviors, we have to first understand their nature and motivations; we have to step back from being fixated on human expectations and instead focus on who they are and what makes them feel whole. From this starting point, we can guide them in a way that keeps the whole house happy.

Ultimately, kids will be kids, and kittens will be kittens—they aren't for everyone or every home. While we can guide kittens toward healthy habits, there's little we can do to change the fact that for the first year of life, they tend to be very hyper. It's important for foster parents and adopters to have a realistic expectation and a healthy attitude when bringing home a kitten, and to opt for a calmer adult cat if they aren't ready for their home to be buzzing with kinetic energy!

Pouncing. Biting. Climbing. Scratching. Butt wiggles. As kittens go through the growth spurt of adolescent cat life, their bodies experience a surge of energy and an instinctive drive to practice their hunting prowess. As cat guardians, we must acknowledge and honor the fact that we are raising micro-panthers, and to cultivate those instincts. After all, cats never asked to be domesticated, and if we've decided to bring tiny hunters into our homes, the least we can do is nurture their natural inclinations!

Pouncing may be a natural behavior for kittens, but what we don't want is for them to be attacking *your bare feet*. Biting can be fine and dandy, but not when they're chomping on *your hands*. Climbing is cool, but not when they're scaling *your pants* like a tree trunk! We want to encourage kittens to practice these behaviors with an appropriate target . . . i.e., not your skin. Fortunately, kittens are adaptive and can learn with a little assistance!

For their mental and behavioral health, we must let the kitten be a kitten—but we don't need to let these crazed carnivores attack at our own expense. By creating an enriching environment and play routine with your kittens, you'll teach them to behave in a way that is both natural to them and comfortable for us. As my friend Jackson Galaxy wisely discusses in his brilliant book on cat behavior, *Total Cat Mojo*, cats thrive when provided with a natural rhythm: "Hunt, catch, kill, eat, groom, sleep." We can begin creating a positive routine for our kittens by providing them with activities that allow them to practice the hunt and the takedown, to feel rewarded by food, and to feel safe and secure enough to clean up and reenergize with a catnap.

Our rescued kittens might not be living in the wilderness, but they do thrive when they're given opportunities to express their wild side daily. As their guardians, we need to provide an enriching indoor experience for these tiny hunters. By envisioning a wildcat's psychological needs, we can start to see how a play routine, a toy collection, and a customized home base can work together to help our little micro-panthers experience the jungle right from the comfort of home.

Over the years, I haven't exclusively worked with little kittens. I've also worked quite a bit with big cats . . . and I'm not talking about ten-pound tabbies! For three years, I was a dedicated volunteer at a big-cat sanctuary in North Carolina that was home to rescued lions, tigers, leopards, cougars, and smaller wildcats like servals, caracals, ocelots, and bobcats. Most of the eighty-plus individuals were surrendered from the cruel exotic pet trade or the heartless entertainment industry, and sadly none of them were releasable, having spent their entire lives in captivity. Fortunately, the sanctuary offered them a safe, nonexploitative space to live out their lives as naturally as possible, and it was an honor to assist them in doing so.

One of the primary ways that sanctuaries provide a natural and positive experience for wildlife is through enrichment programs. Enrichment is any activity that provides captive animals with stimuli that enhance their psychological well-being. These activities are generally species-specific and target the senses and natural behaviors of the captive animals, helping them express their wild nature in an enclosed setting. Enrichment can be anything from a habitat designed to support the needs of the animal to activities and playtime that keep the animal physiologically engaged.

In practice, enrichment at the big-cat sanctuary was a fun and often funny experiment of the senses. Some of the most memorable enrichment activities I did were . . .

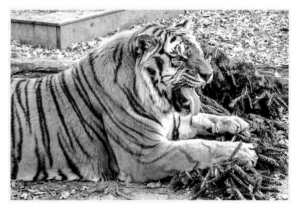

Vincent the tiger plays with a fragrant Christmas tree, sticking his tongue out. This "Flehmen response" is a biological mechanism used by both big cats and small cats to investigate an interesting smell.

- 🐱 Hiding cubed meat in giant piles of wood chips (for the lions to "hunt")

- 🐱 Giving out discarded Christmas trees (for the tigers to smell, roll on, and play with)

- 🐱 Spraying high-end colognes and perfumes onto paper towel rolls (for the ocelots to rub their faces against and explore their scent-driven instincts)

🐱 Playing bird sounds over a boom box (to engage the auditory prowess of the servals and caracals)

🐱 Giving fresh herbs and catnip (for the bobcats to roll in and enjoy)

We would also create enriching environments with each species' needs in mind. For instance, ocelots love climbing into trees, so we'd provide tubes and walkways that led to arboreal platforms. Tigers love water, so we'd provide them with giant water tubs in the summer where they could swim and lounge. Occasionally, we'd move the cats to a new enclosure so that they had an exciting new world to explore. That's the central tenet of enrichment: providing a varied experience to keep the cats' minds curious, their paws busy, and their lives full.

Without enrichment, captive wildlife suffer deeply; their psychological health declines, and they may engage in self-harm or stereotypical behaviors like pacing. This is often seen in animal-testing laboratories, zoos, circuses, and other captive environments, and is a devastating reminder that when we keep animals captive for our own purposes, we forget that they, too, are complex beings with wants and needs. Truly being alive is about more than having food and water; it's about being active, fulfilled, and emotionally whole.

Working with big-cat enrichment programs had a major impact on my understanding of kittens' psychological needs as well. After all, kittens and domestic cats are not all that different from their larger relatives! I'd get home from a day at the sanctuary, look at my little ones, and ask myself, *What can I do to give them an enriching experience today?* Suddenly I'd find myself doing things like hiding treats

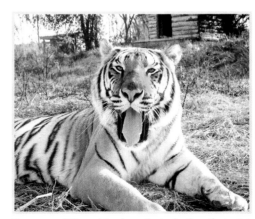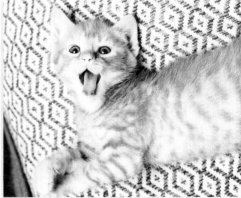

Roscoe and Numpkin show that whether their stripes are big or small, all cats are biologically similar!

for them to hunt, introducing them to new fragrances, and building them castles out of cardboard boxes.

Now enrichment has become an important part of my rescue routine! I play my kittens video clips of fish swimming and birds flying. I give them tunnels, hideaways, and perches, and fill them with treats to encourage exploration. Instead of tossing out that cardboard box full of crinkly paper, I give it to them for a few days and watch them have a party. I take them on scent tours throughout the house to give them an olfactory adventure. I've found that when you get creative, there's no shortage of ways to entertain a feline, big or small!

I LIKE THE WAY YOU MOVE

I'm often asked why kittens like to bite hands and feet, and how to decrease this behavior. The reason kittens bite us is simple: they're predators, and they want to practice their attack on a moving object! Attacks are almost always prompted when the kitten spots movement. If you break the hunting process down, it would start with the realization that something is moving, then the stalking of that moving object, and finally the pounce. Now consider what a kitten sees when they see your fingers reaching out, or your foot stepping by. They're thinking . . .

. . . *ATTACK!!!*

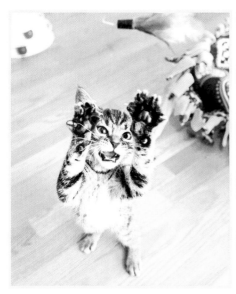 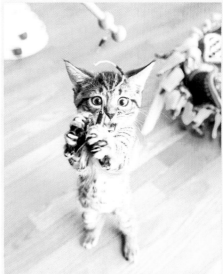

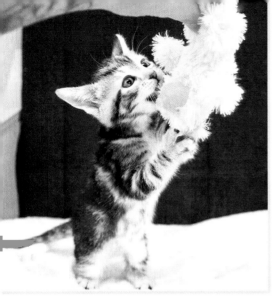

Kittens are biologically predisposed to attack an object that moves, so it is of utmost importance that we teach them how to play with toys from a young age. Think of it this way: if you never dangle a feather toy to mimic a bird in flight, or you never toss a stuffed mouse for them to fetch, then the only potential prey they ever see moving is *you*.

In the absence of actual prey, we must simulate the hunting experience through playtime in order for the kittens to be emotionally and behaviorally sound. Small plush toys, crinkle balls, wands, and other toys each offer enticing qualities, such as a zipping motion through the air, a tempting sound, or a chewable texture. Offer various kinds of kitten-safe toys to provoke their natural instincts. Teach kittens that when it comes to chewing, that's what toys are for!

It's important not just to give kittens toys, but also to actively play with them. Those toys aren't going to move themselves! Actively playing multiple times a day before mealtime is a great way to help kittens develop their motor skills, learn appropriate habits, and get their energy out. Move the toys in an engaging fashion, encouraging them to stalk, chase, pounce, and catch. Once the kitten catches the toy, let her take out her aggression through biting and bunny-kicking before mov-

ing it again. After the kitten has had a nice play session, congratulate and reward her with a treat or meal to simulate the satisfying experience of eating after a kill.

I suggest introducing play to kittens around three and a half to four weeks of age, and focusing playtime around appropriate targets—not your hands. As tempting as it is to rub bellies or wiggle your fingers to get their attention, this teaches kittens that it's okay to

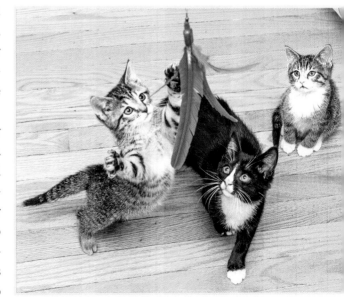

hunt people, and as they grow up, it gets a lot less cute. Even if you don't mind having your hands munched on or your legs clawed, prospective adopters likely will. If you're noticing lots of attacks on feet or hands as you move, don't get grumpy—just disengage. Quickly redirect the kittens to a more suitable object.

One of the great benefits of kittens being raised in litters is that they teach each other good boundaries when it comes to play aggression. Mom cats and littermates might enjoy a bit of a tumble, but if bitten too hard, they'll let out a forceful yap that pierces the kitten's ears and tells them "No!" Kittens quickly learn from other cats about where the line is, and how to have fun without crossing it. That's just one of the many reasons kittens do better in pairs, which I'll talk more about on page 141.

KITTEN PLAYTIME DOS AND DON'TS

Do	Don't
Use plush toys, wand toys, crinkle balls, tunnels, and other enrichment items to play.	Use your hands to taunt and play.
Actively play with the kitten using toys you can move, multiple times throughout the day.	Expect the kitten to play on her own all the time.
Allow the kittens to catch the toys and bite/kick.	Tease the kittens by withholding toys.
Reward kittens after playtime with a treat or meal to simulate the satisfaction of eating after a kill.	Engage in the hunt without letting them experience the fruits of their kill.
Redirect aggressive behaviors toward an appropriate target.	Strike, spray, or yell at kittens who play too rough.

KITTEN TOY SAFETY PRECAUTIONS

Toy Type	Precautions
Plush toys and kickers	These are a great option for chewing, kicking, and hunting! Just make sure that there aren't any small pieces that can be bitten off and swallowed, such as beads or buttons, and avoid feathers that can be chewed and swallowed. Catnip-filled plush toys are fun, too, but most kittens won't react until they're about four months or older.
Crinkle balls	Wonderfully crunchy, these toys make an enticing sound when tossed! These are generally safe, but if you see that the kitten is shredding or swallowing a piece of it, opt for something sturdier like a plush with a crinkle inside of it.
Tubes and tunnels	Kittens love hiding, and these enrichment items make a great place to do just that! Just be sure there are no hanging strings where the kitten could get hurt.

Toy Type	Precautions
Ropes, wands, and fishing-pole toys	Toys that dangle from a string make really great trainers for hunting, but beware— only let kittens have these toys when a human is supervising. Kittens can get seriously hurt if a string wraps around a neck or limb, and just a few rolls can get them tangled up, resulting in strangulation. Only use these with supervision.
Feather toys	These avian amusements are definitely enticing, but use feathers sparingly and only if you're actively playing with the kitten. A feather can get chomped in half and lodged in the kitten's throat or stomach, leading to choking or blockages. When it comes to cat toys, it's best to leave feathers for the birds.
Yarn and string	Don't believe what the cartoons taught you: yarn is not a safe toy for cats. Yarn and string are common culprits at the emergency clinic, as they can be easily swallowed in large quantities. Due to the barbed structure of the feline tongue, it's easier to swallow than to hack objects up, so once yarn enters the mouth it can quickly lead to disaster.
Peek-and-play toys	There are many toys on the market that contain holes or slots where a cat can reach in and move a ball around. While this can be fun for the kitten, I would avoid any items that a kitten can reach into and get stuck. Because kittens' limbs and bodies are so small, it's easy for them to get an arm trapped or a head stuck. Instead, you can opt to put a ball in a shallow box, which allows the kitten to roll it around in a contained space without risking getting hurt.
Ball toys	These come in lots of different styles such as felt, plastic, or rubber, and they're great for kittens because they're fun to chase! Many have bells inside, which make for an amusing sound, but just make sure that the small pieces can't be swallowed.
Household items/DIY toys	We all know that sometimes the best cat toys aren't toys at all. However, you want to avoid household items that can hurt kittens. Twist ties and rubber bands can easily be lodged in a throat, and paper bags can be dangerous if a head gets stuck in the handles. There are many DIY toys such as cardboard boxes and crinkled paper that are safe and fun, so just be mindful about what you choose to let them play with!

CATIFYING YOUR SPACE

In addition to toys and playtime, it's also important for kittens to have an enriching home. Whether you're building a nursery room for fosters or bringing home a newly adopted companion, nothing is more fun and rewarding than catifying your living space. By providing them with perches, structures, and beds that are made just for them, you can help kittens feel a sense of pride and ownership from an early age. After all, cat behavior starts in kittenhood, so when it comes to helping kittens

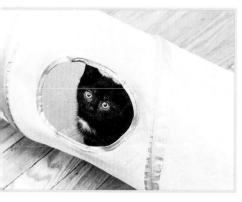

appropriately express themselves in the home environment, it's never too early to start!

When we don't provide an appropriate space, kittens will make their own enrichment out of what they have. By setting up an enriching home base, we help them establish good behaviors from the get-go. Instead of having to say, "Stop climbing my pants" or "Get off the cabinet," we can simply recognize up front that kittens need to climb and access vertical space in order to feel whole. Instead of losing the kittens underneath the couch, we can give them a safer way to burrow with a cozy hideaway. This allows us to focus on the positive rather than the negative—to give rather than to take away. Here are some of my favorite ways to catify your space for kittens:

- Huts and hideaways
- Hammocks and lounges
- Vertical and horizontal scratch posts
- Window perches
- Tunnels and tubes
- Cat cubes

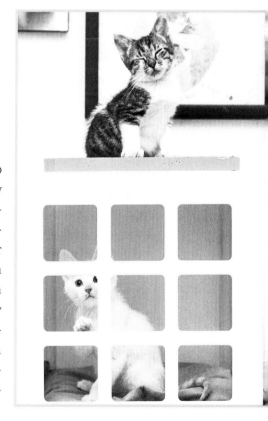

You don't have to sacrifice your personal style to create an enriching environment for your kittens. My friend Kate Benjamin, founder of Hauspanther and coauthor of *Catification* and *Catify to Satisfy*, does a beautiful job of showing how cat enrichment and interior design can go hand in paw. Kate tells us, "Catification should take your style into consideration, too! You can give your cat plenty of places to climb, scratch, play and rest without creating an eyesore. There are endless designer cat products available today, more than ever before, or if you're a do-it-yourselfer you can create something unique that both you and your new kitten will love."

If you're working with foster kittens, be mindful of using enrichment items that can be either sanitized or discarded in between litters so as not to spread illness. Cat trees are wonderful for newly adopted kittens, but may not be the best idea for a foster room since they're quite large and a challenge to disinfect. However, many cat beds and loungers come with washable covers that can easily be disinfected in the laundry, or are made from nonporous materials that are easy to spray down. Tunnels and tubes can be disinfected. Cardboard scratchers are a great disposable starter item that can be tossed or sent home with the adopter. Give your foster an enriching space, and he'll be prepared to be the king of the castle in his forever home!

MY KITTEN NURSERY

In my late twenties, my friends began to move to the suburbs so they could have baby rooms for their kids, so I decided to do the same—with kittens! While I've fostered in studio apartments and shared homes, my rescue game definitely leveled up when I made the move into a home with a dedicated kitten room. Now I live in a home with multiple rooms designed specifically for the care of kittens, from a sterile neonatal ward to a super fun socialization room where kittens can learn to pounce and play. Here's an inside peek at my nonprofit kitten nursery, Orphan Kitten Club!

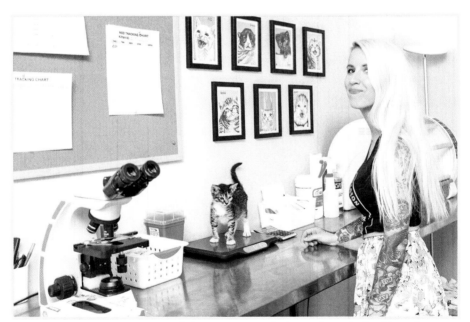

Having a dedicated treatment area helps me monitor the kittens' weight, health, and progress. A stainless steel table offers a simple, sanitizable surface for everyday kitten care.

Neonatal kitten Topanga peeks out from an incubator, a contained unit that helps regulate temperature and humidity for the youngest babies.

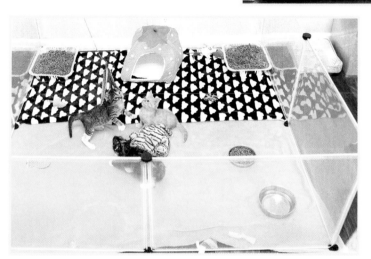

These babies have everything they need in their adjustable playpen: food, water, toys, shallow litter boxes, a comfy bed, and a snuggle companion!

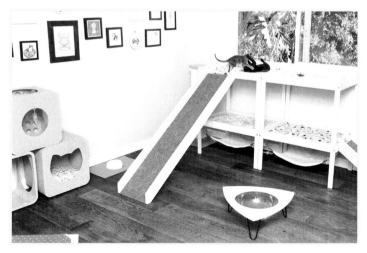

In my socialization room, the older kittens have plenty of space to play and climb! This custom Kitten Activity Center was designed by Kate Benjamin of Hauspanther. Complete with ramps, beds, hammocks, and hanging toys, it is also entirely sanitizable.

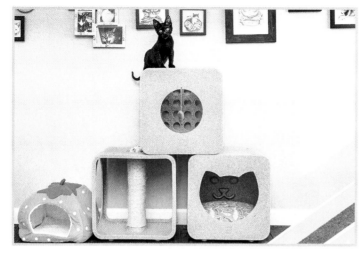

Deep Dish climbs on a set of Kitty Kasas and shows off our kitten art wall.

These lounge chairs are made from plastic, making them easy to wipe down and sanitize between groups of kittens.

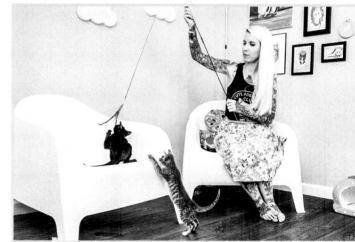

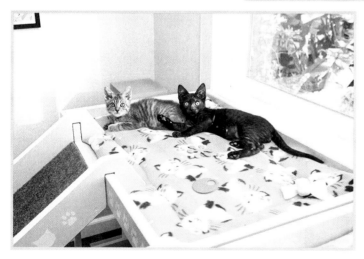

A window seat is a perfect place to curl up for a catnap!

Perhaps the most important way to support the behavioral and emotional development of a kitten is to provide them with a friend. Many people think of cats as solitary animals, but they are, in fact, incredibly social beings who thrive when provided with feline companionship from an early age. While an adult cat may have developed preferences for living alone, a kitten is a blank slate and can develop a friendship with just about anyone! For this reason, I highly recommend adopting a kitten only if you have another cat at home, or if you plan to adopt a pair.

Now, before you furrow your brow and accuse me of trying to upsell kittens to you like a used-car salesman, hear me out. It may come as a surprise to hear this, but two kittens are actually *half* the work of one! Having a duo doesn't just improve the life of the cats, but it also makes your life easier. Here are six ways that kitten friendships are beneficial:

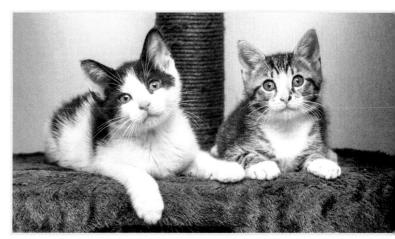
Bud and Twig aren't just brothers—they're also best friends!

🐱 Kittens learn through observation, and are more likely to pick up knowledge if they have another cat or kitten to teach them. Friends can show each other useful skills like using the litter box or grooming, and they'll both be better off having learned from one another.

🐱 Let the kittens pick on someone their own size! Having a friend means they can take out their play aggression on one another, and they'll even teach each other good boundaries about biting and scratching.

🐱 Kittens can feel lonesome or bored without a buddy. By having a playmate, you ensure that the kittens are entertained, active, and enriched. A happy cat makes a happy home!

🐱 You know what they say about idle hands . . . and the same applies for idle paws. One kitten can get destructive if left unattended, but two kittens will tend to keep each other occupied and out of trouble, even when you are asleep or away at work.

🐱 An older cat may have an easier time accepting two new kittens than one. While a solo kitten can nag an older cat, two kittens will keep each other company while the adult cat watches from a distance. This allows the adult to choose when to participate, without being obligated to play along. Two kittens can actually reenergize an older cat, putting some extra pep in his step without the pestering of a solo kitten.

🐱 Having a pal helps to ease the transition into a new home. Just like humans, kittens have an easier time feeling comfortable trying something new if they've got a friend to do it with them. Think of it as a buddy system for baby cats!

THE ODD COUPLE

I was driving down to Richmond, Virginia, to teach a workshop about kitten care, kittenless at the time. Unbeknownst to me, I wouldn't be kittenless for long! I was pulling off the highway when I got an unexpected phone call from my friend Grace, who just happened to live in my destination city.

"There's a little white kitten stuck at the bottom of a stack of cinder blocks, and he's screaming his head off," she told me, looking for help. She was working on getting him to safety and had no idea that I was in town.

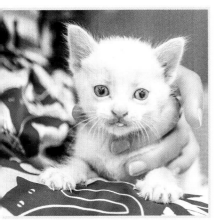

"This is crazy, but I'm actually driving to Richmond right now," I told her. "If you can get him to my event, I'll help him. I have all my teaching supplies with me, so I'm already set up for kitten care!"

Within twenty minutes, we were meeting up at the event space, where I was setting up to teach. I peeked over the large cardboard box she was carrying and saw the cutest little weirdo staring back at me. With snowy white fur, big pink ears, and a pointy face, he looked like an adorable cat-shaped mouse. He gazed up at me with bright blue eyes, opened his mouth, and let out the most bizarre, screeching meow I've ever heard. *What an oddball!* I thought, laughing as I prepped a bottle for him. As the attendees started to come in, everyone couldn't believe that I'd just gotten a new kitten. His surprise appearance was a testament to the fact that rescuers always have to come prepared!

It was impossible not to smile around Fizz. Interacting with him was like interacting with a space alien; he was a kitten who didn't know the first thing about how to be a cat. Instead of lounging on his comfy plush beds, I'd find him sleeping in the weirdest places, like inside a tissue box or stuffed in a candy bucket. He'd stand in front of a full bowl of food, screaming like a banshee because he couldn't figure out

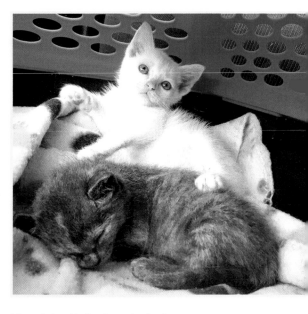

how to eat unless he was hand-fed, bite by bite. After doing his business in the litter box, he didn't know how to cover it; instead, he would scratch at the wall for minutes on end, looking quite perplexed about why his waste was still visible. This little guy clearly needed some direction from a fellow feline.

After I'd been raising my little space cadet for about two weeks, a colleague told me that her foster kitten, Wednesday, was lonely after losing her brother. Although Wednesday was two weeks younger than Fizz, they were actually exactly the same size . . . just completely different shapes. Both under a pound, Fizz was scrawny and lanky with big doofy ears, and Wednesday was plump and pudgy, like a dense little

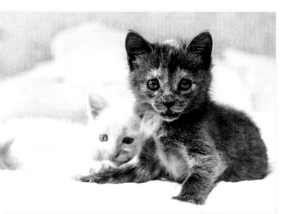

loaf of banana bread. Willing to give it a shot, we introduced the two babies to see if they might like having a friend.

The kittens were an odd couple, but they absolutely loved each other. He brought out her playful side, and she showed him how to, well, be a normal cat! Having a goofy big brother gave Wednesday the confidence to come out of her shell, and in return she taught Fizz everything he needed to know about how to eat, how to cuddle, and, yes . . . even how to cover up his poop. These unlikely companions were adopted into a loving home together, and now they'll be lifelong friends. Fizz and Wednesday were like puzzle pieces: totally different shapes, but they fit together perfectly.

CRITTER FROM ANOTHER LITTER

Kittens do best with a buddy, but before you start meddling with matchmaking, let's talk about how to integrate kittens from different litters safely. When introducing a little one to a brother from another mother or a sister from another mister, you'll want to do so with their health in mind. It might be tempting to quickly place two animals together, but no one should be booping noses or licking faces until the time is right.

If you've just rescued a kitten, it's possible she could be carrying a parasite or virus that is transmissible to others. The first weeks after rescue should therefore be spent stabilizing her health and watching for signs of illness. While kittens are initially receiving preventative care (such as dewormer and vaccines) and being treated for medical conditions, they should be separated from unknown animals in order to prevent the spread of disease. Think of it as primping for a first date . . . but on the microscopic level!

Keeping kittens separated protects their own health, too. Given their immuno-compromised state and their small stature, it can be a good idea to keep kittens in a contained space until they've bulked up a bit, both in health and in size. If you're bringing home a kitten who has already been in foster care for several weeks, you may not need to be as cautious about introductions, as long as she's already received preventative care. Of course, littermates can stay together since they are a package deal, but they shouldn't be introduced to anyone new until their little bodies are ready for forming friendships!

It's up to you how careful you want to be, given your space, resources, and specific circumstances. Some rescuers will introduce animals right away, but take it from me: this can lead to disaster if it turns out that one of them is carrying a serious transmissible illness. Other rescuers may choose to be very careful, waiting until the kittens have had a clean fecal exam, an FVRCP booster shot, and a negative leukemia test. Personally, I err on the side of caution when introducing kittens to ensure that it's a happy meeting. At a minimum, I recommend keeping your kittens separate for two weeks to monitor for serious viruses and prepare the kittens for success.

Once your kitten is ready to meet her new friend, here are some tips for the first introductions:

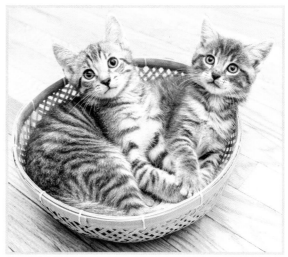

Rizzo and Cole might look like twins, but they're actually from two different litters! These boys met in foster care and became best friends.

🐱 If introducing two kittens from different litters, try to make sure they're as close in age as possible. Kittens are rough when playing, and it isn't kind to put a wild two-month-old with a wobbly one-month-old who can't defend himself.

🐱 Monitor the interaction and help guide them through appropriate play. Showing them a new toy can be a great way to help kittens feel excited by and comfortable with their new playmate!

🐱 Food can be fun, but be cautious about expecting them to share right away. When you're first integrating kittens, try giving them separate bowls so they don't feel that their feast is under threat.

🐱 Most of the time, young kittens will hit it off right away. However, if you see that a kitten is fearful or aggressive, keep the pair limited to monitored visits until they've become more comfortable with one another.

MATCHMAKER, MATCHMAKER

I got the call about Bruno when he came into my local shelter along with dozens of other animals from a hoarding case. At just five days old, Bruno's eyes were still closed, but he'd already experienced more trauma than anyone should ever have to bear. His mother and siblings were nowhere to be found, he was living in filthy conditions, and he had a large abscess on his back. My heart ached for him, and I set out to help him heal.

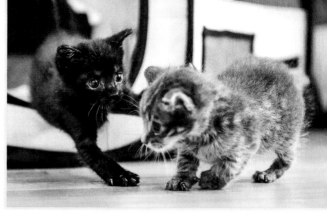

A week passed, and Bruno was looking better. Bottle-feeding had plumped him up, and antibiotics had helped his abscess to heal. His blue eyes were open, and as he peered into the world for the first time, I was his only friend—that is, until Boop arrived.

Boop was discovered outdoors in the trash, and tragically, he was found curled up alongside a dead littermate. Boop was underfed and dehydrated and smelled rotten when I took him in, so I made it my mission to clean him up and get him looking healthy, too. Both Bruno and Boop were about two weeks old, and while they were the same age, I knew that I couldn't introduce them until they were both healthy enough to safely comingle. They just had too many cards stacked against them.

For two whole weeks, I cared for the kittens separately. Everything I did, I had to do twice: making separate bottles, providing two playpens, using different supplies, bringing them with me in two carriers, and even washing my hands in between caring for them. In the interest of protecting these vulnerable beings, I knew they each needed to be quarantined, but my goal was that they'd eventually overcome their hardships and get to be best friends. Knowing that their eventual first playdate would be absolutely darling, I contacted a professional animal photographer and asked if he'd be willing to come photograph my two orphaned kittens meeting each other at their first playdate. As I booked the appointment, I heard Andrew's voice for the very first time.

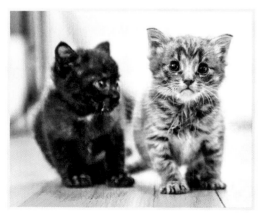

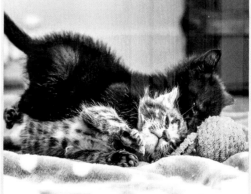

The kittens' big day came, and as I opened the door for the photographer, something told me that this day would really be a special one. We sat on the floor, giggling and "aww"-ing as Bruno and Boop clumsily rolled around, discovering each other with absolute glee. There's something deeply endearing about watching two kittens who have never known friendship discover what it's like to have a buddy, and my heart was wide-open as I chaperoned their very 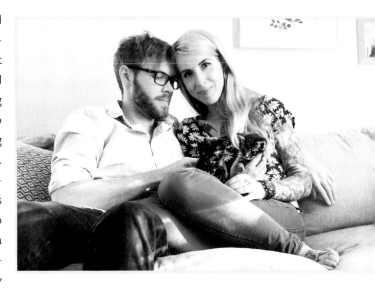 first playdate. Andrew's photos beautifully captured the fresh, fun spirit of that afternoon; his snapshots are a time capsule of the bliss, awkwardness, and excitement of meeting your new best friend.

As the day went on, it became clearer and clearer to me that Bruno and Boop were not the only ones who had met their match. Just like the little kittens, Andrew and I simply didn't want to leave each other's side . . . and I suddenly realized, *I think this might kind of be a date.* We talked for hours, and by the end of our visit, we had made plans to see each other the following weekend at a cat café. For our third date, I invited him to come help me TNR a colony of cats in my neighborhood, and by our fourth date, he was my new boyfriend, helping me prepare Bruno and Boop for their forever home.

It turns out that kittens and humans aren't so different after all. We may be able to live just fine as solitary creatures, but we thrive when we have a companion. Even when we've been through hardships, we can overcome them with time, love, and support. And once we're healthy enough to meet our match, we can discover great joy in having someone to experience life with. Bruno and Boop are now lifelong companions, and I'll always be grateful that just as I brought them together, the kittens ended up being matchmakers for me, too.

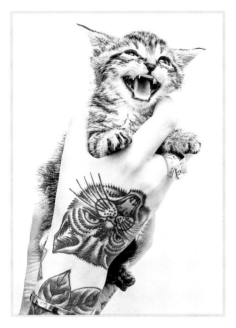

Helping kittens hone their confidence and cattitude is a blast. But what about when you have a five-week-old who already growls like a ferocious lion? Sometimes, you may encounter kittens who are exhibiting feral behaviors, and you're going to need to know how to help them, too. With a little patience and know-how, these hissy, spitty kitties can be guided toward socialization success.

Maybe it sounds crazy, but hear me out: some of the kittens I love the most are those who like me the least. There's something really respectable about a one-pound fuzzball hissing and asserting herself against a giant hairless beast like a human being. Feral kittens aren't so sure about us, and why should they be? To a tiny feline, we are suspicious until proven innocent. There's nothing quite as gratifying as gaining trust by working with a hissy feral kitten and helping her melt into a comfy, cozy companion animal.

Why might a kitten exhibit feral behavior? Just like humans, cats establish their worldview and disposition during the critical developmental period of childhood. All cats are born with innate defense mechanisms that protect them from danger, and the introduction of any new stimulus can bring these behaviors to the surface as the kitten calculates whether a threat is present. That's why even a one-week-old kitten with her eyes still closed may hiss at me when newly rescued; the introduction of a new smell or sound feels scary until she gets used to it! It's a fight-or-flight response, and while more mobile kittens will always choose flight, defenseless neonates have no option but to make themselves look as threatening as possible when scared. While it might be a very endear-

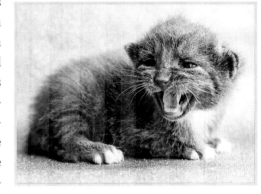

ing experience to have a toothless palm-sized panther threaten to gum me to death, I try to remember that I'm a hundred times bigger than she is. It's my duty to help that kitten have a good experience so that she can feel safe in human hands.

SOCIALIZATION IS A SPECTRUM

People have an innate desire to classify others into groups, but we do this to the detriment of truly understanding each individual's full complexity—including felines! While it's common to group cats into categories such as "friendly" and "feral," the truth is that socialization is a spectrum, and cats exhibit a wide range of behaviors just like we do. There are owned indoor cats who don't want to be touched, and there are outdoor community cats who will jump right into your lap! Behavior is linked with experience, and those who have positive experiences with humans at a young age will behave with trust and affection. While an adult cat might be set in his ways, young kittens' social behaviors are still malleable; they can shift from feral to friendly through experience, time, and proven socialization techniques.

Here are some telltale kitten behaviors to help you determine which side of the spectrum a kitten falls on. Note that these behaviors are contingent upon the presence of a human, as many feral kittens will exhibit plenty of social behaviors around other cats but may be completely unsocialized to humans.

Socialized Kitten Behaviors	Unsocialized Kitten Behaviors
Meowing, vocalizing, or purring	Growling or silence
Mellow when approached	May hiss or pop when approached
Body relaxed and comfortable	Body tense and cowering
Tail upright or relaxed behind body	Tail wrapped tight against body
Fur flat against body	Fur may be poofed out
Ears upright	Ears flattened ("airplane ears")
Pupils normal	Pupils dilated

It's always a bit of a mystery when I open a box of kittens for the first time; I never quite know what I'm going to get! The element of surprise makes it all the more fun and exciting, like unwrapping a gift. I've been handed many a cardboard box in my day, but on one sunny afternoon I was brought a box that clamored and shook in my hands. "What's in here?" I asked. "A baby dinosaur?"

I lifted one of the cardboard flaps, and commotion ensued. Two feisty felines popped like popcorn and bolted like lightning, and they looked like they'd been struck by it, too—their fur stood up on its end and poofed out like a round Koosh ball. Knowing that I'd inherited quite a handful, I decided to name the disgruntled duo Riff and Raff. I didn't know much about where they'd come from, but I did know right away that they'd probably never seen a person before. To them, I probably looked like a giant alien from outer space, or a hungry beast ready to chomp down and turn them into a meal. At six weeks old, these two were totally feral, but I knew that with a little TLC I could get them acclimated to me.

I came home and set them up in a playpen in my living room. I knew that if I was going to have any success turning these two into lap cats, they'd need as much exposure to human activity as possible. For the first day, I let them have their space and settle in. They'd observe me as I went about my day, hissing hot tuna breath in my

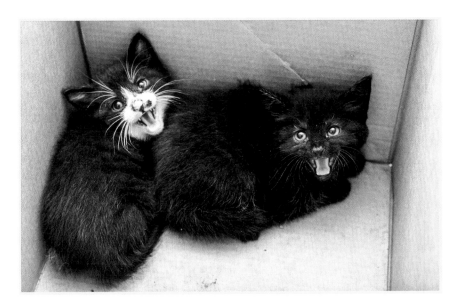

direction any time I got within a few feet. Although tense, they would eat wet food in front of me, looking up with suspicion every few seconds and grumbling as they munched.

By day two, I was able to get the kittens to accept baby food from my fingers. Chicken puree is irresistible to kittens, and as they licked my fingers clean, they looked at me with curiosity, as if trying to calculate my intentions. *How could a bad guy have such good treats?* At each feeding, I'd scratch their heads with one finger, and after a while they started to reflexively lean in. I couldn't help but giggle watching these grouchy goobers wrestle with their emotions. They wanted so badly to hate me, but at the same time, chin scratches just felt *so good.* Over the next few days, they slowly began to give in.

Day five rolled around, and I walked into the living room in the morning to find that not only were they no longer hissing and avoiding me . . . Riff was actually climbing the inside mesh of the playpen, anxiously await- ing my presence. He let out the most pa-

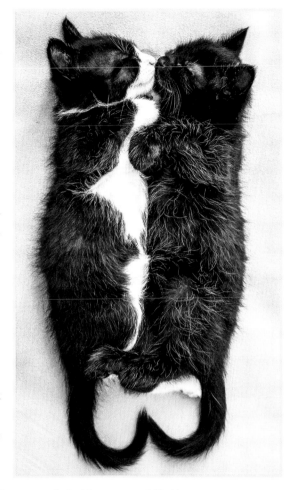

thetic little squeak, and my heart melted. Riff was actually inviting me over! *Aha!* I was in. The more Riff and Raff had begun to associate me with petting and snacks, the more they determined that I actually wasn't so bad after all.

Just one week into knowing them, they were completely different kittens. They napped in my lap without hesitation. They played and pounced with my other foster kittens. They continually begged for baby food. Most of all, they loved each other to pieces and would curl up in the most incredibly angelic snuggle sessions I've ever seen. Looking at them before and after, you'd hardly believe that they were the same pair! Riff and Raff were adopted into a home by a loving couple and their little hedge- hog friend, Prickles, and they are now cuddly, spoiled house cats.

Hissing is a defensive behavior that all cats instinctively do when threatened. Kittens don't have to see this behavior in order to understand it—in fact, I've had kittens hiss at me at just one day old. Hissing is a warning sign, telling the threat to back off . . . or else!

Hissing can be provoked by new and frightening stimuli, such as unfamiliar scents, sights, or sounds. In some cases, a hiss may occur when a kitten is in pain and feels that her body is under attack. Then there are play hisses, which generally occur when a kitten is roughhousing with another kitten—and these hisses tend to be much

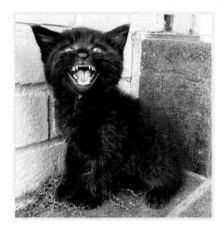

shorter and less drawn out. In general, hissing occurs when a cat or kitten has a burst of adrenaline due to feeling startled and vulnerable. Think of it as a stranger-danger alert system!

When a kitten hisses, her mouth will become wide and she will force a big gust of warm air past her tongue. The ears will generally fall flat against the head, the fur may stand up on end, and she may appear to crinkle her nose as she lets out the warning sound. The sound of a hiss closely mimics that of a hissing snake; this mimicry can be a valuable survival tool to warn opponents to stay away.

THE SOCIALIZATION WINDOW

Before you go starting a social club for hissy kitties in your living room, let's talk about the right conditions for such a venture. Kittens are most physically and emotionally adaptive during the weaning period, when their dependence on a mother is waning. During this time, they are inclined to accept change, seek new experiences and food sources, and develop a sense of independence. This makes sense, because as their mother begins to push them away from nursing, they have a biological requirement of adaptability. They must rapidly learn new lessons in order to survive. Thus, feral kittens who are at weaning age are the most impressionable and willing to accept humans, given time and exposure.

Around two months of age, the window for socialization starts to close, and by three months it may be entirely shut. Once kittens are fully weaned, they are no longer predisposed to accept change; in fact, experts agree that kittens older than ten to twelve weeks will generally be steadfast in their impressions of humans and thus quite challenging to tame. It's important to be totally realistic about what is possible, as it's all too common for people to misjudge the capacity of a kitten to be socialized, or to underestimate what it will take to help the kitten truly transition. In order to be properly socialized, the kitten must be an appropriate age, *and* you must be set up to provide effective support, hands-on. Feral socialization is a two-way street: both the kitten and the human must be capable of making it happen. Forcing such a feat on an animal who will not be able to adjust is not only terrifying and unkind, but it can actually completely diminish his chance at a full life.

I can't tell you how many times I've met kittens who were far past the socialization window, but were being pressured to "warm up." In one case I'll never forget, a local shelter had taken in a pair of three-month-old feral kittens and kept them in a kennel for nearly two months, trying to help them adjust to humans. This was clearly a losing battle; the kittens were far too old to be socialized, and a shelter is typically not an appropriate environment for this effort. By the time I met them, they were five months old and still completely terrified of humans—and now they were at risk of being euthanized because there was nowhere for them to go. On the one hand, they'd been away from their colony for so long that they couldn't be humanely returned, and on the other hand, they weren't candidates for adoption. Their story reflects why it is so essential for us to be pragmatic in our approach; it's far more humane to TNR a kitten than to place her in a cage where she will never have a chance.

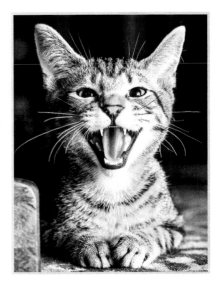

In the case of these two little ones, they lucked out. I found them a barn home out in the country, and a friend and I swooped in just in the nick of time. They were sterilized and eartipped, and driven out to their new rural home in a big pickup truck full of supplies to help ease the process. We set them up in a temporary transition cage in the barn, where they could adjust to the new surroundings and take a peek at their new digs. After several weeks of adjusting, the kittens were able to exit the transition enclosure and make their way around the barn—mingling with goats, climbing the rafters, and sleeping on hay bales. Lucky for these two, their new family loves them just how they are! They may not be homebodies, but now they have a home where they can receive care from a comfortable distance. Sadly, many others don't have the same opportunity—it's a massive effort to relocate a kitten, and a barn home is not an option much of the time. It's therefore important to accept if a kitten isn't a candidate for socialization and opt for TNR instead when necessary. Remember that there are many ways to be a cat, and that as advocates we must meet and accept them exactly where they are.

THE TAMING OF THE MEW: HOW TO SOCIALIZE FERAL KITTENS

The primary principle of socializing feral kittens is gradual, humane desensitization. By helping them associate human presence with a pleasant stimulus, we slowly condition them to feel that we aren't so scary after all. If you're planning to socialize kittens, it's important that you're committed to seeing the process through to its completion. Taming kittens requires frequent interaction throughout the day, a dedicated process, and a lot of patience, but through a series of persistent positive experiences, we can make a lasting impression.

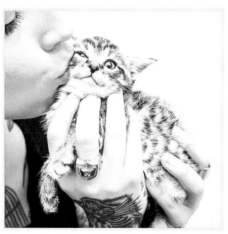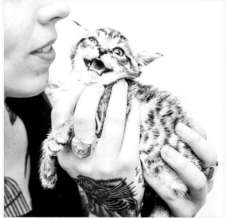

Provide Suitable Shelter

🐱 First things first, make sure that the kitten is sheltered in an enclosed space such as a large crate, a playpen, or even a small bathroom. Ensure that the space is adequately kitten-proofed and free of places where the kitten can escape or get hurt. Never let feral kittens loose in your house, lest you lose them under a dresser and never see them again! Keep the kitten safely contained somewhere that you can easily access him.

🐱 Consider keeping the kitten's crate lifted off the ground, perhaps on a coffee table. Kittens will often feel more comfortable and confident with a higher vantage point.

🐱 Provide a good hideaway—but not *too* good. It's kind to give feral kittens someplace where they can feel safely tucked away, but you do want to ensure that they're able to look around at their new surroundings so they can begin to adjust. I like to use a small fabric tent, a covered bed, or even a cardboard box to help kittens feel like they have a bit of a safe escape, but also so they can see me and the room around them.

Incentivize with Food

🐱 Unsocialized kittens may be too scared to eat in front of people at first, so a good first goal is to get them to eat something yummy while you're in the same room. Place the food in the kitten's space, then give distance so the kitten can learn that it's safe to eat in front of you. Each meal, move closer to the kitten until he is able to eat with you fairly nearby. Once you're close to the kitten during mealtime, you can slowly inch the dish closer to you until the kitten is able to eat right next to you, perhaps even while you hold the dish.

🐱 Once the kitten is confidently eating in front of you, it's time to start using food strictly during socialization time. Don't free-feed; instead, use mealtime as an incentive for the kitten to interact with you. You may want to try feeding the kitten on a wooden tongue depressor or a plastic spoon to help him start associating food with you. Once the kitten is able to eat from a utensil, you can gradually move to letting him lick food off your finger or even eat from your palm.

🐱 It's important to use a very desirable, highly palatable food for this. The classic feral-kitten treat is meaty baby-food puree, as it's often impossible for them to resist licking it off your fingers (just make sure you're using a product that doesn't have any garlic or onions!). Any stinky wet food will be a good option for getting kittens interested in what you've got to offer.

Introduce Gentle Touch

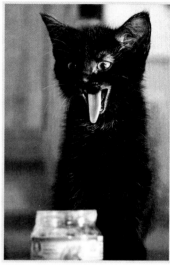

🐱 As the kitten becomes more comfortable with hand-feeding, you can add gentle touch to the routine. Using a finger or a toothbrush, gently pet the kitten's head while he eats. Eventually he may start to lean into your pets, and you can begin exploring petting the back, or gently rubbing the cheeks or chin.

🐱 As the kitten gets more comfortable with petting, he may even begin to lean into your hands as if to ask for more. Once the kitten is actively interested in pets, you can start introducing other touching like gently grasping his sides to lift him. Over time, you can desensitize the kitten to the idea of being picked up.

Raff can't resist chicken baby food!

🐱 If the kitten is able to be safely held, you can try the "feral-kitten wiggle," my patented technique for helping soothe grumpy babies. I take the kitten in my arms, hold him stable, and gently wiggle him back and forth, side to side. This rocking motion seems to have a truly mollifying impact on tense kittens, and when done in tandem with head scratches, this often elicits their very first purr!

Use Your Voice

🐱 As much as you want to desensitize kittens to the sights and touch of humans, you also want to help get them used to your voice. In between your hand-feeding sessions, you can spend some time with the kittens, speaking softly to them or maybe even reading a book aloud. The more they hear your voice, the less jarring it will become.

🐱 Every time you feed kittens, it's a good idea to gently talk to them during their meal. This helps associate the sound of your voice with something they really love, and eventually the sound of your voice will sound just like a dinner bell to them!

🐱 Not at home for a little bit? Consider leaving a television or radio on low so that the kitten still hears human sounds.

Divide and Conquer

🐱 If you have the mama and she is feral, you will want to separate the kittens from her as soon as they are weaned. Kittens will look to their mother for cues that help guide their understanding of the world around them, so if she is scared of you, she will teach them to be scared of you, too.

🐱 Kittens can be socialized in pairs or in a group, but in some cases you may want to separate the most fearful of the litter and work with him one-on-one. This places the more sociable kittens on the fast track to friendliness, while increasing the more fractious kitten's feelings of dependence on you.

🐱 Once the kittens are all comfortable and social, you can reunite them. Having a friend is a wonderful form of enrichment for baby cats, and once they see that everyone is feeling comfortable and confident, you'll find that they'll be melting into a cozy cuddle puddle!

Expose to Play and People

🐱 Introducing play to feral kittens too quickly may be frightening to them, so start slow and avoid any fast movements with toys until they've acclimated to your presence. You want to ease them into feelings of safety around humans, so try to limit the number of people they interact with until they've started to open up a little bit.

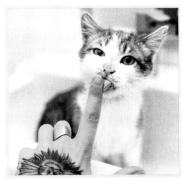

🐱 Once the kitten is comfortable with being handled, you can start introducing toys. A wand toy is a great option that allows kittens to practice playing while being safely distant from your hands. Experiencing fun in front of humans will teach them that they can move freely without fear.

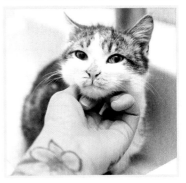

🐱 As the kittens' socialization improves, it's time to expose them to more people! You want to ensure that they know it's not just you who is safe, but that all humans are safe. Invite friends to pet them, hand-feed them, and play with them so that they can become friendly toward newcomers.

Oh, little ones—they grow up so fast! Now that you know how to help little kittens learn to eat, play, and interact like big kids, you'll be able to give them the best head start they can possibly get. In a perfect world, they will be behaviorally and physically healthy, and well on their way to adoption! But what about kittens who experience illness along the way? In the next chapter, we'll talk about the health conditions you might encounter as a rescuer, and how to help sick kittens recover and feel their very best.

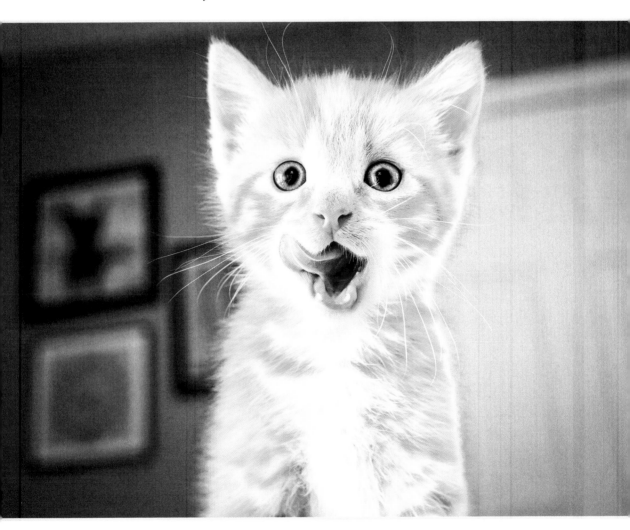

CHAPTER SIX

IN SICKNESS AND IN HEALTH

ROOTING FOR THE UNDERCAT

I f you're someone who enjoys rooting for the underdog, then just wait until you meet the under*cat*—under*age* cat, that is! Young kittens are prone to illness due to a unique set of vulnerabilities, and it's therefore essential for caregivers to have a basic understanding of the medical needs of pediatric felines. Their first weeks can feel like a battle for life, but with the right combination of dedication and knowledge, it's a battle we can help kittens win.

Caring for sick kittens might seem daunting, but it's something that anyone can learn to do with time, patience, and determination. In this chapter, I'll share how you can help kittens through early intervention, strong supportive care, and a working knowledge of common diseases and how to combat them. It's important to always work with a veterinary professional when treating kittens, so I'll also share tips for finding veterinarians who understand feline pediatrics and communicating effectively with those in the veterinary field. Of course the best way to fight disease is to prevent it from starting in the first place, so by the time this chapter is finished, you'll have a tool kit full of preventative-care tactics to help keep kittens protected and healthy.

If you're anything like me, you'll find that when you do become tasked with caring for sick kittens, it's extremely rewarding to walk them through the healing process. Each ailment is a puzzle that must be solved. A kitten falls ill, and suddenly I'm a detective searching for clues in the litter box, rummaging through my notes and trying to connect the dots and solve the mystery. I become a partner in

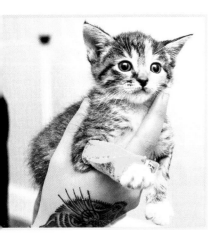

the struggle, and together, the little kitten and I team up in a fight for her life. I supply the supportive care, and she supplies the will to live. By guiding her through this fragile state, we can elicit a truly profound transformation.

My favorite kittens are often those who have conquered these impossible odds, whom I've sat alongside day and night as they heal. I feel close to every kitten I raise, but there's no bond quite like the one you make when you struggle together in a battle for life. Each purr is that much sweeter; each playful moment is a victory.

YOU HAVE WHAT IT TAKES

When I tell people I'm caring for a sick kitten, one of the most frequent questions I receive is: "Did you go to vet school?" It's a common belief that veterinarians are the only people who can help sick animals, but they're actually just one piece of the puzzle. Veterinarians play an essential role in the health of kittens in the same way that doctors play an important role in children's health: through their research, guidance, and knowledge, we obtain diagnostic information and treatment plans. But just like doctors, veterinarians are limited in the amount of time they can spend with each patient, and they don't physically do the majority of the hands-on care. While a vet can provide medical direction and medication, it's up to the everyday caregiver to see it through. And that means people like you and me!

I'm often surprised by how many people wish they could help animals, but assume they must obtain an advanced degree to become qualified to do so. This misconception should be challenged, as it keeps compassionate community members from stepping up and lending a hand. By working *with* a vet, anyone can gain the experience and skills to be a caregiver for sick kittens. Rescuers, shelter coordinators, and veterinary staff are all pieces of the same puzzle, and every piece is essential in order to complete it.

In the spirit of empowering others to see their capacity to help, I want to emphasize that I am not a medical expert and that everything I share in this chapter is based on my own personal experience, combined with knowledge and hands-on training I've acquired from professionals I respect in the veterinary field. I encourage all kitten caregivers to work in collaboration with veterinarians and to believe in their ability to make a difference. You have what it takes to save them.

AN ARMY AGAINST ILLNESS

Kittens are immunocompromised, and in order to understand their medical fragility, it's helpful to first understand how their immune systems work. The immune system is the body's natural defense against disease, and is present in all animals, including humans and cats. Think of it as an army that protects against foreign invaders like viruses and bacteria. This army is small and weak at birth, but grows stronger through age and vaccination. By four months of age, most kittens can be fully armed to fight the most common bacterial and viral agents. Prior to that, kittens must make do with what weakened immunity they currently have.

The moment a kitten is born, she has a very immature immune system as there is minimal transplacental antibody transfer from a mother to her young. She must therefore borrow some assistance from her mother in the form of maternal antibodies. Rather than obtaining these antibodies in the womb, kittens receive them only by consuming colostrum, a natural component of breast milk rich in immunoglobulins, which delivers passive immunity to the kitten. This acts as a temporary defense loan from the mother's immune system; the army won't be there forever, but it'll protect the kitten for the first few weeks of life.

There are some problems with this system. Colostrum is produced only at the start of lactation. Kittens absorb colostrum and all the precious antibodies it contains through their gut. The catch is that the gut is only permeable to these antibodies for the first eighteen hours of life.[1] After that, the gut forms a barrier, and the ability to gain any more antibodies from colostrum is lost. It's therefore critical that kittens nurse and consume these antibodies within the first few hours after birth. The second problem is that there isn't an endless source of colostrum—once it's lapped up, it's gone. By the time the last little baby is born, all the other siblings will have been nursing for hours, and there may be a low supply of colostrum.

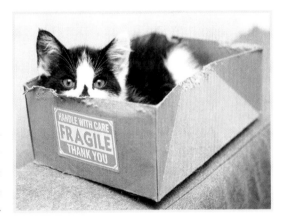

When you understand this process, it's easy to see why many kittens on the streets and in shelters are at risk of low immunity. Those kittens who are weak, such as preemies and runts, may not suckle effectively during the first hours of life. Those who are taken from their mothers at birth will have no opportunity to obtain her antibodies. Those who nurse from a sick mother may fail to obtain proper antibody transfer. And finally, even those who do obtain maternal antibodies will still become vulnerable as those antibodies begin to wear off. Even healthy kittens may become susceptible to disease as their maternal antibodies taper if they're not promptly provided with vaccination on an appropriate timeline.

If this sounds like a losing battle, don't fret. There are several important things we can do to help protect kittens with weakened immunity. Aside from vaccination and transfusion, the single most important way we can help immunocompromised animals is to get them out of the shelter and into a safe environment.

EXITING THE WAR ZONE

In any close-quarters environment, there are invisible threats to our well-being. Now consider a high-volume setting like an animal shelter, where a large number of animals are being cared for in close proximity. This is like sending a little kitten into a war zone with no armor! It's no surprise that even the best shelters in the country struggle with kittens contracting communicable diseases—a shelter is simply not a suitable environment for an unarmed baby cat. This is why a foster home is truly a sanctuary of hope for a baby kitten. Shielded from the contagions of the shelter, kittens are able to recover in the safety of a home environment.

SMALL FRY: THE TINIEST TATER

On a winter morning, I got a call from the DC shelter asking if I'd like to take on a sick kitten who was failing to thrive. A week earlier, she had been surrendered to the shelter along with her mother, a gray-and-white tuxedo cat, and four other littermates. Since arriving at the shelter, the siblings had grown and thrived, but the littlest one was steadily declining. By the time I got the call, it wasn't clear if the little kitten would survive at all.

When I first laid eyes on her, I was gutted. While she was visibly thin, her downy kitten fur belied how severely emaciated she was. When I picked her up, she was brittle and lighter than air—like holding a pile of matchsticks. She felt to me like she could break at any moment. Small Fry looked almost cartoonish, with sad, sunken eyes and a body too small for her head. As she floated in my hands, her breath crackled through a crusty nose as she wheezed for air. "She won't nurse," I was told by a shelter employee. "She won't take a bottle, either." It was clear this kitten hadn't eaten in days and was rapidly fading away.

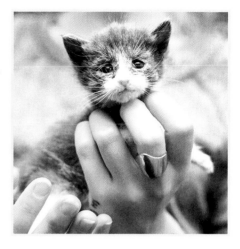

Not wanting to separate her from the only family she knew, I agreed to take her home along with her mama, brother, and sisters. The whole crew looked like their mother, with beautiful gray and white fur, and they were perfectly portly compared to their starving sister. Side by side, they looked like a bunch of plump little potatoes all lined up to nurse. I decided to call them the taters, with each being named after a potato product: Mama Latke, brother Chip, and sisters Yam, Gnocchi, and Poutine. The littlest one I named Small Fry, and I set out on a mission to save her life.

Small Fry's diagnoses were copious. After a visit with my vet, she was confirmed to have an upper respiratory infection (URI), a collapsed lung, a heart murmur, anemia, and emaciation. She was experiencing severe dehydration and muscle wasting due to starvation, which caused her to look gaunt and frail. On X-ray, she had no food whatsoever in her gut; she was instead full of air from gasping while attempting

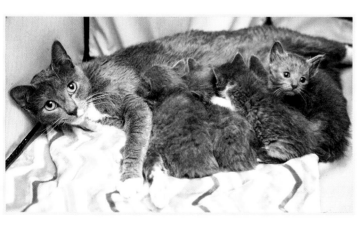

to eat. At just 170 grams (0.37 pounds), she was less than half of a healthy weight for her age. She was bone-dry and withering away.

Her condition is a prime example of the tragic domino effect that can occur when a kitten becomes sick and is not provided with proper care. The runt of her litter, she was likely the most immunocompromised of her siblings, making her susceptible to the upper respiratory infection she caught at the shelter. Left untreated, this URI stuffed up her nose, and her inability to smell had led to inappetence. Furthermore, the blockage of the nasal passage prevented the critical task of being able to breathe through her nostrils while eating—so she had stopped eating altogether. Not eating had led to dehydration, emaciation, and anemia. The URI progressed into her lungs, and her heart struggled to keep up with a body that was fading. The cards seemed stacked against her, but there she was, looking at me with big doe eyes and a strong will to live.

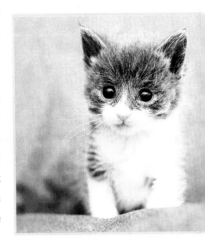

Our first week together I cared for her with obsessive frequency, canceling all my commitments to focus on her care. Subcutaneous fluids three times a day to combat dehydration. Two antibiotics twice a day to fight her respiratory infection. Saline nasal drops as needed to break up congestion. Iron and B12 supplements to combat anemia and reenergize her. Plasma therapy to boost her immunity. Daily pain medication to keep her comfortable. Tube-feeding every four hours. Constant monitoring of weight and symptoms. Frequent physical affection and comforting vocal tones to let her know that she was safe.

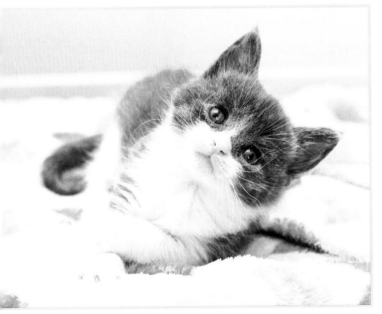

Caring for a starved animal takes patience and time. Small Fry's body was so frail that it couldn't handle a normal meal, so I started slowly, tube-feeding just a tiny amount of diluted formula to ease her stomach back to a proper feeding schedule. Over the course of a few days, I increased the frequency and the concentration of the formula until she was prepared to tolerate a regular meal. Her belly began to slowly puff out as she started to regain mass. One week into her time with me, she had doubled in weight and was finally breathing well enough to eat without a tube. My little Small Fry was transforming into a loaded baked potato!

Meanwhile, Mama Latke was caring for her other little taters with ease. Her little milk-fed babies were developing at a normal rate, starting to pounce and play with toys as they fattened up, and it was sweet to watch Small Fry cock her head with curiosity as she watched them from my lap. Eventually, she was strong enough to integrate back into the family, but her growth and development were stunted and I knew she'd be with me long after the others had gone to their forever homes.

Even with her small stature, Small Fry had a spunky spirit. She quickly bonded to her sister Poutine, a sweet gray poofball with green eyes, and the two of them spent their days chasing each other around the kitten room, their paws pitter-patting at all hours. When Chip and Mama Latke found a home together, followed by Yam and Gnocchi, I knew that I wanted to hold on to Poutine until Small Fry was big enough to be adopted . . . and send them home together.

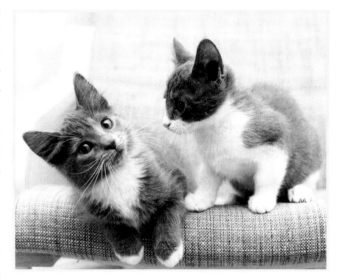

Weeks passed, and suddenly Small Fry wasn't very small at all! I found a fantastic young couple who would make the perfect parents for this little duo. Two months after her life had nearly ended, Small Fry's life was finally truly beginning: she was going to her forever home!

I'll admit, I teared up at her adoption, but I also beamed with pride at this brave little tater's success. A few weeks had totally transformed her future, and now she'd get to be someone's best friend. Touched by Small Fry's life, her adopter decided to begin volunteering at the animal shelter she had come from . . . and she hasn't stopped since! Small Fry's inspiration now carries on to give other shelter kittens the same gift she was given: a chance at a brighter future.

If you're caring for a sick kitten who just won't eat, here are some things you can try:

🐱 First, make sure it's safe to feed the kitten. Is the kitten responsive? Never attempt to feed a kitten who is extremely lethargic or unable to swallow. Seek medical advice for serious medical conditions that prevent eating.

🐱 Make sure the kitten is an appropriate temperature. Is the kitten cold? Never feed a hypothermic kitten. Instead, warm her up gently and gradually for thirty to sixty minutes before attempting to feed.

🐱 Don't feed a full-strength meal to a very sick kitten. Dilute the formula and gradually increase the concentration over the course of several feedings.

🐱 Feed appropriately for the age. If a kitten doesn't have all her teeth, don't expect her to understand meaty foods yet—she may still need to nurse or bottle-feed.

🐱 Switch up the food. Some kittens may refuse one brand but accept another. Others may refuse wet food but accept dry. Occasionally, a kitten won't accept solid food at all but may still accept formula—even if she's beyond weaning age. The important thing is that the kitten is getting calories and nutrition, so try different options until you find something she'll accept.

🐱 Try baby food. Chicken or turkey baby food is often irresistible to kittens! Just make sure the food is free of onion and garlic, which aren't safe for cats.

🐱 Change the way you're feeding them. If you're feeding them in a deep bowl, try a flat plate. If you're feeding them canned food, try adding a little water and smushing it up to change the texture. Sometimes little changes can make all the difference.

🐱 Hand-feed. I can't overstate how helpful it is to hand-feed kittens with low appetites. Pick up a pea-sized amount of wet food with your thumb and index finger, and bring it to the kitten's mouth. If she's not interested, try using your middle finger to gently press into the side of the kitten's mouth and place the food in her mouth. Sitting with the kitten and bringing the food from the dish to her mouth might sound tedious, but sometimes a few monitored meals like this can get the kitten back on track. Sometimes just dropping the food onto the kitten's tongue a few times can prompt her to begin eating on her own, but if this doesn't stimulate her to eat, don't continue to force food into her mouth; seek help from a veterinarian.

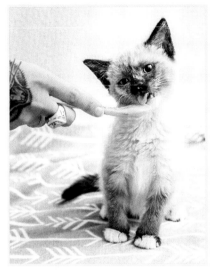

🐱 Tube-feeding should be considered a last resort, as it comes with risks and requires special tools and training. That said, if you're caring for a kitten who is so sick that he cannot safely be fed, don't shy away from asking a trained professional to teach you this skill. In extreme cases, tube-feeding can be a lifesaver. Talk with your vet about the kitten's physical condition and whether tube-feeding is advisable.

Offering palatable food on a spoon or finger can help encourage a kitten to eat.

DEEP BREATHS: FIGHTING UPPER RESPIRATORY INFECTIONS

Crusty muzzles, oozy eyes, and sneezy snouts . . . if you're working with rescued kittens, chances are you'll be dealing with your fair share of upper respiratory infections (URIs). Symptoms of an upper respiratory infection are much like the common cold, but for kittens, they can become life-threatening if left to progress. Fortunately, it's not too hard to kick URIs to the curb with early intervention and a little know-how.

Upper respiratory infections are often viral in nature, and most of the time occur when an immunocompromised kitten is exposed to a virus such as rhinotracheitis or calicivirus either in the environment or in the womb. Early symptoms may include sneezing or discharge from the nostrils and eyes that appear winky or wet. As the infection progresses, the kitten may have a severely stopped-up nose, goopy eyes, and difficulty breathing and eating. Secondary bacterial infections can accompany a viral infection, resulting in yellow-green mucus from the eyes and nose. If these symptoms are present, the kitten needs to be taken to a

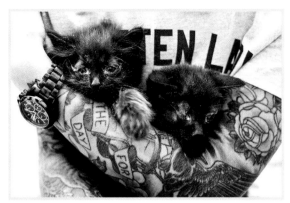

Rescued from a hoarding case, these little ladies had severe URIs and secondary bacterial eye infections. With TLC and medication, they fully healed.

veterinarian immediately and put on an appropriate antibiotic. Caregivers should not delay treatment until the symptoms progress.

If you're caring for a kitten with a URI, take swift steps to start supportive care early. The nasal passage should be kept clean by gently wiping away any visible mucus with a warm, wet cloth. Congested kittens may benefit from saline nasal drops, or even a nebulizer treatment. Nebulizers are affordable, compact machines that can be very useful for delivering saline or a prescription medication to the kitten via inhalation, but in a pinch, congested kittens can also be placed in a steamy bathroom near a hot shower or a warm humidifier for fifteen minutes to help open the airway. An appropriate oral antibiotic may be essential to helping fight most URIs, so talk with your veterinarian. Eyes should be kept clean and free of mucus, and a topical eye ointment should be applied if swelling, redness, or discharge is present. In more extreme cases, additional supportive care may be necessary, such as supported feeding or fluid therapy for kittens with decreased appetite or dehydration. Note that kittens with blocked noses can't smell their food, which may cause decreased appetites—so try using extra-stinky foods or adding some tuna juice on top to stimulate their appetites.

SEE THIS THROUGH: HEALING EYE INFECTIONS

If a kitten is winking at you, don't be too flattered. Eye infections are prevalent in young kittens and can cause inflammation, redness, discharge, and a lot of discomfort. Although these ocular symptoms are common with the little guys, they should be treated seriously and addressed right away in order to prevent ulceration or blindness. Fortunately, while they can look pretty gnarly, most eye infections are easy to treat if caught early, and you can often get the kitten looking bright-eyed in a matter of days.

The most common reason that a kitten develops crusty eyes is because she already has an upper respiratory infection. Herpesvirus, calicivirus, and even bacterial agents that cause respiratory distress often additionally target the conjunctiva (the mucous membrane that coats the eye and eyelid), so if a kitten's nose is goopy, chances are pretty good the eyes will be, too. Mild, uncomplicated cases of crusty or irritated eyes can generally be treated with three simple steps:

- Use a warm compress to soften any dried crust and gently wipe away discharge.
- Administer a saline eye solution to clean out the eye.
- Apply a topical ophthalmic antibiotic ointment.

Most of the time, treating kittens' eyes is easy-peasy! In some cases, however, you may witness more severe eye conditions that will require further examination and a different treatment path. If a kitten's eyes are cloudy, oddly shaped, or severely swollen, it's important to go to a veterinarian and get the kitten checked out for ulcers and other conditions that can cause damage to the eye. While some kittens with severe eye conditions can recover fully, others may develop lifelong scarring, and some may even require enucleation to surgically remove a damaged eye. It's best to see a vet as soon as possible if you're concerned about a kitten's eyes.

Don't forget that newborn kittens' eyes are closed for the first eight to twelve days of life, so it's important to let them naturally open their eyes on their own. Caregivers shouldn't mistake a newly opening eye for an infected one; it's totally normal for kittens to look a little silly as their eyelids slowly unseal and reveal their eyes to the world! That said, if a newborn kitten has severe swelling or discharge leaking even from a closed eyelid, it should be examined by a veterinarian and possibly gently opened so that appropriate steps can be taken to clean and medicate it.

MY CAT ELOISE: THE ONE-EYED ONE I LOVE

I told myself I wasn't going to foster another kitten just yet. I was twenty-four years old and living in a small cabin in North Carolina, and after a huge batch of foster kittens got adopted from my house, I was ready for a little break from rescue. So of course that's when my friend called me from the mobile spay/neuter clinic where she worked. "Hey, I know you're taking a break, but would you be interested in helping this little white kitten someone just dropped off here?" she asked. "She's just got

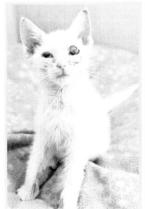
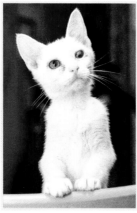

Eloise one week after rescue and one month after rescue. Amazing improvement!

an eye infection, but she's a super cute, fluffy white kitten. I bet you could find her a home in no time."

Rats, I'm such a sucker, I thought. I had been trying to learn the virtue of boundary setting, but alas, I failed. "Okay. Why not. Sounds pretty easy. I'll be right there."

"Just an eye infection" turned out to be the understatement of the century; hers was literally the worst one I'd ever seen. One eye was sealed shut, while the other was so swollen that you couldn't even see her eyeball underneath the bright red conjunctiva, which burst forth from her eyelid like a chunk of raw meat. *Ah! God, that looks so painful.* I tried to dull my horrified facial expression, momentarily unclenching my jaw to say, "Hi, lil' sweetie." To my surprise, this blind little baby, who must have been in so much pain, was loudly purring and kneading the towel with her dirty paws.

I took her home and put her in my tiny bathroom, the only room in my loft-style cabin with a door. First things first: a comfy cat bed with a fresh baby blanket. She kneaded and kneaded on the plush, unable to see where she was, but seemingly happy to be somewhere soft. I applied a warm compress to her right eye, and her eyelid slowly began to open. Underneath the lids, she was swollen and red, but— *aha!*—I could see one little eye peering back at me. "There you are! I see you in there!" I rinsed her eyes as best as I could with saline solution, then applied a topical ophthalmic antibiotic to each. That night I didn't want to leave her side, so I dozed on the bathroom floor with her in between feedings and head scratches.

Eloise was a lot of work. She wheezed badly from a severe upper respiratory infection, which was treated with antibiotics and by setting her near steamy showers to break up the snot. Her ears were completely crusted with mites, which had to be cleaned out daily. She was so starved that she could only handle small bits of food fed by syringe. Her eyes needed frequent medicating, and while her right eye seemed recoverable, the left one was a mess for weeks. But she and I became a team, huddled up by the toilet, working hard to turn her life around. And slowly, she made progress.

A few weeks into her time with me, she started to lengthen into a cute, lanky preteen with one normal eye and one kinda wonky one. She was as healed as she was going to get: her respiratory symptoms had passed, her ear mites were gone, and her eye wasn't swollen anymore; it was just scarred. My vet explained that her eye had totally ruptured, and that the lid had fused to her cornea and healed over it like a bandage. Underneath, the eye was unrecoverable, but she wasn't in any pain and could safely keep the blind eye. Satisfied that she was as healed as she would ever be, I put her up for adoption.

It was alarmingly hard to find her a home. She was a bright white, beautiful, affectionate young kitten, but so many people were turned off by her blind eye because it was cloudy with the scar tissue of the fused inner eyelid. Weeks passed, and Eloise and I grew closer and closer as she failed to find a home. She'd sleep in my bed and wake me up in the morning with biscuits (not real ones, but she'd try her best by kneading the pillow). Eventually, a woman responded to a flyer I'd made about her, and she was adopted. I was thrilled for her! I kissed her furry head with congratulations and sent her to her new home.

A few months had passed when, seemingly out of the blue, her adopter called. "She's too hyper; it just isn't going to work out." She was being returned for being too energetic (sigh . . . *all* kittens are energetic), and just like that, she was back in my little cabin, but this time she was three times the size as when I'd last seen her! She climbed into my lap and kneaded my belly. She was always a kneady girl, and still is.

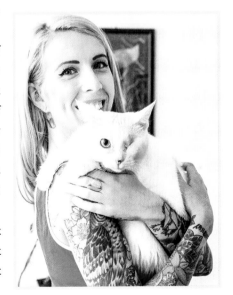

Adoption is a serious decision, and one that should of course be made with the intention of providing a home for life. Knowing the dedication I felt to my cat Coco, it was always hard for me to understand how a member of the family could be given up, but I will always accept my kittens back—no questions asked. In this case, it turned out that Eloise was returning right around the time I was considering my own big decision . . . of adopting a second cat to be friends with Coco.

Once Eloise was returned, the idea of putting her out there for others' disapproval again just made my heart sink. She'd been through so much, and I hated the thought of having to prove to someone else that she was worthy of keeping for good. She fit in so nicely with my home and had become fast friends with Coco, so I did the only thing I could to ensure that her next home would be forever: I adopted her myself!

Best decision ever. Now I get biscuits in bed every morning and purr therapy every night. I get a loyal companion who begs for affection all day, demanding to perch on my shoulder or get a hug. (She's not just kneady; she's also needy!) Though her left eye did eventually need to be enucleated, she gets around like a champ, and she's still perfect to me. As the years have passed, Eloise has watched hundreds of rescued kittens come and go through her one eye. But she knows that at the end of the day, she'll always be the one I love forever.

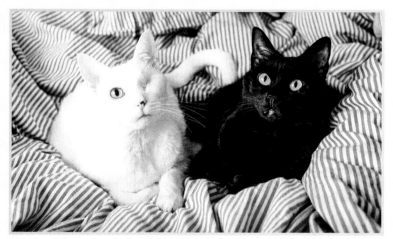

Eloise and Coco, best friends forever!

STOP THE SPREAD: UNDERSTANDING COMMON VIRUSES

Just like humans can suffer from viruses, so, too, can cats and kittens. A virus is a contagious, microscopic infectious agent that replicates inside the body of a host. While you can rest assured that your kittens won't pick up a cold or flu from you, cats have their own special viruses that impact them as a species . . . and of course, it's often the little guys who get hit the hardest. It's important to understand what the most common viruses are, how they are spread, how to prevent them, and what to do when they do happen.

The two greatest actions you can take when working with virally infected kittens are to provide individual supportive treatment and to prevent future spread of disease through quarantine and sanitation. Because viruses typically can't be stopped in their tracks, the most important thing to know is how to treat each symptom as it arises and support the kitten until these symptoms have passed. While it might sound overwhelming to battle a virus with a name you maybe

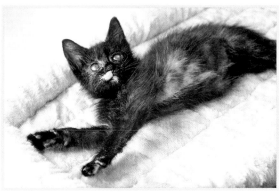

Annie, a kitten with calicivirus. With care, Annie made a full recovery!

can't even pronounce, just remember that what you're dealing with are individual symptoms, and it will start to feel feasible. One animal at a time, one symptom at a time.

Most viruses are spread through direct contact (from one cat to another), but also may be spread through contact with contaminated objects in the environment, such as shared bedding, dishes, or even unwashed human hands or clothing. Viruses can spread from your fingertips onto other items you touch. Respiratory viruses are aerosol and can spread through the air. Understanding how each virus is spread will help you proactively avert illness through establishing good prevention measures so that other animals aren't at risk. Remember that the animals who are most likely to fall ill with a virus are those who are young or immunocompromised, so your healthy adult cats are not at the same degree of risk as the kittens you may save in the future. That said, it's of course important to keep your cats up-to-date on their FVRCP vaccines and to take action if they do show symptoms of a virus.

If you're a cat person, you've probably heard of FVRCP, which stands for feline viral rhinotracheitis, calicivirus, and panleukopenia. It is considered a "core" vaccine, meaning it is essential for all kittens and cats, as these three common viruses are highly contagious.[2] If you're rescuing kittens from a high-volume setting such as an animal shelter or a community cat colony, it's quite likely that you'll encounter at least one of these three viruses at some point. Let's take a look at what each of these viruses is all about, and how to fight them.

Name	Rhinotracheitis
Symptoms	Upper respiratory symptoms impacting the eyes, nose, and throat may be observed, including sneezing, coughing, and ocular/nasal discharge. Kittens are likely to appear crusty and congested. In some cases, conjunctivitis or corneal ulceration can occur, causing the eyes to look inflamed, red, cloudy, or otherwise damaged.
Incubation period	Most kittens are symptomatic two to five days after exposure.
Active infection	Symptoms can last up to three weeks.
How it's spread	Through direct contact via saliva, discharge, and aerosolized fluid through sneezing, or to a lesser extent through contact with contaminated items in the environment, such as food dishes and bedding. The virus can survive in the environment if kept moist, such as in a food dish or cleaning cloth, but will die when dried up.
How it's diagnosed	Typically by a veterinarian by physical examination of symptoms.
How it's treated	Each kitten will be treated based on the specific symptoms present. An oral antibiotic may be warranted for kittens with upper respiratory infections with a secondary bacterial infection. Kittens should have their nasal passage kept clean by gently wiping away mucus with a warm, wet cloth. Congested kittens may benefit from saline nasal drops, nebulizer therapy, or being placed near a steamy shower to help thin out mucus and open the airway. Eyes should be kept clean and free of mucus, and a topical eye ointment should be applied if swelling, redness, or discharge is present. In more extreme cases, additional supportive care may be necessary, such as supported feeding or fluid therapy for kittens with decreased appetite or dehydration.
Preventative measures	Unvaccinated kittens should be kept separate from large volumes of animals; from nonvaccinated, undervaccinated, or immunocompromised cats; and from those who are ill or have been ill in the last three weeks. Avoid sharing food or water dishes with symptomatic animals. Sanitize items that have come into contact with infected animals using a disinfectant or soap and water, and dry completely. Wash and dry hands after handling infected kittens. Once an appropriate age, kittens should receive an FVRCP vaccine. Adult cats who are regularly vaccinated are at less of a risk of contracting this virus.

Name	Calicivirus
Symptoms	Upper respiratory symptoms such as nasal congestion, sneezing, fever, conjunctivitis, and discharge from the eyes or nose. Cats with calicivirus often also exhibit oral symptoms such as ulceration of the tongue, lips, and gums, a painful condition that can impact their ability to comfortably eat. In some cases, kittens may experience painful joints or even temporary limping or lameness of the limbs.
Incubation period	Most kittens are symptomatic two to six days after exposure.

Name	Calicivirus (cont.)
Active infection	Symptoms can last two to three weeks.
How it's spread	Through direct contact between cats, through the air, and through objects that have been contaminated by saliva or mucus. Once outside the cat's body, the virus can live in the environment for roughly one week, continuing to seek a host.
How it's diagnosed	A veterinarian will make a diagnosis based on symptoms, especially if ulceration is present. In some cases, more extensive laboratory testing may be advised to confirm a diagnosis of calicivirus.
How it's treated	Each kitten will be treated for the specific symptoms present. Depending on the degree of the infection, an oral antibiotic may be essential to fight a secondary bacterial infection. Kittens with nasal or ocular discharge should be kept clean of any mucus with a warm, wet cloth. Congested kittens may benefit from saline nasal drops, nebulizer therapy, or being placed near a steamy shower to help open the airway. If eyes are infected, a topical eye ointment may be prescribed depending on the severity of the conjunctivitis. Anti-inflammatory drugs or pain medications may be prescribed by a veterinarian to combat limping or lameness. Feverish kittens can be offered a cool ice pack in their bed, covered with a soft blanket.
Preventative measures	Unvaccinated kittens should be housed separately and given separate food dishes and bedding from cats who currently have or have had calicivirus in the past, as some may asymptomatically continue to shed the virus. A disinfectant should be used to sanitize items that have come into contact with infected animals. Thoroughly wash hands after handling infected kittens. Once an appropriate age, kittens should receive an FVRCP vaccine. Adult cats who are regularly vaccinated are at low risk of contracting this virus.

Name	Panleukopenia (commonly referred to as feline distemper or parvovirus)
Symptoms	This highly infectious virus has severe symptoms of nausea, liquid diarrhea, dehydration, lethargy, high fever, anorexia, and sudden death. Because the virus attacks rapidly dividing cells, the gut and bone marrow are most impacted in kittens, who often experience ulceration of the GI tract and the temporary inability to make and keep white blood cells. Panleukopenia is a serious and potentially fatal disease, and many kittens die due to dehydration, anemia, sepsis, or other secondary conditions. According to the American Veterinary Medical Association (AVMA), roughly 90 percent of cats with panleukopenia pass away without supportive care.[3]
Incubation period	While symptoms can occur as quickly as three days after exposure, this virus can have an incubation period of up to fourteen days.
Active infection	Extreme symptoms generally last three to five days, with some symptoms lasting up to a week or more.

Name	Panleukopenia (commonly referred to as feline distemper or parvovirus) (cont.)
How it's spread	This highly infectious virus is spread easily via contact with feces, urine, saliva, and microscopic molecules that contaminate any objects that come into contact with the infected animal. Known for its hardiness in the environment, panleukopenia can survive on contaminated objects for up to a year without proper sanitization.[4]
How it's diagnosed	Due to the severity of the illness, rapid diagnosis of panleukopenia is critical. For this reason, a fecal parvovirus test is preferable, which will show either a positive or negative result in a matter of minutes. Although the fecal test is a canine parvovirus test, studies show that it is effective for the diagnosis of panleukopenia.[5] Your veterinarian may also choose to do confirmatory blood testing, which is sent out to a laboratory.
How it's treated	While no treatment exists to fight the actual panleukopenia virus, kittens can respond well to intensive supportive care to ameliorate symptoms and get them through the illness. A veterinarian may prescribe an antibiotic that will help fight secondary infection and decrease the risk of sepsis. Oral or subcutaneous fluids can keep the kitten hydrated and replenish lost electrolytes. Vitamin B12, probiotics, and other supplements can help support the kitten through this challenging time. A veterinarian may also prescribe antinausea medication to decrease vomiting and plasma therapy to boost the kitten's immune response. Kittens with panleukopenia should be carefully monitored and given highly palatable diets, with supported feeding by hand or, in extreme cases, by tube. Even with treatment, it's important to note that many kittens with panleukopenia will lose their lives to this horrible virus.
Preventative measures	Unvaccinated kittens should be kept separate from unfamiliar animals for a minimum quarantine period of fourteen days to reduce the risk of this virus. If panleukopenia does occur in your home, all items that came into contact with the animal should be either thoroughly disinfected or discarded. Gloves should be worn when handling these animals, or if none are available, caregivers should thoroughly wash hands with warm water and soap. It's important to be especially mindful of exposing other animals via shoes, clothing, cleaning tools, or anything else that may accidentally spread the virus. Once an appropriate age, kittens should receive an FVRCP vaccine. Adult cats who are regularly vaccinated are at low risk of contracting this virus.

BEATING THE ODDS: HANK'S FIGHT AGAINST PANLEUKOPENIA

I'd raised Hank since she was just a writhing wiggle worm who fit perfectly in my palm, so minuscule that I could cover her whole body if I cupped it with both hands. She'd been dropped off at a pet store inside a tissue box, and I'd picked her up when she was just four days old. Babies like these always end up as my little sidekick, like a temporary bestie. After many weeks of waking up in the middle of the night to fill

Hank's belly, I'd watched her transform into this teensy tiger, buzzing with energy. She was growing up so beautifully.

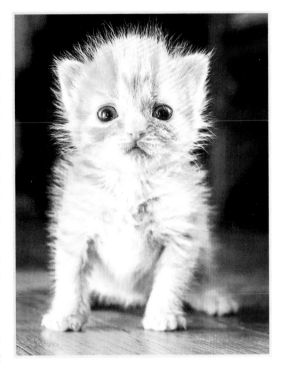

But one day, she looked different. She was sitting on a soft blanket looking up at me, but instead of the usual connection we'd make, I felt like she was almost looking past me. Her eyes were glassy and dull, and her face shape looked thinner and more triangular. She just looked *off*. For a day or two, her stool had been pretty loose, but I had shrugged it off, thinking it had to do with the digestive changes that can sometimes accompany weaning. Over the next few hours, I noticed that she hardly moved an inch. Her typical playful behaviors had dissipated, leaving behind a lethargic shell.

When a kitten's behavior or appearance changes like this, it shouldn't be ignored. *It's better to be paranoid than regretful*, I thought, and I went into my supply cabinet to look for my parvovirus tests (most people don't have these at home, but you can get this test done at a veterinarian's office). I was certain the test would be negative, but since she had symptoms of diarrhea and lethargy, I wanted to rule it out for my own peace of mind. I opened the test kit, swabbed a bit of her poop on the end of the pipette, mixed it with the diluent, and dropped three drops in the sample well. The test itself looks like a rectangular pregnancy test, and you have to wait patiently for either one or two lines to pop up and give you a result. If there's just one C line, it's negative and the kitten doesn't have the virus. If there's a C line *and* a T line, that means both the control and the test are positive, and the kitten has the virus.

Almost instantly, two lines appeared. I couldn't believe it. *No*, I thought. *No way. No. Nope. No.* I looked over at her. She looked back at me, listless and vacant. I looked back at the test. Two lines. No!

Panleukopenia, also called feline distemper, is a rescuer's worst nightmare. If left untreated, panleukopenia has about a 90 percent mortality rate in cats, and kittens are most severely affected by the disease due to their immunocompromised state.

To make matters worse, not only is it one of the deadliest diseases a kitten can get, but it's also one of the most contagious. The microscopic organism is famously hardy, hiding for up to a year in your floors, furniture, toys, bedding, walls, and anything else that comes into contact with an infected kitten if not properly sanitized. This means you don't just have to worry about the kitten you're caring for now, but you also have to worry about contaminating your house and putting future animals at risk, too.

Okay, time to put on your game face, I thought. By this point, I knew my whole nursery room was contaminated. I grabbed Hank. I grabbed a playpen. I set her up in my bedroom at the farthest corner of the house. I washed my hands and took a deep breath. Then I grabbed another playpen and set up my other kittens (who were not symptomatic and, thankfully, never got the virus) in the living room. I washed my hands again. Now that it was empty, I shut the door to the nursery and declared it a no-entry zone. I'd worry about sanitizing it later . . . Right now I needed to worry about saving Hank's life.

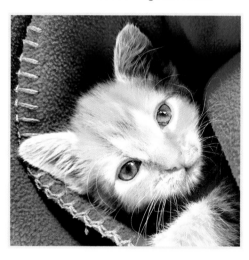

Back in my bedroom I looked down into the playpen and Hank's condition was already worsening. Hunched over in the litter box, she defecated yellow liquid. *Ugh.* It felt like it was happening so fast. I called my vet and told them she needed to come in immediately—panleukopenia progresses quickly, and these kittens can't wait. I heated up a bag of fluids, knowing I'd need to start her on subcutaneous fluids right away. I'd also need to get her an antibiotic, add electrolytes and a few supplements to her food, and carefully ensure that she was eating enough to keep her blood sugar up. I'd do everything I could to keep her stable. After all, the panleukopenia virus cannot be cured outright, and the only way to beat it is to keep the kitten alive long enough for it to pass. The only way out is through, as they say.

I started calling around and talking to friends and colleagues, searching for any tidbits of information that could save her. One friend I knew through my local animal shelter had gotten so sick of euthanizing panleukopenia kittens that she had made it her mission to figure out how to save them, and she had some great tips and encouraging words. She reminded me that years previously, I had sat in the shelter with her, holding four dying panleukopenia kittens in my hands as she put them to sleep. After, I had sobbed in her office, looking for any answers about what I could do differently in the future. She reminded me that I'd learned so much in the years since that happened, and this was my chance to beat the odds. I swallowed hard. The thought of going through that again with Hank didn't just make me sad . . . It made me livid. *I am not doing that again. Heck no.* My fire was fueled.

I got out a piece of paper and made a grid, writing across the top everything that I wanted to monitor: temperature, weight, poop, energy, appetite, treatment. I'd sit with her every two to three hours, taking note of how she was doing, hand-feeding her, and giving her supportive care to help keep her body alive long enough for the virus to pass. When I wasn't sitting with her, I was researching the disease online, trying to understand what was happening to her body at each step. I knew that if I could decode what her body was trying to tell me, I'd have a better chance at helping it change course.

And so, for five days, I was consumed by this battle—engaged in combat with her virus like a game of chess. Each time the virus made a move, I'd try to counteract it. She'd have diarrhea; I'd give her a fiber supplement. She'd have dehydration; I'd give her fluids. Her temperature would drop; I'd keep her warm. She'd lose her appetite; I'd find something more palatable for her to eat. With each action and counteraction, I felt more and more driven to defeat this thing once and for all.

I was up at all hours, obsessing over Hank's poop. Late one night, I talked with a vet friend on the West Coast, Dr. Rachel, who suggested giving her a micro-dose of an acid reducer, and I got so excited to try something new that I didn't want to wait until morning . . . so I found myself driving around DC in my pajamas at 1 a.m., trying three different twenty-four-hour drugstores before I found what I needed. *I sure know how to have a wild Friday night*, I told myself, but I wouldn't have had it any other way.

Another night, I video-chatted with my licensed veterinary technician (LVT) friend Ellen, and she taught me a super gross (but amazing!) trick to check if Hank had blood in her stool. I smeared her poop (which by this point was black and tarry) across a white sheet of paper, then dropped a few drops of hydrogen peroxide on it. It fizzled like an icky, effervescent science project. "Aha!" I exclaimed. The fizzle was a sign that blood was indeed present, due to the ulceration of her GI tract. "I feel like a wizard. I'm like the Hermione Granger of poop." Maybe it sounds gross, but knowing and understanding each of these details gave me more tools to fight back. Anticipating the virus's next move, I was able to avert excess damage . . . and, eventually, start to win.

You know you're a kitten rescuer when a solid poop makes you shout for joy. On the fifth day of Hank's battle against panleukopenia, I finally had a sign that she was slowly overcoming the virus, and I was beaming from happiness and exhaustion. I kept up the supportive care strategies all the same, not stopping her care routine until I knew she was out of the dark. Slowly, her dim light started to glow a little brighter, and brighter still, until eventually, she was glowing.

Hank recovered just a few days before Christmas, and having her with us for the holidays was the best gift I could have ever asked for. Regaining her playful spirit, Hank played with bows and wrapping paper, ate many treats, and was spoiled rotten

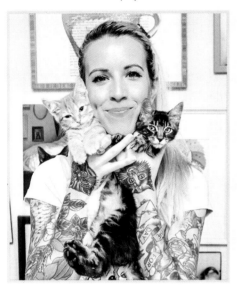

with toys. Now that she had conquered a deadly virus, Hankie was stronger than ever!

Hank's transformation was a sight to behold. From being left at a store in a tissue box to surviving a deadly virus to bounding around the house like a jungle cat—she had earned every moment of joy she experienced! Hank became best friends with another little kitten in foster care, Kodiak, and together they explored the nursery, played with toys, and developed what would be a lifelong relationship. They were adopted together and are now best friends for life, living in cat paradise with a loving family.

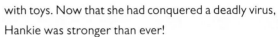

GIVE 'EM A BOOST: KITTENS AND VACCINES

Vaccination is an essential part of caring for cats and kittens. Every new kitten should receive a series of FVRCP vaccines as part of their routine care. Typically, the kitten will receive an initial FVRCP vaccine, then a series of booster shots over the second to fourth months of life. If you're a private rescuer or a new adopter, you'll want to bring your kitten to be vaccinated at either a vet's office or through a low-cost vaccine clinic, available in many communities. Foster programs will typically provide all vaccines to kittens being fostered through their organization at no cost.

There are several schools of thought about the most appropriate age for the first vaccine, and choosing when to begin and how often to boost depends entirely on the kitten's circumstances. For instance, an animal shelter may elect to vaccinate as young as four weeks of age and to boost every two weeks, due to the high risk of exposure to viruses. A private practice vet, on the other hand, may recommend waiting until the kitten is closer to eight weeks and boosting every three to four weeks, as they're at lower risk of picking up an illness. In most cases, animal rescuers will want to give their first vaccine around six weeks of age and provide booster shots in three-week intervals until the kitten has reached fourteen to sixteen weeks of age, but this can vary depending on the situation.

It's important to understand that maternal antibodies can also interfere with the effectiveness of a vaccine, so depending on how much passive immunity the kittens obtained from their mother, vaccines may not be entirely effective until kittens have reached twelve to sixteen weeks of age. Vaccination of young kittens is an essential component of preventative care, but to be certain that there has been no maternal antibody interference, adopters should continue boosters until the kitten has reached sixteen weeks. After that, it's just an annual booster shot to help keep the cat protected.

The rabies vaccine is generally given as a single shot at twelve weeks of age, which is then boosted one year later, and then in three-year increments thereafter.[6] Even if you think the kitten is at extremely low risk of contracting rabies, this isn't something to overlook. Feral kittens and even socialized kittens who are scared or in pain may bite, and if that occurs, you'll need a proof of rabies vaccination in order to protect the animal. Having proof of rabies vaccination is legally required in many parts of the United States, and might be required if the cat becomes lost and is impounded at the shelter. Even if you don't live in a state where rabies vaccination is mandated, it's still a good idea to get a vaccine so that the cat is protected. Of course, make sure you're keeping good records of your vaccines!

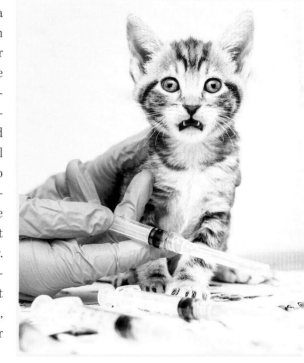

Feline immunodeficiency virus is a slow-acting infection that weakens the immune system of a cat, making him more susceptible to illness. For a long time, FIV was considered a death sentence for cats and kittens—not because the virus killed them, but because a positive diagnosis often meant that they were preemptively euthanized. After the virus was discovered in 1986, misconceptions pervaded our understanding of the disease for many years, with deadly consequences.[7] Many organizations and veterinarians erroneously feared that the virus would cause immense suffering, or that it would be easily spread. Fear of the virus meant that FIV-positive cats were often not considered adoptable. This led to many adult cats and even young kittens being overlooked, or even killed, simply for testing positive.

In recent years, cat advocates and veterinary scientists have proved that our previous assumptions were wrong. It's now understood that many cats live long and normal lives with FIV.[8] Animal shelters and rescue organizations are working hard to dismantle outdated fears about the virus and encourage people to consider adopting an FIV-positive cat; after all, these cats are every bit as capable of love—and as deserving of life—as their FIV-negative friends. As studies have been published showing that FIV is not as easily spread as once thought, it's also becoming more accepted to adopt an FIV-positive cat into a multi-cat household. These cats pose little threat to playmates unless they are in a truly aggressive fighting or mating situation and the bite wound is deep; the likelihood of this is extremely low in households where all cats are spayed and neutered.

Unfortunately, change happens slowly, and the stigma against FIV still exists to some degree, which can have a devastating impact not just on cats but on kittens in particular. As horrible as it is that so many lives have been unnecessarily lost due to misunderstandings about FIV-positive cats, I find it additionally tragic that a positive test can result in euthanasia when the majority of young kittens who test positive for FIV are, in fact, negative. It's time to put an end to euthanizing based on FIV testing, and to shed a light on kittens, false positives, and false assumptions.

In order to understand why kittens often have false positives, it's helpful to first take a look at how FIV is transmitted. Because the virus is contracted primarily through deep bite wounds, cats typically must engage in serious fighting behaviors in order to spread FIV. These fighting behaviors are commonly associated with mating: either tomcats fighting over a mate or tomcats biting females during the mating process. It therefore makes sense that the virus is disproportionately represented in unsterilized adult cats, especially intact males who live (or have lived) outdoors and females who are (or have been) pregnant. It is essentially a disease of fighting and breeding.

Now consider where kittens come from. Because the majority of rescue kittens are born outdoors to unsterilized community cats, there is an elevated chance that they will be born to a mother who is FIV-positive. But does this mean the kittens will have the virus? Most of the time, the answer is no. True transmission of the disease from mother to kittens is actually rare; it's much more common that an FIV-positive cat will give birth to FIV-negative kittens. That said, kittens born to a mother cat with FIV may test positive on an FIV test, even if they do not truly have the disease; a mother is more likely to pass FIV antibodies to her kittens than the actual virus. When a kitten tests positive, these results can unfairly weigh against that kitten when it comes to adoptability.

"About 25 percent of kittens with an FIV-positive mother will test positive," says Dr. Marcus Brown, leading cat veterinarian and owner of Nova Cat Clinic. This is due to the presence of maternal antibodies, which can be passed from the mother to the kitten through nursing and can linger in the body until the kitten is up to six months of age. This complicates the test results because the test looks only for the presence of antibodies, not the disease itself. Dr. Brown continues, "Most kittens who test positive do so because of maternal antibodies, but the odds are that they will retest negative at six months. Very few kittens get FIV from their mothers."

If a kitten tests negative, it is considered a true negative. If a kitten tests positive, this is considered a potential positive, with a plan to retest at six months of age. My recommendation is to not let this weigh against them or delay adoption. Kittens should be spayed or neutered, and placed into a home with a low risk of fighting. Prospective adopters should simply be informed of the positive result, and should agree to a retest. Of course, in the unlikely event that these kittens do remain positive, they can still live a wonderful life and are at low risk of spreading the virus so long as they are sterilized and not biting each other. But most of the time, you'll find that as the maternal antibodies fade, the kitten will be FIV free.

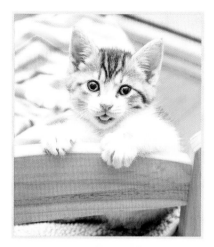

Blossom was found outdoors on the streets of Philadelphia, along with her siblings, Sprout, Twig, and Bud. As tiny as they were at just two and a half weeks old, Blossom was definitely the biggest of the bunch, with a rotund pink belly and a chunky, round face. From the moment I brought her home, this little girl was a silly little goober who loved cuddling and sticking out her bright pink tongue. She was certain to be a cherished companion for someone, someday.

As the kittens reached adoption age, I brought them in for their final vet visit, a routine appointment that involved spay/neuter, vaccines, and, finally, an FIV/FeLV test. Each kitten gets a quick prick with a needle to draw blood, which is then dropped onto a small plastic tray called an ELISA test. It works kind of like a pregnancy test: if the test is negative, only the control will have a line. If it's positive, you'll have a control line *and* a test line. With the four tests in a row, I watched as all the control lines popped up, and then sighed with disappointment. There was a light line showing a positive result on one of the tests. Of the four kittens, Blossom was the only one whose blood tested positive for the FIV antibody. Ugh.

"It makes sense; their mother was probably FIV-positive, and one in four kittens born from positive cats will have her antibodies . . . so here's our one." Dr. Brown assured me that this was likely just an antibody response, and not a true positive. I knew that it was quite likely these antibodies would leave Blossom's body over the coming months, but it broke my heart to know that potential adopters might not look at her the same. When the public doesn't have all the details, one little line on a piece of plastic can be enough to turn them away in fear.

So I made it my mission to help people understand. I shared very openly about her FIV-positive result, and had discussions about her potential status with each prospective adopter. I made the decision to adopt Blossom out with her sister Sprout, knowing that even if she truly had FIV, she could still live safely with her favorite little friend. As the months went on after Blossom and Sprout's adoption, I hoped for the best and waited for more news from her adopter.

When the news came, I celebrated! Blossom's retest came back negative, just as we had hoped and expected. Our pudgy little girl was FIV free!

Feline leukemia virus (FeLV) is a serious retrovirus that can infect cats and kittens. The virus attacks the body's natural defense system and bone marrow, and can make cats more prone to other diseases, including anemia, bacterial infections, viruses, and even cancer. Unfortunately, it is typically considered a terminal illness, especially in kittens, whose bodies are less able to fight off the disease. Still, the cat's life span can vary dramatically. While some kittens will live only a few months with FeLV, others will grow to adulthood and live normal lives for several years.

FeLV can be transmitted via saliva, nasal secretions, blood, urine, feces, or even breast milk. Although it is most often spread to adults through fighting or prolonged grooming, kittens are much more likely to obtain the virus in utero or by nursing on an infected mother. After the kitten has been exposed, it can take a month or longer for the virus to show up on a diagnostic test.

Testing for the feline leukemia virus is a standard part of a kitten's early life, and the most common way for vets and shelters to test is through a combination test that looks for both FIV and FeLV. Unfortunately, testing kittens for leukemia is not always reliable, as the test shows only one snapshot in time, and that snapshot can change. Both false negatives and false positives can occur in young kittens depending on a number of circumstances, including when the kitten was exposed and whether the body is able to fight off the virus. If a kitten tests positive for FeLV, it should not be considered an absolute diagnosis unless she is symptomatic—she should receive a second test (called an IFA) that confirms the diagnosis, and a follow-up test at least thirty to sixty days later.

Many veterinarians and animal shelters still euthanize those who test positive for leukemia, but it's my belief that euthanasia should be reserved only for those who are symptomatic, suffering, and truly in untreatable condition. If a kitten is asymptomatic or recoverable, it's of course the most ethical decision to let that kitten live—though special precautions should be taken when choosing an adopter. FeLV-positive kittens should be adopted into loving homes that provide close monitoring for signs of illness, routine visits to the vet, and a safe environment where the kitten will not expose others to the virus or be exposed to potentially dangerous conditions for an immunocompromised cat. Whether an FeLV kitten lives for three months or three years, she can still experience joy, comfort, and companionship just like any other cat . . . and she certainly deserves a chance to do just that.

When I brought Beignet home, she was a mess . . . and no one could figure out why. She and her five littermates had been saved by a local rescue organization, and had been perfectly healthy up until now. They'd been named after French pastries and prepared for adoption. Four of the six siblings were already in their forever homes

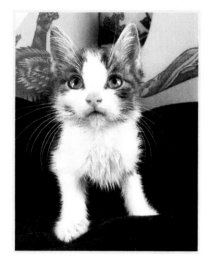

when Beignet and her brother started to get sicker and sicker. By the time I found out about Beignet's condition, her brother had died by her side, and she was on death's door herself; she was a frail, skeletal nine-week-old cat weighing less than one pound. My heart broke for her, and I offered to take her home and see what I could do.

It was a rough first night. She was so dehydrated, so skinny, and so lethargic that I wondered if she would survive another day, and contemplated whether euthanasia was the most humane decision. But when I looked at her, she looked right back at me with big, loving eyes and purred—in spite of her condition, she was still "in there." She had already tested negative for panleukopenia, FIV, and FeLV, and while it was unclear why her body was withering away, I knew that I wanted to fight for her.

For the next two weeks she was by my side, getting fluid therapy, hand-feeding, and TLC. Her brittle body soaked up fluids like a dry sponge begging for moisture. Each meal she'd eat a little more, and her weight gradually increased. At night, I'd lie with her bony body against my chest, petting her as she vibrated with purrs. "I need you to live, Beignet. Someday, you're going to be somebody's very best friend." I know, I know—cats don't understand English, but they can comprehend a gentle voice of encouragement, and I truly believe that they benefit from comfort during illness. Of course, as I said the words, I knew I was saying them as much for my own comfort as for hers; I wanted badly to believe them. Beignet listened, cocking her head, her body rumbling and gently purring.

Just a few weeks later, my wish came true. Beignet plumped up and recovered, and she did become someone's very best friend. She was adopted by a young woman from Delaware, and it was instant love. We had a small adoption party to celebrate her success, and her adopter glowed with adoration for her new companion. There was so much to celebrate!

But a few weeks later, Beignet's adopter contacted me with shocking news. "I took Beignet in for her first appointment with my vet, and she tested positive for feline leukemia." My heart sank. How could that be? She had tested negative just a few weeks prior, but there is always the possibility that it hadn't been long enough since her exposure for the test to have given an accurate result. My mind reeled trying to grasp this diagnosis, and I wondered if her battle with illness had actually been her body's response to the incoming retrovirus. I talked with the adopter, suggesting that we get a confirmatory test and then retest her in sixty days. The adopter expressed her undying commitment and love for Beignet no matter what the outcome was, and we both crossed our fingers and hoped the test had been wrong.

All future tests confirmed that Beignet does, in fact, have feline leukemia. While this was devastating news, her adopter's perspective was ultimately one of gratitude. She was grateful that for now, Beignet was in good health, and she'd continue to be grateful for every single day that Beignet could enjoy her life on this earth. After all, none of us know how long we have, so we can and should live life to the fullest. I felt such relief for Beignet, knowing that she'd found the best home ever. She had found unconditional love.

And thank goodness she did, because more than three years later, she's still doing great! Beignet is still as strong as ever, living a life of love every day. She's transformed into a healthy and hilarious cat who loves to chase toys, stick her tongue out (*blep!*), and cuddle with her mama. By having an attitude of hope and thankfulness for each day, her adopter has given Beignet the opportunity to live a full life—one where every single day is a celebration.

SPOTLIGHT: PROTECT YOUR KITTENS, PROTECT YOUR CATS

If you have a pet cat at home with FIV or FeLV, you can still foster—but you'll want to take extra precautions to keep both your cats and your foster kittens healthy. Keep in mind that these are transmissible illnesses that can potentially be passed to your kittens, *and* that your kittens may carry illnesses that can harm your vulnerable cat. Because these illnesses can make your cat more susceptible to disease, it is advisable to keep your kittens separated and quarantined from your cats, especially if they are new to the home and have an unknown health history or if they are exhibiting any signs of illness (learn all about how to quarantine a kitten on page 191).

If your kittens have been through a quarantine period and are healthy, they can be introduced to a friendly FIV-positive cat with supervision; however, if any aggression is witnessed, it's best to keep them separate due to the risk of transmission via bite wounds. When it comes to FeLV, you'll do best to keep them totally separated, as this disease can be more easily spread between cats, such as with grooming. Finally, if you do intend to introduce kittens to your adult cat, talk to a veterinarian first about vaccinating against FIV or FeLV. While vaccines do exist, they are not given unless specifically requested. When in doubt, I recommend keeping your cats and kittens protected by keeping them separated.

UNDERSTANDING FELINE INFECTIOUS PERITONITIS

Feline infectious peritonitis (FIP) is a fatal viral disease caused by a mutation of certain strains of the feline coronavirus. This aggressive disease is known for quickly sneaking up on kitten adopters and resulting in rapid decline. While coronavirus is prevalent in multi-cat households, not all cats infected with the coronavirus will develop FIP; in fact, about 95 percent will not.[9] In most cases, the cat will never have symptoms. However, a small portion of immunocompromised cats—typically young kittens—may eventually develop FIP over time, sometimes months or even years after exposure to the virus. It is believed that stress and overcrowding may also contribute to the mutation, making FIP more common in kittens living in a high-volume setting such as an animal shelter. Most kittens with FIP will develop symptoms after three months of age.

If the coronavirus progresses and becomes FIP, it will infect the kitten's white blood cells, which are then transported throughout the body by her own immune system. Symptoms of noneffusive "dry" FIP can be varied, including a slow decline in weight, appetite, and energy, or even neurological symptoms. Many kittens with FIP additionally present with a chronic low-grade fever and unkempt coat. Symptoms of effusive "wet" FIP are generally more rapid; while an afflicted kitten may experience similar weight loss and lethargy, this form of the disease additionally causes an accumulation of fluid in the abdomen or chest that can make it challenging for the kitten to breathe. Tragically, symptoms can be subtle or go unnoticed until the kitten is in critical condition, making it even harder for caregivers, who must quickly cope with the loss of a life.

If FIP is suspected, it's essential to work with a veterinarian who can make a diagnosis. While supportive care has the potential to help in the short term, there is devastatingly no cure for FIP at the time of this writing; the disease is progressive and is inevitably fatal. For this reason, caregivers often make the decision to humanely euthanize kittens before their suffering becomes too much. This decision should be made case by case with the kitten's welfare at heart.

As we await new research about FIP treatment, we can always take steps to reduce the risk of the disease.[10] By keeping a sanitized environment, reducing overcrowding, and limiting stressful events, we can greatly decrease the risk of FIP. This is one of the many reasons that offering up our homes to foster animals can save more lives! We reduce the density of animals in the shelter and allow kittens to grow up in a stress-free, safe environment.

RINGWORM: THERE'S NOTHING FUN ABOUT FUNGUS

Here's a ring that no one wants to wear: ringworm! Ringworm is a condition that causes hair loss and ring-shaped, patchy circular lesions on the skin. Despite its confusing name, ringworm isn't a worm at all; it's actually a fungal infection, and it's contagious to cats, dogs, and even humans. This funky fungus primarily affects those who are young or immunocompromised, making kittens especially prone to picking it up if exposed.

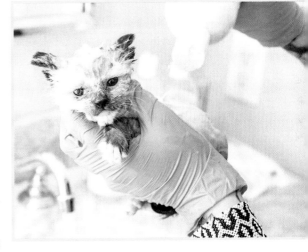

The good news is that ringworm is a totally treatable condition if given a strict care regimen and a bit of time. The bad news is that because kittens with ringworm require this extra care, many of them are euthanized in shelters, even though they would have a bright future if given the opportunity to be treated. This demonstrates the incredible opportunity that foster parents have to make a lifesaving impact on a kitten; by fostering little ones who have ringworm, we can give them the only chance they might have to survive, to heal, and to get the fungus-free future they deserve.

If a kitten has bald patches or dry, flaky skin, you'll want to get her examined right away. A veterinarian can do a fungal culture to confirm the presence of ringworm, but since these confirmatory tests can take time, it's often good to go ahead and get started with your treatment if ringworm is suspected. The other common method for diagnosing ringworm is to examine the skin and fur under a black light, or a Wood's lamp. Certain strains of ringworm will glow under a black light, so when you shine it on the kitten, you may see that their patchy parts look bright purple! Just be careful using this method, because not all strains will glow, and some things will glow that are not ringworm, like certain fibers or food residue.

Treatment for ringworm is typically a multimodal approach that may include a prescription oral antifungal medication, a topical antifungal ointment for the lesions, a twice-weekly medicated dip or bath, or some combination of these treatments. One of the most commonly used treatments by rescuers is lime sulfur dip, a stinky yellow liquid (seriously, it smells like rotten eggs) that acts as a powerful antifungal agent. Kittens being treated with this method will typically need to be dipped twice a week in the smelly stuff, which is then left on the fur to dry. This smelly dip is effective and affordable, but can be caustic and drying as well—so it's good to know that other options do exist, including antifungal shampoos that you can obtain from a vet. The most common topical treatment is miconazole, which can be purchased over the counter. Talk to a veterinarian about the best treatment methods to suit your situation and needs. Consider supporting the kitten's overall skin health during treatment by providing a small dose of omega-3 fatty acids (fish oil) in the food once daily; while this won't fight ringworm, it will keep the skin healthy so that it can better defend itself and heal.

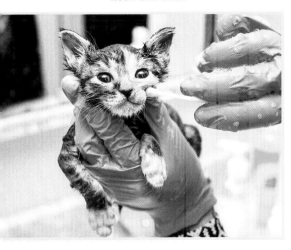

Since ringworm can be highly contagious, you'll want to ensure that your kittens are quarantined from other animals and children in the home, preferably in a playpen, a kennel, or a room that can be easily sanitized such as a bathroom. Wearing gloves, tying up long hair, and rigorous hand washing will help decrease the risk of you contracting ringworm yourself. Because the spores can be spread via items in the environment, you'll also want to thoroughly disinfect toys and bedding twice a week, every time you bathe or dip the kittens. Be mindful of sanitizing all items that come into contact with the kittens' area. Practicing good sanitation means you'll pull the plug on the spores' ability to spread, and soon you'll be exiting the fungal jungle for good!

As tempting as it is to bring home a boatload of kittens and let them run rampant around the house, it's safest for everyone if some degree of separation exists . . . especially if you're dealing with sick or potentially sick kittens. "When taking in a kitten with an unknown history, in-home quarantine is important for the health of both the kitten and your resident pets," says Jackie Noble, manager of the kitten nursery at the San Diego Humane Society. To quarantine means to keep the kittens contained in such a way that they don't have access to other animals, or to general items in the household, until it's confirmed that they are not at risk of exposing themselves or others to disease. Depending on the situation, there are different levels of quarantine that may be appropriate.

General Quarantine

- In general, it's safest to keep all new kittens isolated from others for a minimum period of two weeks in order to ensure that they don't have a surprise illness that can be spread. Not everyone does this, but trust me—if a virus pops up, you'll be glad it's contained! During this two-week period, you'll be deworming them, vaccinating them (if old enough), FIV/FeLV-testing them, and monitoring them for any symptoms that arise.

- After two weeks, healthy, asymptomatic kittens can be cleared to access other parts of your house if desired, though in many cases it's easiest to keep them in one area for the duration of their early weeks. If you're introducing them to other animals, it's best for the kittens to have received at least one FVRCP vaccine and to have obtained a negative FIV/FeLV combination test.

- During general quarantine, keep kittens in a playpen, kennel, or sanitizable room such as a bathroom (carpeted areas are discouraged). Avoid sharing litter boxes, toys, bedding, or food dishes with other animals in the home until the general quarantine has passed.

Isolation (Strict Quarantine)

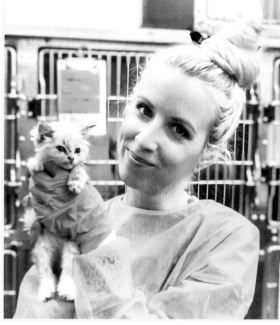

- If a kitten has, or is suspected to have, ringworm or panleukopenia, strict quarantine procedures should apply. Keep the animal contained and completely separated from other animals unless paired together with others with the same diagnosis.

- Strict quarantine areas should be free of carpeting, wood, furniture, or other porous surfaces (a metal kennel is ideal). Use only items that can be sanitized or discarded. Be mindful of any items that come into contact with the area such as cleaning tools, care supplies, cell phones, and even your hands and clothing. Any item that has potentially been exposed to the contagion should be sanitized.

Working with a kitten in a ringworm quarantine area.

- Because both ringworm and panleukopenia can be easily spread via environmental contact, it's highly advised that you wear gloves and a gown/smock, tie your hair up, and wash your hands immediately after handling the affected kittens.

CLEANUP CREW: SANITIZING 101

It's important to keep a clean space for animal care, but it's even more important to sanitize . . . and to understand the difference between cleaning and sanitizing. To clean is to remove dirt and debris so that an area looks and smells fresh, but to sanitize is to clean on a molecular level. Sanitizing destroys organic material, typically through extreme heat or contact with a chemical disinfectant. Because kittens can shed viruses, fungal spores, and parasites that aren't visible to the human eye, it's critical that rescuers know how to truly decontaminate living spaces, bedding, and other supplies.

You should clean as frequently as you need to, but sanitizing should take place any time you're helping a kitten recover from an illness, and always in between litters. Any time a new animal is going to be coming into contact with the space or supply, it should be sanitized.

Not all disinfectants are created equal. Each product has different properties, so it's important to get to know the disinfectant you're working with. In general, there are two disinfectants that are advisable:

Product	Pros	Cons	Additional Info
Household bleach	—Affordable and easy to find —Effective against panleukopenia, ringworm, and other contagions —Works well for sanitizing laundry and toys	—Inactivated by organic material; thus, extensive cleaning is required beforehand —Only effective for twenty-four hours once diluted —Not appropriate for furniture or upholstery —Irritating when inhaled by humans or animals —Must be rinsed after use	—Dilute with water at a ratio of 1:32 (half a cup per gallon of water) to kill panleukopenia and ringworm —Contact time of ten minutes in order to effectively sanitize —Rinse after use
Rescue disinfectant (accelerated hydrogen peroxide)	—Concentrate is effective for ninety days once diluted —Mild detergent activity makes it stronger against organic material —Effective against panleukopenia, ringworm, and other contagions —Safe for use around animals —Can be used on furniture and upholstery —Does not require a rinse after use	—More expensive than bleach —Typically must be purchased online	—Dilute concentrate with water at a ratio of 1:32 (half a cup per gallon of water) to kill panleukopenia and 1:16 (one cup per gallon of water) to kill ringworm —Contact time of ten minutes in order to effectively sanitize —No need to rinse after use

HOW TO SANITIZE EVERYTHING

🐱 **Bottles and food dishes:** First, use hot, soapy water to scrub away all visible debris. Follow up with a hot dishwasher cycle to kill remaining antigens. If no dishwasher is available, a bottle sterilizer can be used, or boiling water.

🐱 **Hard floors and walls:** Sweep to remove any visible debris. Use a spray bottle or mop bucket with your chosen disinfectant and completely saturate the area where contamination occurred. Ensure that the area is completely dry and aerated before introducing new animals.

🐈 **Carriers, kennels, and playpens:** Wipe down the area with an all-purpose cleaner to remove any visible debris. Use a spray bottle with your chosen disinfectant and completely saturate the item. After ten minutes, wipe down any remaining liquid.

🐈 **Soft furniture and carpets:** Large porous items should be avoided when possible, as they can be more difficult to sanitize. Use a vacuum to remove as much debris as you can, and use a steam cleaner to sanitize the item.

🐈 **Toys and bedding:** Toys and bedding can be washed in a washing machine with hot water, detergent, and half a cup of bleach, Rescue disinfectant, or a laundry sanitizer. Dry on high heat.

YOU'RE NOT INVITED: WHY PARASITES ARE FREELOADERS AND MUST BE STOPPED

Rescuing a kitten should be between you and the feline. When you invite this wondrous new individual into your house, you really only want to be providing a home to that one being . . . not a few hundred additional living organisms! Parasites are disgusting little invaders that can infest a kitten internally or externally, living off of the body's nutrients at the kitten's expense. That means when you bring Fluffy home, you could also be bringing home a whole party of nasty little freeloaders.

Almost all rescued kittens are bound to have some kind of parasite. Fleas, ear mites, worms, and other microorganisms exist abundantly in the environment, and even though many are imperceptible to the human eye, they can pose a serious health risk to kittens if left to thrive. It's essential that we pull the plug on the parasite party, and send those little ingrates packing. Being so small, kittens don't have spare blood lying around to give to a ragtag gang of fleas, or excess nutrients to share with a bellyful of deadbeat roundworms. They need it all for themselves!

Parasite control is typically a two-part process: prevention and proactive treatment. Certain parasites are so prevalent in kittens that they should be preventatively treated no matter what, while others should be treated only if their presence is confirmed. Either way, it's important to know that parasites do not go away on their own—they will stay and party as long as you'll let them, living off the kitten until they've virtually depleted her life force. Let's learn how to kick those nasty buggers to the curb.

THE PARTY IS OVER: GETTING RID OF FLEAS

A flea is a small insect that survives by consuming the blood of a host animal. As ectoparasites, fleas live on the outside of the animal's body, taking up residence on the skin and underneath the fur. Their bodies are perfectly designed for the devious task of blood sucking, with flat bodies that can easily glide through the fur, long frog-like legs for jumping onto hosts, and vampiric mouths. Fleas are commonly found on animals who have been living outside or in close quarters with others, so all kittens should be assumed to be at risk and should be checked for fleas.

Unlike many parasites, fleas are large enough to be visible to the human eye—they're about the size of a pencil tip. While they're big enough to see, they're also stealthy, and you might not even notice that the kitten has them just by looking. But fleas are messy guests, and they leave behind something called flea dirt, which is waste that looks like black specks or coffee grounds. Flea dirt is the waste fleas produce after consuming blood—it's small, dark, bloody poop flakes.

Here's how you want to check the kitten for fleas:

- Use a flea comb. These small, affordable combs are perfect for brushing through the kitten's fur, and will reveal if fleas or flea dirt are present. Comb through the kitten's fur, especially down the back and by the base of the tail, where fleas are likely to hang out.

- If you don't have a flea comb, you can run your fingers through the kitten's fur and see if black specks are present. Look for dirt or live fleas through the fur at the base of the tail, around the groin and hind legs, and around the ears and face.

- If you've found dirt but aren't certain it's from fleas, you can put the dirt onto a paper towel and add a few drops of water. If it looks like a small red blood-stain, it's flea dirt.

Fleas might be small, but they're a big deal. You might know that fleas can cause itching and skin irritation, but did you know they can also spread viruses, bacteria, and tapeworms, and even cause anemia and death? If you've found fleas on a kitten, don't delay in evicting their unauthorized party. Here's what you need to know about killing fleas:

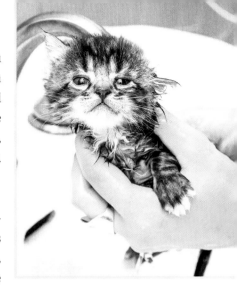

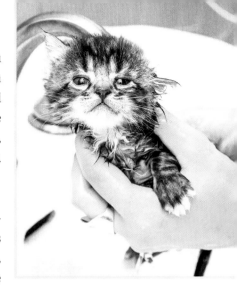 Don't assume that you can safely use a flea topical treatment on a kitten. Many flea treatments for kittens are only safe for a certain weight, usually one and a half or two pounds. Some over-the-counter products can be toxic or ineffective in kittens, so talk to a vet about getting the right product for your kitten's age and weight. *Flea products for dogs should not be used under any circumstances. Avoid any product containing pyrethrin/pyrethroid ingredients, which are toxic to cats.*

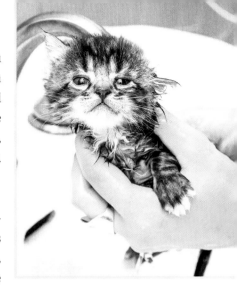 Don't use flea collars or sprays. These products aren't approved for young kittens, and can overdose even older kittens. The last thing you want to do is poison the kitten, so avoid these products.

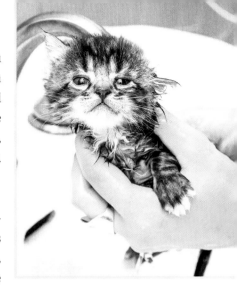 If the kitten is under two months, the safest way to treat the fleas is by bathing. A baby soap or fragrance-free dish soap will work great—as long as it's unscented and has a sudsing agent, it'll be safe for the kittens but deadly for the fleas. Follow my tips for safely bathing kittens on page 198, and they'll be flea-free in no time.

SPOTLIGHT: FLEAS SUCK

Fleas suck, both literally and figuratively. An infestation of fleas can steal so much blood that it can cause anemia, and this happens especially quickly in the minuscule body of a kitten. Caregivers should be concerned about anemia if a kitten has had a severe flea infestation and *also* has signs of lethargy, low appetite, breathing difficulty, or pale gums. You can help some kittens survive flea anemia simply by removing the fleas and providing supportive care, but kittens with severe blood loss may require a blood transfusion in order to survive.

I'll never forget the first severe flea infestation I ever saw. My friend and I were riding bikes down a city street in West Philadelphia, when our path was obstructed by a little kid who lay sprawled across the road next to his bicycle. The little boy was maybe eight years old and seemed to be peering underneath a car, though I couldn't quite tell what was going on until we began to talk.

"You okay?" I asked as I hit the brakes, hoping he wasn't hurt.

"Yeah, but there's a little cat under this truck! A really dirty one!" the boy responded.

We pulled over to the sidewalk. On my hands and knees, I pressed my face toward the hot pavement, and sure enough, I saw a dusty figure with large ears and a coat so unimaginably dirty that it's hard to put into words. I could hardly detect her coat color through the thick layer of grime that cloaked her body. I offered an outstretched hand for her to sniff, then pet the top of her crunchy little head, then wrapped my hand around her belly and lifted her. Within seconds, I felt a crawling sensation run up my arm.

Ack! I looked, and I already had several fleas zipping around my skin. Her fur was absolutely swarming with little brown bugs that darted over the bridge of her nose, around her eyes, and all across her back. The dirty little kitten clearly had a gnarly infestation. Knowing that this was a temporary state, I shook it off and looked back at the kid. "Thanks for helping her!" I said with a smile to the little boy. I looked up at the street sign, which read DEARBORN STREET. "I'll name her Dearborn! She'll be safe with me."

I knew there was no way on earth I could safely ride all the way to my home in South Philly while holding a flea-covered kitten. Fortunately, my friend lived within walking distance, and had grown used to my street-kitten shenanigans, so he was willing to let me bring Dearborn over to his house and clean her up. Holding her tightly on our walk to his house, I could feel that her coat was coarsely textured from mud, motor oil, fleas, flea dirt, and other general filth that caked her fur. Tiny pests hopped on my hand, my arm, even my neck. I tried to ignore it, and walked quickly alongside my friend, with my bike in one hand and Dearborn in the other.

As soon as we got to his house, it was time to clean her up. We ran warm water in the sink, and I made a ring of soap around her neck. As we washed her body, the water ran dark crimson; the fleas had been bleeding her dry. Once . . . twice . . . three times we washed her, and each time we rinsed her, the water was a little less red.

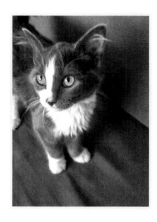

More friends came into the bathroom, and before I knew it, we had a crew of four of us spot-cleaning her head, combing and picking through her fur, and removing any remaining fleas. I couldn't believe the beautiful cat who was emerging: a pretty, long-haired gray-and-white fluffball with majestic ear tufts. Who'd have known what beauty lay underneath the city grime?

And really, that's all it took. One afternoon of crud and suds in a West Philly bathroom with some friends, and Dearborn's entire life turned around. She grew into a flea-free, ultra-fancy, sophisticated, wispy poof and was adopted by a friend of a friend, who cherishes her to this day.

RUB-A-DUB-DUB: BATHING KITTENS

Bathing a kitten might sound super cute, but it's something you should do only in cases of necessity. While having a bath is a relaxing activity for humans (seriously, bubble baths are my number one self-care activity!), it can be a terrifying or traumatic experience for kittens. Limit the amount of time they spend in the bath, and proceed with caution and care.

Kittens should receive a bath if they have fleas, or if they are extremely dirty from feces, mud, or any other filth. In many cases, baby wipes are enough to clean up a small mess, but if wipes aren't cutting it, you'll need to do a bath. Here's a ten-step guide to bathing kittens safely:

1. First, set up a heating pad where the kitten can get warm after her bath. Then set up your bathing station next to a sink. You'll want a fresh towel and a fragrance-free liquid soap (baby shampoo or dish soap are both fine—I prefer using a natural, cruelty-free brand). If you need to clean the kitten's face, you'll also want a washcloth or some cotton pads. Another thing you might want to have on hand is a friend who can help you out!

2. Run the water until it is comfortably warm. If it feels too cold or too hot for your

skin, it's definitely not the right temperature for the kitten. Kittens can chill very easily, and it's extremely important to keep them warm throughout this process.

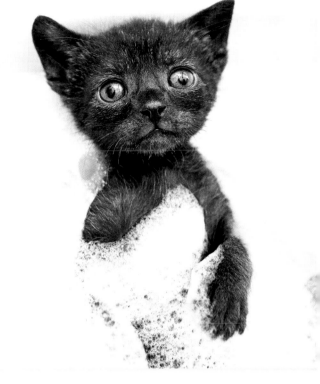

3. Hold the kitten in your nondominant hand. You'll want to hold them the entire time, helping to completely avoid getting water in the eyes, ears, nose, mouth, or anywhere else on the kitten's head. Your dominant hand will be used for applying soap, sudsing the kitten, and rinsing.

4. *If the kitten has fleas*, create a ring of soap around the neck before bathing the kitten. Use your fingers to create a sudsy collar. This soapy ring will act as a fence, preventing fleas from crawling up onto the head, where they can avoid being killed. By cutting off access to the head, you'll seal their fate and be able to kill every flea from the neck down.

5. Use the liquid soap and warm water to quickly bathe the kitten from the neck down, or where needed if the kitten is only dirty in one area (butt baths, anyone?). Remember that while you may want to be thorough, you also want to be speedy. I generally recommend trying to keep this entire process under two minutes.

6. Rinse the kitten thoroughly, avoiding the head.

7. Immediately towel-dry the kitten, getting her as dry as possible. Purrito the kitten by wrapping her in a dry towel while you complete this process.

8. *If the kitten has fleas*, you'll need to carefully rid the head of fleas at this time. Comb through the fur around the head and cheeks with a flea comb. Tweezers or fingers can be used to pull off any visible fleas around the face, and fleas should be disposed of in hot soapy water.

9. If necessary, carefully spot-clean the kitten's head with a washcloth or cotton pad. Avoid any contact with eyes, nose, ears, and mouth. Rather than rinsing the face, use a warm, wet washcloth to get rid of excess soap or waste.

10. Keep the kitten warm and dry her completely. Young kittens can't regulate their body temperature easily, and it's dangerous for them to be chilly. Towel-drying a kitten is fine, or you can very carefully use a hair dryer to dry her more quickly. If using a hair dryer, set it to a low setting, hold the device at least two feet away from the kitten, and oscillate the dryer so that it doesn't get too hot. A toothbrush can also be used to back-comb the kitten's fur and speed up the drying process. Once the kitten is dry, always offer her a warm heating pad to help get her core temperature to a comfortable place.

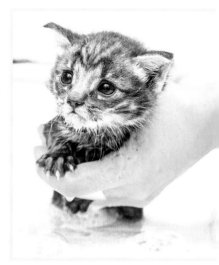

TINY BUT MITEY: BANISHING EAR MITES

Ear mites are minuscule crawling arachnids that take up occupancy inside cats' ears. These parasites typically occur in kittens found outdoors, though they are less common in newborn kittens due to the ear canal being closed during the first week of life. Ear mites crawl onto a host animal and make their way toward the ear canal, where they can feed on wax and begin propagating. Kittens with ear mites experience an itchy, uncomfortable feeling, so they may scratch at their ears, wiggle their heads back and forth, or in some cases tilt their head or ears at an odd angle. While

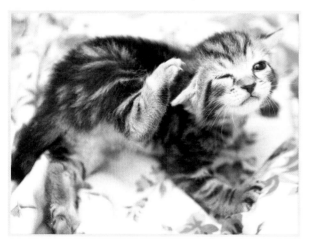

a cocked head on a curious kitten might look cute, there is nothing cute about an infestation of ear mites!

If you witness a kitten with ear discomfort, take a peek inside and see if there is evidence of mites. Like fleas, ear mites also leave behind dark, crumbly debris that's a telltale sign of their presence, and any dark residue should be cause for concern. Though ear mites are extremely small, their movement can be perceived by a discerning eye or with magnification at home or at a vet's office. Left untreated, ear mites can migrate even deeper into the kitten's ear, and can cause more than just discomfort—they can even cause permanent damage to the eardrum. Inner ear damage can result in hearing loss and problems with balance and equilibrium, so it's important to stop ear mites in their tracks before they migrate too deep.

Ear mites are treated through a two-step process that involves cleaning out the ears and applying a topical prescription medication that kills both the mites and their eggs. To clean, use an ear-cleansing solution to remove as much of the dirt, wax, and residue as possible. Do so by placing a few drops of the solution into the ear, then gently rubbing the ear for ten to fifteen seconds to allow the solution to break up the discharge. Use a dry cotton ball or gauze pad to gently swab the moist residue out of the ear and repeat as needed. Never use a cotton swab to clean a kitten's ears, as this can rupture the fragile eardrum. After cleaning, apply a topical prescription medication labeled for killing ear mites to ensure that they don't continue to hatch.

NO VACANCY: EVICTING INTERNAL PARASITES

Even more cunning than external parasites, internal parasites are especially devious because they can take up occupancy inside a kitten's body without making themselves seen at all. Because of their ubiquity, every kitten should be assumed to have some kind of parasite, especially if his poop isn't looking quite right. It's extremely common for kittens to pick up parasites either from their mother's milk, from the outdoors, or from being in close quarters with other animals. Left untreated, parasites can reproduce perpetually inside of kittens, whose young age and immunocompromised state make them especially defenseless.

Because some parasites, such as roundworms and hookworms, are so commonplace, it's recommended that you treat for some of them prophylactically—meaning you should always preventatively treat for them no matter what. Other parasites like coccidia and giardia are often treated only if they are present, though some programs will treat for these parasites preventatively as well. Kittens generally can begin receiving dewormer as young as two weeks of age, and treatment is repeated two weeks later. Caregivers can decrease the risk of parasitic infection by keeping kittens indoors, keeping them away from high volumes of animals, and keeping a clean litter box and a sanitized environment.

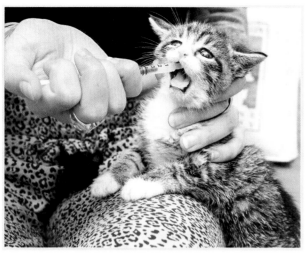
Yuck! Patty isn't the biggest fan of dewormer.

Any kitten with ongoing bowel issues should get a fecal exam from a veterinarian, who can look at the stool under a microscope and tell you if parasites are present and, most important, which ones. Don't fear—treatment is typically a breeze once you know what you're dealing with and how to fight it! Each parasite will have slightly different symptoms, and different medications that will end their reign. Let's take a look at the most common parasites in kittens.

GI PARASITE CHEAT SHEET	
Name	Roundworms
What it is	These three- to five-inch worms live in the intestines and eat the food ingested by the cat. As they are the most common intestinal parasite in felines, it's estimated that up to 75 percent of kittens will have roundworms.[11]
How kittens get it	While adult cats typically get roundworms by ingesting eggs or larvae from their prey, kittens typically get roundworms by nursing. The larvae of the *Toxocara cati* roundworm can be passed from the mother through breast milk, often infecting kittens shortly after birth.
Symptoms	Some kittens with roundworm may have no symptoms at all, while others may have diarrhea, constipation, or lack of appetite. In more advanced cases, the kitten may be nauseated, and may vomit worms that resemble thin pieces of spaghetti.
Treatment	Due to the high prevalence of this parasite, roundworm dewormer should be given to all kittens. Deworming can begin as early as two weeks of age, and should be repeated every two weeks until twelve weeks of age. There are several prescription medications used to treat roundworms, as well as over-the-counter medications like pyrantel pamoate. All dewormer should be properly dosed to the kitten's weight.

Name	Hookworms
What it is	These small, thin worms attach to the intestinal lining and subsist off the kitten's blood. Though less common than roundworms, hookworms are still seen in a number of kittens.
How kittens get it	Hookworm eggs are passed through stool, where they hatch into larvae and then seek a new host via ingestion or through the skin. In kittens, hookworms can be transmitted via the breast milk of a mother cat.
Symptoms	Kittens with hookworms may experience weight loss, bloody diarrhea, black or tar-like stools (indicating blood), loss of appetite, or sometimes labored breathing or wheezing due to the presence of hookworms in the lungs. In extreme cases, kittens may become anemic due to blood loss from hookworms, which can lead to death if not treated.
Treatment	There are several over-the-counter and prescription medications used to treat hookworms; these drugs are typically the same ones used to treat roundworms, including pyrantel pamoate. Hookworm treatment is part of the standard preventative care of any kitten and can begin as early as two weeks of age. All dewormer should be properly dosed to the kitten's weight.

Name	Tapeworms
What it is	These long, segmented worms anchor themselves to the small intestine, where they absorb nutrients from the kitten. As the tapeworm grows, small egg-bearing segments of its body break off and are passed in the stool.
How kittens get it	Cats and kittens get tapeworms by ingesting an infected flea, so any kitten with a flea infestation may be at risk of tapeworms. In order to pass tapeworms to a cat, fleas must first ingest tapeworm eggs during their larval stage. These fleas then mature and bite cats and kittens, who may respond by licking or consuming them. This allows the tapeworm to be released inside the kitten's body.
Symptoms	Kittens may have tapeworms without showing any symptoms at all, though some may show general unthriftiness and low weight. The most common visual symptom of tapeworms is the presence of tapeworm segments in stool. These segments may look like a small piece of white rice, which may move around throughout stool found in the litter box.
Treatment	There are several prescription medications that treat for tapeworms, including praziquantel. You'll want to talk to a veterinarian about the best one for your kitten.

Name	Coccidia
What it is	Unlike some parasites, coccidia are not worms; they are microscopic single-celled protozoa. Coccidia has a high prevalence in cats, and it can cause serious illness in kittens.
How kittens get it	Kittens cannot be born with coccidia, but many are exposed to it when they come into contact with their mother's feces and ingest the microscopic cysts, or by sharing a litter box with an infected animal. Once inside the kitten's body, coccidia can reproduce abundantly.
Symptoms	Coccidia damages the lining of the intestines, causing watery or mucousy diarrhea, abdominal distress, dehydration, and occasionally nausea. Because it takes nearly two weeks after infection for symptoms to occur, caregivers should look for these signs in any kittens older than two weeks of age. Left untreated, coccidia can be fatal to young kittens.
Treatment	There are several prescription medications that treat coccidia, including ponazuril. You'll need to talk to a vet about the right medication for the kitten. You'll also want to carefully sanitize the kitten's environment to avoid reinfection.

Name	Giardia
What it is	Like coccidia, giardia are single-celled protozoa that infect the intestinal tract. You may have heard giardia referred to as "backpacker's disease" due to its reputation for infecting hikers who drink from contaminated water sources. Giardia has several strains, and the type of giardia infecting kittens is different from the one infecting humans, making the risk for transmission from cats to humans very low.[12]
How kittens get it	Kittens typically get giardia by coming into contact with the contaminated feces of the mother cat or other animals in the environment, often through use of a shared litter box. Once the cysts are inside the intestinal tract, they can mature and attach to the intestinal wall.
Symptoms	Kittens infected with giardia will typically have extremely foul-smelling, yellow-green diarrhea that may be frothy or greasy. It's also common for these kittens to experience weight loss, dehydration, gassiness, and bloating. Left untreated, giardia can be fatal to young kittens.
Treatment	Several medications exist that are effective against giardia, including fenbendazole and metronidazole. Talk to a vet about the right medication and dosing. You'll also want to carefully sanitize the kitten's environment to avoid reinfection.

It's a common assumption that all big bellies are wormy bellies, but caregivers should be aware that there are many causes for round tummies in kittens aside from parasites. Congenital abnormalities, bacterial infections, FIP, and even overfeeding can cause this symptom, so if you're not sure what's going on, always talk to a veterinarian.

Of course, many kittens are simply chunky in the middle and perfectly healthy! If you notice that most of your young kittens have an avocado bod, this is because their abdominal muscles are underdeveloped, so their bellies aren't well contained, making them look quite rotund. Ultimately, the size of the gut matters less than the firmness of the belly does. "A kitten needs to have a body shaped like a pear or a lightbulb with a soft abdomen," says Ellen Carozza, LVT. If the kitten feels firm at the core, that's when it's time to see a professional.

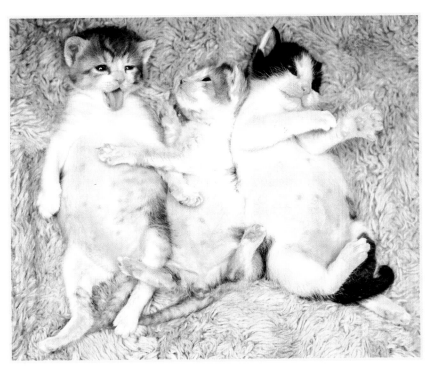

Ugh. It's the worst, right? Diarrhea is a common, crappy (pun fully intended) experience for kittens during the first weeks of life. But just because it's common doesn't mean it's normal or okay, and it's important not to assume that it will pass on its own. Diarrhea is like a stinky alarm system: it is *always* a sign that something has gone awry. It's up to caregivers to determine what the problem is, to address the root of it, and to treat kittens' symptoms until they're back to their regular selves.

Unfortunately, diarrhea can have many causes, including viruses, bacterial infections, food intolerance, premature weaning, stress, or other medical conditions . . . so finding the cause might feel like trying to solve a mystery. The most common causes of diarrhea are parasites and bacterial infections, so that's always a good place to start! Getting a fecal exam from a veterinarian will help to diagnose and treat any unwanted inhabitants in the gut, or to determine other potential causes and remedies.

Loose liquid stool should be addressed quickly if it occurs. Diarrhea might not seem like an emergency, but it can indicate something more serious, and its side effects can quickly lead to decline or even death in young kittens. When dealing with diarrhea, you'll always want to rectify the associated symptom of dehydration, which can cause a domino effect of medical issues if left unaddressed. Kittens experiencing ongoing diarrhea should receive oral electrolytes and, in some cases, fluid therapy (read more about dehydration on page 213). A probiotic should also be used to help create a healthier gut environment as the kitten recovers.

While it's way more common for a kitten to experience diarrhea, it's not unheard of for the opposite malady to occur: constipation. Kittens vary in how often they go to the bathroom, but any kitten who hasn't pooped in more than forty-eight hours should be seen by a vet to determine the cause of their constipation. Left untreated, constipation can cause severe discomfort, suppressed appetite, and even permanent damage to the colon.

Causes of constipation can include dietary issues, dehydration, blockages, and even congenital defects that can make it challenging or impossible for the kitten to pass stool. Of course, if a kitten is three weeks or younger and hasn't pooped, it's because they may not be physically *capable* of pooping without help. Young neonatal kittens require stimulation from their mother's tongue in order to defecate, and orphans under three to four weeks old must be manually stimulated by a caregiver (see page 100).

To treat kittens with constipation, caregivers should first rule out serious medical conditions by getting a physical exam and an X-ray from a veterinarian. A medical professional can also help manually remove blocked waste, or provide an enema to help the kitten's bowels start moving. Once it's known that the kitten isn't suffering from an underlying defect, caregivers can help by providing small amounts of laxative supplements and probiotics, by keeping the kitten well hydrated, and by helping the kitten stay active and moving to stimulate bowel movement.

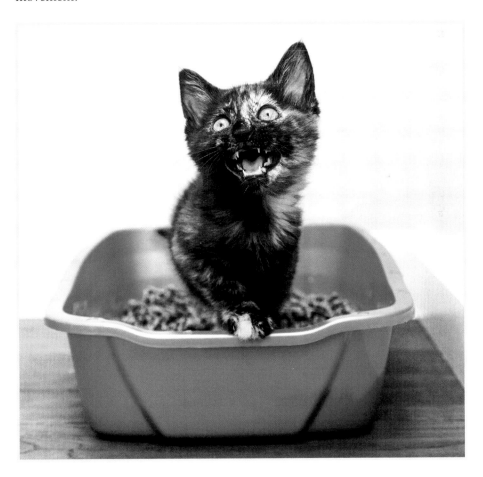

Marlin came to me with a batch of three feral littermates, but something was different about him. He was literally half the size of his brothers, and almost immediately I noticed that something about his butt looked odd. (Yes, I know, it's a fun skill to be so familiar with staring at kitten buttholes that you can tell when one looks different; try not to be jealous.) He went to the vet, who gave him an enema and sent him on his way. But in spite of the enema, his little butt was just not performing. He literally could not poop.

A few days into having him, I became scared for his life. Marlin's butt was misshapen and distended. He strained over the box and screamed the saddest little screams in the world. His pain from not being able to poop was unbearable to witness, and it became clear that his life was in danger. Fortunately, a specialist was able to identify the problem: Marlin had atresia ani. Atresia ani is a rare congenital deformity in which the lower gastrointestinal tract is malformed, essentially making it impossible for the kitten to pass stool. Marlin's condition also caused him to be abnormally small in stature. Without treatment, Marlin would have no chance of survival.

Here's the best way to describe Marlin's condition: It was like he was given the wrong butt at the butt factory. They were supposed to give him a kitten butt, but instead, they gave him a mouse butt. What he needed was to trade in his mouse butt for a kitten butt so that he could have a normal, functional bowel movement. But how do you obtain the right-sized butt for a kitten born with the wrong one?

Many kittens with atresia ani die without ever being diagnosed, and those who are diagnosed are often euthanized. But Kitten Lady don't play like that. So instead, at just a few weeks of age, Marlin had a series of sedated procedures with a veterinarian in which a surgical balloon was gently inflated in his rectum, helping it expand to a normal size. Marlin was treated with steroids, stool softeners, and other drugs to help him maintain muscle tone and stay comfortable. With each procedure, his butt troubles improved and he became able to pass stool all by himself. I've never seen a kitten so happy and so proud to poop!

As his condition improved, Marlin became a totally different kitten. He began to purr incessantly, to eat voraciously, and to learn how to play and hunt his toys like a little lion! With the pain of the past fading into the distance, Marlin could finally discover what it was to be a normal cat. Once he was a healthy weight, he was able to get his final procedure with a specialist: a reconstructive surgery to permanently replace his mouse butt with something that would last him a lifetime. With his fancy new designer butthole, Marlin was ready to find love—and on the day he was adopted into a forever home, he found just that!

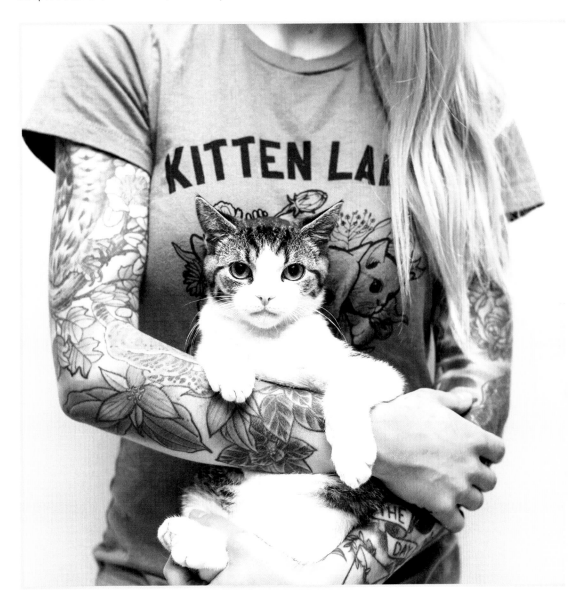

Puzzled by problem poop? Stumped by strange stool? It's important to look at what's coming out of each kitten and make sure everything seems normal. It might sound gross, but when you want a kitten to be well, you get extremely invested in what comes out of his bum. I sometimes joke that I'm like the Sherlock Holmes of kitten poop, because if there's something amiss, I'm on the case! When it comes to the health of kittens, my number one concern is number two.

Poop is an important indicator of health, and I recommend monitoring it closely—it's like a smelly progress report that tells you how the kitten is doing. A fecal exam from a veterinarian is the essential method to get to the bottom of your troubles, but here are some visual indicators that can help to lead you in the right direction.* I now present to you . . . the color wheel of poop.

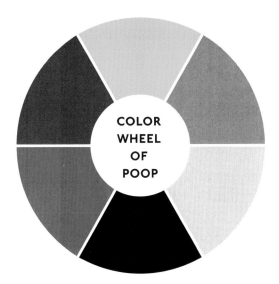

---

*Please note that while this chart can lead you in the right direction, it is not a replacement for a fecal examination. If a kitten is experiencing poop problems, please get her diagnosed by a vet ASAP. Be sure that your veterinarian is doing a thorough fecal exam and looking for all common culprits that affect kittens. Don't delay—problem poop can become a *big* problem very quickly, but with diagnostic information, you'll be able to get the kitten on the right track.

Colors

BROWN

Solid, formed brown stool is normal for a weaned kitten. If the poop is well formed and looks like a miniature cat poop, that's the goal! Woo-hoo!

Loose, smelly brown stool can indicate an internal parasite. Get a fecal exam and obtain a prescription medication if needed.

YELLOW

Mustard-yellow stool is normal for kittens on kitten formula or their mother's milk. Once they're weaning, it will transition to brown.

Super stinky or loose yellow stool can be an indication of a parasite. You'll want to go to the vet for a fecal exam and medication.

GREEN

Green stool may indicate a bacterial infection; if so, you'll need to see a vet for a prescription antibiotic to clear this one up. Don't forget to give a probiotic, too!

Yellow-green stool may also sometimes be a sign of giardia.

BEIGE

Pale poop is often a sign that the kitten is failing to absorb nutrients from her food. A probiotic or predigestive enzyme can help support kittens with malabsorption concerns.

Beige poop can also occur with premature weaning. If the kitten has recently been weaned, consider scaling back and giving her a liquid formula diet until her tummy settles.

Overfeeding may also cause this issue.

BLACK

Black, tarry stool typically indicates bleeding in the upper GI tract, which can occur for a number of reasons, from parasites to viruses. You'll want to talk to a vet immediately to figure out what is causing the bleeding and how to treat it.

The very first poop after a kitten is born will be a dark, tarry stool called meconium. If the kitten is just born, you can expect his feces to look black-green.

RED

Red blood in the stool usually means the kitten is experiencing problems in the lower GI tract, which could be caused by anything from colitis to bacterial infections. You'll want to let a vet know that something is troubling the kitten's gut.

Textures

MUCOUSY Mucousy, slimy, or oily stool is often a sign of a protozoan parasite such as coccidia or giardia. Make sure the kitten is dewormed and receives a fecal exam to determine if any additional parasites are present.

CURDLED Curdled-looking stool can occur when a kitten has indigestion due to a parasite, bacterium, or difficulty absorbing the fats and proteins in his food. Ensure that the food is fresh and not spoiled, be sure the kitten is being treated for parasites, and consider providing a probiotic or digestive enzyme.

LIQUID Liquid stool indicates severe distress and should be addressed immediately. This often accompanies panleukopenia or an untreated serious parasitic infestation. Seek immediate veterinary support for kittens with liquid diarrhea, and ensure that you are also replacing lost hydration by providing oral or subcutaneous fluids.

SOFT Loose, unformed poop that looks like soft serve is a sign of a moderate GI issue. Ensure that the kitten has been dewormed, and if the issue persists, seek veterinary support.

HARD Hard, dry stool can be a sign that the kitten is severely dehydrated or suffering from a motility issue. Make sure that the kitten is adequately hydrated, and if chronic constipation occurs, seek assistance from a veterinarian to determine if there is a systemic cause that can be addressed.

FORMED A healthy kitten's poop will be solidly formed. If that's your kitten, celebrate! Woo-hoo!

BE A PROBIOTICS PRO

With all these tummy troubles, kittens sometimes need a little help getting their GI tract back on the right path. Probiotics are gut-friendly bacteria that help regulate the kitten's intestinal health, and they typically come in a gel or powder form that can be purchased over the counter or from a veterinarian and easily added to food. Once inside the kitten's body, each strain of bacterium takes the lead on a different useful job, such as easing digestion or maintaining the health of the colon.

Make sure you're purchasing a probiotic that is specifically designed for cats and that contains multiple strains of healthy bacteria so you can maximize the benefits.

According to Dr. Rachel Wallach, a veterinarian with a practice in Agoura Hills, California, "Probiotics aren't just useful for maintaining the health of your colon; they're important to full body health. As weird as it sounds, the majority of a kitten's immune system exists in the gut. Making sure the gut is healthy, happy, and has the right amount of 'good bacteria' in it really enables kittens to fight infections effectively and thrive. Many kittens are put on antibiotics, which can wipe out multiple strains of bacteria in the gut. Probiotics help to replenish the 'good bacteria' and, if possible, should be incorporated into your kitten's health plan."

RUNNING DRY: THE DANGERS OF DEHYDRATION

Just like humans, kittens need to be well hydrated in order to function properly. Kittens have a decreased ability to conserve water until their kidneys mature, and their small bodies can quickly run dry. To maintain a healthy body, kittens should have a body water content of about 80 percent, which is much higher than adult cats, whose fluid content is about 60 percent. Because of the myriad ways that kittens can quickly lose fluids and decline, dehydration is especially common and risky for them, and it is considered one of the primary causes of death in young kittens.

So how does it happen? Dehydration occurs when kittens lose fluids through diarrhea, vomiting, or hyperthermia (overheating), or when they are not consuming enough fluids to begin with.

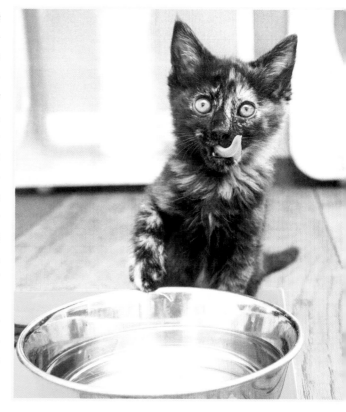

Caregivers can support good fluid intake by providing frequent age-appropriate meals that are rich in moisture content, such as formula and wet food, as well as access to clean and fresh water at all times once the kitten is able to drink on her own. Fluid intake is especially important to consider when kittens are weaning, as they're coming off of a liquid diet and moving on to solids, but they may not quite "get" how to drink water yet. Adding a bit of water to a kitten's food during the weaning process can be a great idea so that her fluid intake remains sufficient. Any kitten experiencing diarrhea should be considered a risk for dehydration, and fluid intake should be carefully monitored and increased as needed.

Knowing a kitten is dehydrated is the first step to addressing the issue, so here are four ways you can test hydration at home:

- For kittens four weeks and older, a skin turgor test is a common method that involves manually testing the elasticity of the skin. With the kitten seated comfortably, gently grasp the skin behind the neck, called the scruff, and lift it momentarily. Once released, the skin should snap back to its normal form; but as the kitten becomes more dehydrated, it will take longer and longer for the skin to return to its place. "Tenting," or skin that stays up in a tent position for an extended period, is considered a sign of moderate to severe dehydration. It should be noted that a turgor test is not a reliable method in kittens under four weeks of age due to the looseness of their skin.

- Pale or dry mucous membranes are another indicator of dehydration. The nose should be moist. Gums should be moist and pink. You can test the capillary refill time by pressing against the kitten's gums with a clean finger for one to two seconds. The area pressed should quickly go from white to pink. If a white dot remains visible for any extended period of time, this could be a sign of dehydration.

- Kitten urine should be colorless or very light yellow, but dehydrated kittens will often have dark urine. Urine with a rich yellow color can indicate that the kitten is not sufficiently hydrated.

- In cases of severe dehydration, the eyeballs may appear sunken in. If a gap is visible between the eye and the tissue surrounding it, the kitten will need IV fluids from a veterinarian. Do not delay this care; a kitten with sunken eyes is in critical condition.[13]

Caring for a dehydrated kitten means increasing and balancing his fluid intake. For mild cases, caregivers can simply increase the amount of liquid in the diet, often by adding water to the food or by very slowly syringe-feeding oral fluids (being mindful not to cause aspiration). One fantastic way to increase oral fluids is to give kittens an oral electrolyte either supplementally or mixed into their regular food or formula. Just make sure it's unflavored, as kittens don't appreciate fruit punch! When a kitten in my care is dehydrated, one of the first things I do is switch from mixing his formula or food with normal water to using an electrolyte-rich fluid.

In more moderate cases, caregivers can provide subcutaneous fluids (sometimes called "sub-Q fluids") either at the vet clinic or, once they've been trained, at home. These special fluids are given under (sub-) the skin (cutaneous) via injection with an electrolyte-rich prescription solution and a sterile needle. After you safely inject the kitten with a proper dose of fluids, she will have a small hump on her back, which will dissipate as the fluid fills her body. If that sounds terrifying, I promise it's not! Administering fluids at home is a skill anyone can learn after being trained hands-on by an experienced veterinary professional. Be sure you have proper training about not just how to do it, but how *much* to give, as it is possible (and very harmful) to give too much fluid. If you're rescuing animals of any species or age, this is a great skill to have in your back pocket, so talk to your local clinic or animal shelter about getting trained to do it safely.

Kittens with severe dehydration may require IV fluids, which must be administered on-site at a vet clinic. The best way to avoid this is to know (and avoid) the threats to hydration, and to act quickly when signs of dehydration arise, treating both the symptom and the underlying cause. And hey, while you're at it, make sure you're also caring for the caregiver . . . and drink a big glass of water yourself!

THE SHORT AND SWEET ON LITTLE KITTENS AND BLOOD SUGAR

Another risk for kittens is hypoglycemia, or low blood sugar. Sugars obtained through the kitten's diet are what give her the energy to pounce, play, and even simply stand up. When those sugars decrease, the kitten's energy does as well, leaving her listless and lethargic. Hypoglycemia typically occurs when the kitten fails to attain adequate glucose levels through nutrition, either by not eating enough or by eating a poor diet, but it can also result from diarrhea, vomiting, low temperature, or other medical reasons.

Symptoms of hypoglycemia include low energy, lack of coordination, trembling, and twitching. Any kitten experiencing low blood sugar should be supported without delay. In severe cases, kittens can experience seizures or temporary blindness, or even lose consciousness. While caregivers should bring these kittens in for emergency treatment from a medical professional, they should also act immediately to help any kitten experiencing severe symptoms by giving them supplemental sugars at home.

Fortunately, if you have a sweet tooth like me, you might already have the tools to help a hypoglycemic kitten right in your kitchen cabinet. Corn syrup, honey, agave nectar, maple syrup, and even white sugar are all acceptable products that can be given in small amounts orally to temporarily boost a kitten's blood sugar before rushing to the vet (a vet may also give additional oral or IV medications). I'll never forget the time a friend and I were baking and she asked, "Do you have corn syrup?" to which I responded, "Yeah, but it's in my kitten supply cabinet!" My friends have grown to expect nothing less.

DON'T FADE AWAY

Kittens are delicate beings, and one of the greatest challenges you may be faced with is a baby in critical condition, sometimes called a fading kitten or a kitten who is failing to thrive. There's nothing more gutting than watching an animal crash before your eyes and feeling powerless to help her. We can drastically increase the kitten's chances of survival by taking preventative steps to stop illness from progressing, by monitoring for signs of fading, and by intervening quickly in a life-threatening situation.

"Failure to thrive" or "fading kitten syndrome" are terms often used by animal rescuers to describe the rapidly declining health and subsequent death of a neonatal kitten, but I find that these terms can sometimes cloud our comprehension of the true causes of decline, and discourage innovation and problem solving. Simply put: If a kitten is fading, there is always a reason—and it's up to us to provide a solution. "There is no such thing as fading kitten syndrome," says critical kitten expert Ellen Carozza, LVT. "There is always a reason for death, and our job is to find the cause, not simply give a name to something we don't understand or aren't willing to investigate further."

The decline of a kitten's health is often caused by a domino effect, typically beginning with one or more problems that, left unaddressed, spiral into various secondary conditions and worsening symptoms. There may be any number of initial issues, such as infections, parasites, viruses, or congenital defects, that are specific to the individual kitten and can lead to a series of problems that put the kitten in critical condition. For instance, a kitten may have something as simple as internal parasites, but over time this can lead to seriously dangerous problems with digestion, dehydration,

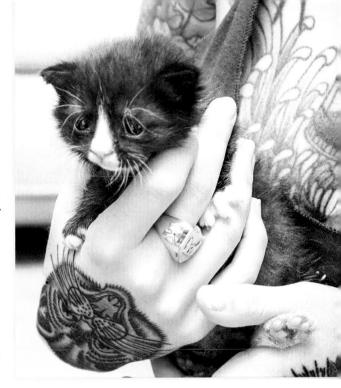

and emaciation. Or she may have an upper respiratory infection that progresses into life-threatening pneumonia. For this reason, it's advised to address all health conditions swiftly, to stop illness from progressing.

If illness does progress and you're faced with a kitten with signs of fading, don't panic or lose hope . . . but do act fast! There are many supportive care measures that can be implemented if fading is caught quickly. By learning more about these fragile felines, you'll be armed with knowledge about what to look for and how to respond with lifesaving support.

Signs that a kitten is fading may include lethargy and listlessness, glassy eyes, constant discomfort, odd vocalizations, muscle wasting, agonal breathing, neck arching, dehydration, emaciation, liquid diarrhea, pale gums or tongue, or weight loss.

Fading kittens may appear less alert, with low energy, and may even show decreased interest in food. Caregivers may notice that the kitten's skin is less hydrated or that the body is losing muscle mass. Muscle wasting is a visual cue that can quickly alert caregivers; the kitten's face may start to look gaunt and triangular. The kitten may begin to lose weight or fail to gain weight, which can be

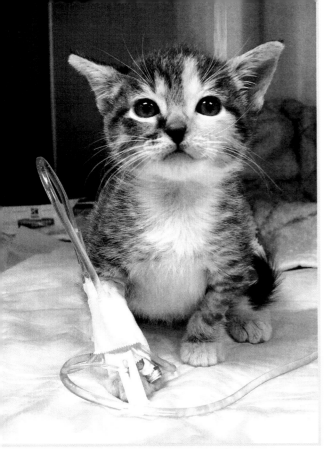

If a kitten has symptoms of fading, don't delay—go to a vet.

determined by monitoring each kitten's weight at least once a day. Kitten caregivers should not wait until a kitten is in crisis to intercede—these early signs should spring the caregiver into action immediately.

If a kitten is showing signs of fading, the best thing to do is to immediately bring him to a veterinarian without delay. Through an examination and diagnostic testing, a veterinarian can identify any illness, such as respiratory infections or internal parasites, and can prescribe an antibiotic, dewormer, or other medical treatment that can fight the root of the problem. Addressing underlying conditions will be a crucial step to ensuring the kitten's survival.

That said, saving critical kittens isn't just about addressing the root cause—it's also about addressing secondary symptoms through supportive care. In almost every case, the kitten will be suffering from related issues such as hypothermia, dehydration, or hypoglycemia, and we must aid him in combating these symptoms as they arise. I find it useful not to think of fading as one big problem but as a series of small, solvable problems, each able to be addressed with appropriate care. The key to saving a fading kitten's life is really to provide supportive care that keeps the kitten alive long enough to survive the underlying condition.

Those who frequently care for kittens, such as neonatal-kitten foster parents and rescuers, will benefit from learning advanced kitten-care skills that can save a fading kitten. Tube-feeding, for instance, may save the life of a fading kitten who is unable to suckle or swallow; a skilled tube-feeder can bypass the esophagus and supply food straight to the stomach. Subcutaneous fluid therapy, when carefully dosed by an experienced caregiver, can help provide essential hydration to keep a kitten's bodily functions working. Plasma therapy, an infusion of plasma from a feline blood donor, can provide the kitten with immune support and replace metabolic proteins that are lost when a kitten is fading. Proper administration of vitamins such as iron and B12 can boost a kitten's energy and combat vitamin loss. Hypoglycemic kittens can quickly bounce back with a small dose of Dextrose 50% or other sugar sources. Each of these lifesaving skills should be learned and provided under the supervision of an experienced veterinary professional, as every kitten's situation will be different and will require specific treatment tailored to her needs.

In some cases, a kitten's condition may unfortunately be untreatable or too advanced, and she may ultimately be unable to survive. Caregivers and veterinarians should make careful decisions about whether a kitten is in treatable condition. In extreme cases of untreatable suffering, euthanasia may be the most humane solution. Through early intervention, caregivers can hopefully avoid this scenario.

The most important thing for caregivers to know is that early intervention plays a critical role in saving kittens who are failing to thrive. "By acting quickly, understanding the symptoms, and working with the right veterinary team, the chance

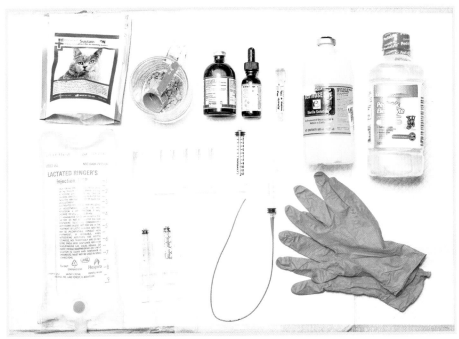

Many supportive-care measures can be taken to support kittens in critical condition.

of survival goes up exponentially. The biggest killer to these little guys is waiting," says Carozza. Caregivers can give kittens the best chance by planning ahead. By studying the early signs, monitoring kittens carefully, treating illnesses swiftly, and providing supportive care as needed, caregivers can lay the groundwork for a high chance of survival.

THE LITTLEST NOODLE, SOBA

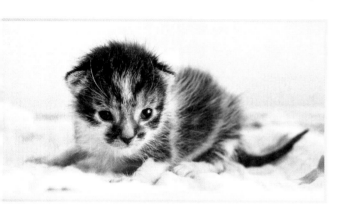

Immediately after I wrapped up a workshop at a cat convention in New York City, a woman approached me frantically, telling me that a litter of orphaned newborn kittens had just come into the local shelter and asking if I would take them. "Oh, wow! Okay. Can I have a minute to think about it?" I asked, taking a sip of water . . . but secretly I'm a sucker and knew immediately what my answer would be. I packed up my presentation materials and walked back to my booth in the convention hall. "Should we take home some kittens?" I asked Andrew, who gave me a knowing look. The truth is, we *both* know the answer is almost always yes. We agreed.

What we hoped would be a happy occasion turned into a long, sad, and trying day. As I pulled each tiny neonatal kitten out of the carrier, I noticed one was ice-cold and suffering from a large, unrecoverable wound to his backside. He was alive, but hardly. For a few seconds I panicked, trying to put my emotions on the back burner and focus on the crisis at hand. *Oh god, oh god, oh god, okay. Okay. Find an emergency vet. Oh god.* As fast as we could, we ran to an emergency vet two blocks away and there we made the decision to humanely euthanize the suffering kitten.

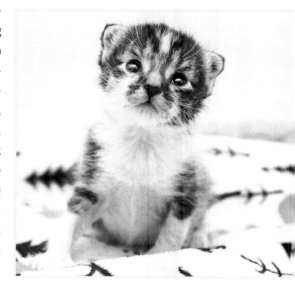

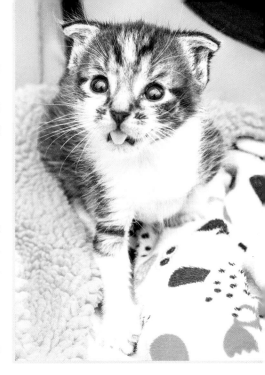

Ugh. One of the hardest parts of working with critical kittens is accepting when they're too far gone to save. Wiping my tears on the walk back to the hotel, I peered through salty eyes inside the carrier at the remaining survivors, whom I'd hardly had a chance to meet. "Hi, little ones, I'm so sorry. I'll feed you soon. I promise."

Back at the hotel, I prepared a bottle for the kittens, each multicolored and squinting through freshly opened eyes. They each ate well, with one exception: the tiniest kitten, whom we named Soba, didn't want much. Soba had an odd look about her. She seemed slow, maybe a little sleepy . . . She was certainly the runt of the litter, but didn't seem ill. I fed her as much as I could and popped a heating pad and baby blanket in their carrier, and we began our four-hour drive back to DC, kittens in tow.

Halfway through our drive, we pulled over in Philadelphia to feed the kittens again. Eager to get back on the road, I quickly made a bottle. Andrew picked up Soba and held her to his eye level. "I don't like how she looks," he said. *Oh no. What now?* She looked drained; her breath was shallow, her head hanging heavy. *Ugh.*

It's crazy how fast little kittens can crash when they have cards stacked against them, and it seemed she had many: she was the frailest, she had been outside in the cold, she had been undernourished. Her brother's severe condition suggested that they'd had a difficult start to life. Looking at her closely, I could see her dry, pale gums indicated that she was clearly dehydrated and hypoglycemic. This condition is often referred to as "fading kitten syndrome," or failure to thrive, but more specifically, it's a set of symptoms that reflect a rapid decline that quickly leads to death. Sitting in a parking lot in Philly with her tiny body sluggish in my hands, I knew it was a bad idea to keep driving. We had to act fast.

We happened to be just blocks away from an animal shelter I'd worked with previously, so I called and begged for their help. We walked right in, and their vet, quite generously, took a look at little Soba. As critical as she had become, her needs were really quite simple: sugar, moisture, warmth. The vet gave her oral dextrose (to increase her blood sugar), an injection of B12 (to increase her energy), and subcutaneous fluids (to rehydrate her). I anxiously watched as the fluids filled her body. *Come on, Soba. You've got this. Please perk up. Come on, girl.* I didn't want to lose a second kitten in mere hours.

I popped her heating disk in the microwave, and as the clock counted down from five minutes, Soba was miraculously already perking up. As fast as kittens can fade, they can also recover quickly if given appropriate supportive care, and she was responding well. She lifted her head and looked around through sleepy eyes. I hugged their staff with deep gratitude for their willingness to lend a helping hand. Split seconds can make all the difference, and can determine whether a kitten is unrecoverable or is able to be saved. Through early intervention, the scales had been tipped in her favor.

The rest of her journey was a breeze. She remained the tiniest runt, and though she was always a little behind her sisters developmentally, she grew into a wonderful little weirdo. I'll never forget how her ears stayed folded for *weeks*—giving her a totally precious and comically pathetic look—and only popped up right before it was time to be adopted. When she made it to her forever home, I hugged Andrew and thanked him for advocating for her that day in the parking lot. Thanks to his keen observation and our split-second decision to intervene, the littlest noodle would get to flourish as a happy house cat.

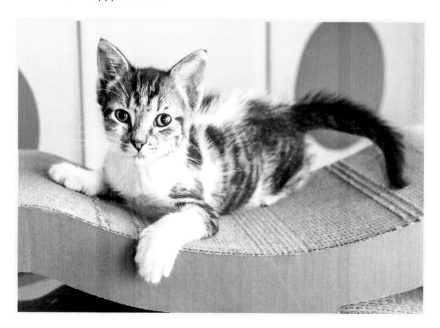

HANNAH SHAW

Navigating the veterinary industry as a kitten caregiver can be surprisingly challenging. I'll never forget one of the first times I brought a young orphan to the vet in search of medical support, and the doctor walked into the room and said with a smile, "Wow, I've never seen one that young!" My heart sank at the realization that I was caring for an animal whose needs were seemingly a mystery. In subsequent years I've worked with dozens of veterinarians and can confirm that feline pediatrics is indeed a rare focal area in the field.

To understand veterinary care for kittens, it's important to first understand that there are two modalities of veterinary medicine for cats: shelter medicine and private practice. Shelter medicine is the field of veterinary care within an animal shelter, and its task is therefore to do the greatest good while dealing with a high volume of animals and a limited budget. Shelter veterinarians are certainly likely to encounter neonatal kittens in their line of work, but because many shelters don't have programs that meet the needs of neonates, some of these vets may have little experience providing them with lifesaving care.

Private practice, on the other hand, is the care of owned animals in a private clinic. In a private practice setting, individual members of the public pay for the cost of their animals' care. Private practice veterinarians are therefore unlikely to see kittens younger than six to eight weeks old, because that tends to be the earliest that adopters bring them in for care (as the youngest age of adoption from a shelter or rescue organization in the United States is typically eight weeks). So it makes sense that the average veterinarian has lots of experience with the standard preventative care that occurs with newly adopted kittens, such as the baby's first vaccines and dewormers, but not so much experience with neonates and young orphans with medical crises. Unfortunately, many clinics are unfamiliar with the needs of fading kittens and may even be resistant to providing treatments that are necessary to save their lives.

The lack of veterinary care for young felines is therefore an issue of supply and demand—there is little demand for the care, so there is little supply of knowledge. This same issue is reflected in the veterinary focus on felines in general. A 2016 study showed that dog owners were six times more likely to have taken their pet to the veterinarian in the last year than cat owners, and that two-thirds of pet parents believe that cats have fewer health needs than dogs.[14] When we mistake stoicism

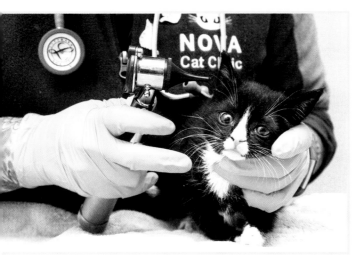

for well-being, we regretfully underestimate the needs of our feline friends.

What does this mean for foster parents? It simply means we have to be strong advocates for the animals in our care, and try to find kitten-friendly vets who are enthusiastic about helping the little guys. All vet clinics are not created equal when it comes to pediatrics, so it's important to find a vet who works well with your needs. If you're fostering a kitten for an animal rescue or shelter, chances are they'll provide you with a vet with experience treating kittens. But if you've rescued a kitten on your own, you'll need to find a private practice vet who is comfortable with the little guys.

TIPS FOR FINDING A KITTEN-FRIENDLY VET

- The first way to know if a clinic has experience with pediatrics is . . . to ask! Don't be afraid to ask about their history of treating young, sick kittens. Are they comfortable prescribing medication to a neonate? Have they successfully worked with kittens with panleukopenia? What's their protocol for helping a kitten who is failing to thrive?

- Try looking for a feline-focused practice. Cats are seen less frequently than dogs at many hospitals, and finding vets who focus primarily on cats will increase the likelihood that they'll be comfortable working with sick kittens, too.

- Find out if they're willing to work closely with you to teach you lifesaving skills. Will they teach you how to administer subcutaneous fluids or B12? Will they allow you to be in the room during exams to ask questions and learn?

- Veterinarians with a background in shelter medicine are more likely to have experience working with sick little kittens, and may be willing to try more outside-the-box treatment to save a life. In some cases, finding a veterinarian who has worked or volunteered with an animal shelter or rescue organization can increase the quality of care the kitten receives.

Sometimes you may not be able to access a veterinarian who specializes in kittens, or may need to work with an emergency vet after hours. Having a basic understanding of your kitten's health needs will help you to be a great advocate for her medically! Don't be afraid to ask questions of your veterinarian and to communicate about your impression of the kitten's needs. Provide as much information as you can, approach your appointments with an inquisitive mind, and document what you learn so that you can become a more informed rescuer. A successful relationship with a veterinarian is ultimately about collaboration and communication.

HANNAH JR., MY HOTEL ROOM FOSTER KITTEN

When I flew to Iowa for work, I had really only planned for it to be a consulting job. I had been hired to train the staff of a local animal shelter, and I headed straight from the airport to their facility to provide a midday course about feline shelter programs. As a professional kitten lady, I bring materials that look a little different from those of your average consultant: instead of a briefcase, I carry a diaper bag full of kitten-care supplies, and instead of clip art and slide shows, I present using real stories and

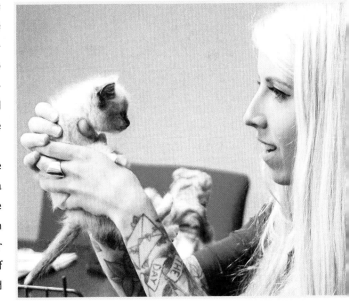

videos demonstrating kitten-rescue techniques. I do my best to encourage shelters not only to implement long-term strategies that save lives, but also to take small steps that make a big impact for animals. It's through individual acts of kindness, after all, that change begins to take place.

As I wrapped up my training in the shelter's conference room, there was a knock at the door. As fate would have it, someone had just found a little kitten outside, and was there to surrender her to the shelter. A little Siamese poof with chocolate points, she clearly would have been quite a beauty if it weren't for her rough condition. Her eyes and nose were crusted shut with yellow pus, and she was so underfed that if you palpated her abdomen, your index finger and thumb could practically make contact through her empty belly. *Of course,* I thought. *Of course a sick kitten would come in while I'm training a shelter halfway across the country.*

"Let's name her after you. She can be Hannah Jr.," the staff suggested. We all had a good chuckle over the sudden appearance of this coincidental kitten, but behind my laughter I was already calculating the kitten's needs.

The kitten needed a level of care that is best provided in a foster home. Knowing we had about 150 people planning to attend my kitten-care workshop at the local university the following day, I felt confident that I would be able to find a foster parent by the end of my trip, but the kitten was already in critical condition and needed help *now.* I knew what I had to do.

"How about this: she can be my hotel room foster kitten," I offered. I already had all my teaching supplies with me anyway, so I had most of the gear I needed in order to get her on the right track, aside from a few medications, which the shelter vet could provide. Besides, this would be a perfect opportunity for me to demonstrate for the workshop attendees how just a few days of one-on-one support from a foster parent can help an animal change course.

Once I was back at the hotel, I snuck in through a side door and discreetly brought the kitten up to my room. I started running hot water and made a warm compress, gently holding a wet washcloth over each eye and wiping away the goop, then clearing her nasal passages so she could breathe. I squeezed an ophthalmic antibiotic into each eye and examined the damage—a bit of swelling to both eyes, and perhaps some permanent scar tissue over one, but they looked recoverable. I breathed a sigh of relief and gave her the oral antibiotic that would help fight her infection from the inside.

Next I needed to weigh her. I plopped her on the small digital scale I carry with me and shook my head. Five weeks old and only 313 grams (0.69 pounds), she was practically caving in from hunger and dehydration. As I warmed some subcutaneous fluids in hot water, she looked up at me from the hotel bathroom floor, curious about my actions but not at all scared. I sat on the tile, steadied her in my lap, and slid the needle under her scruff. Letting out just a tiny peep, she rubbed her face into the side of my leg, a sign of trust and self-comfort. In just a few moments, her body was being replenished with vital electrolytes; I could literally feel her body soaking in the hydration like a sponge.

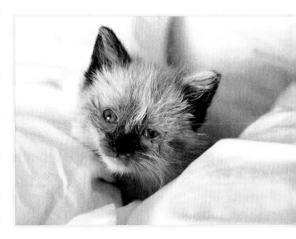

Like many young kittens with respiratory infections, she didn't eat when food was presented to her. It's likely that she couldn't smell the food to identify what it was, and that she may have been too quickly separated from her mother and was not accustomed to having solid food placed in front of her. To help her out, I picked up a bit of kitten food, slid my finger into the gap on the side of her little mouth, and plopped a chunk of the wet meat onto her tongue. She gazed up at me with a knowing look, as if to say, "Oh my gosh, it's food." She munched and munched and looked at me for more. I picked up the food and placed it in front of her mouth, and she gobbled it up. Over and over, I hand-fed her her first healthy meal of kitten food.

It's moments like these that really bring into context the importance of one-on-one care for kittens. A sickly baby like Hannah Jr. may not be able to survive if simply left alone in a kennel with a bowl of food, but having a dedicated human bring each bite to her mouth makes all the difference. To hand-feed a sick kitten is to make a tangible promise to her that she can keep living. As simple as it is, it is a lifesaving gift.

That day, Hannah Jr. and I quickly became besties. She followed me around my hotel room like a baby duck, always underfoot. That evening, an episode of Animal Planet's *My Cat from Hell* was airing, featuring me and Jackson Galaxy rescuing fifty kittens, and now I wouldn't have to watch it alone . . . I'd have a kitten to watch it with me! Just before the airing, I got a video call from Jackson, who asked, "Where are you today?" I lifted Hannah Jr. to the screen and said, "Well, I'm in a hotel room in Iowa, and believe it or not, I've got a little friend with me." We both had a good laugh, knowing that a rescuer's work is truly never done.

The next day, I taught a full-day workshop about kitten care and community cats at Iowa State University. I set Hannah Jr. up in a small playpen at the front of the classroom, and she was a great ambassador for kittens. By the end of the workshop, I had so many offers for foster homes that I was able to find her a perfect placement with a young woman who could continue her treatment and keep her on track for full recovery.

That night, I kept her in my hotel room for one last evening together, and continued to plump her up with wet food and treat her medical needs. I was so proud of her for how far she had come in just two days. We fell asleep cuddling on the white double bed, and as the light came through the window the next morning, the cat who peered back at me looked different. Her eyes were bright and clear, her body was warm and soft, and her little spirit was full of life. As she purred and played, I kissed her fuzzy head, so relieved that just two days had made such a big difference for her.

Hannah Jr. went to a new foster home that continued her care, and I flew home to my nursery where my own kittens were waiting for me. I received many updates about my favorite little Iowa girl until she was adopted by a loving family, and it warmed my heart to know that my little baby duck would get to have a beautiful, full life. We may not have known each other for long, but the impact we made on each other was great. Her story had unfolded in front of a whole community of compassionate people, and through her example, Hannah Jr. became a tiny kitten who inspired others to start saving lives.

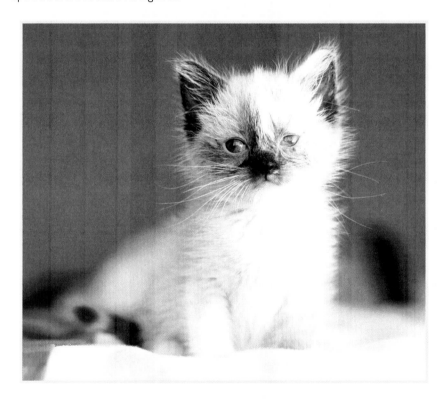

CHAPTER SEVEN

PREPARING FOR TAKEOFF

GOOD-BYE IS THE GOAL

If you're fostering, the ultimate goal is to prepare the little ones for the main event: adoption! Many new foster parents fear their first good-bye, which is understandable since we naturally tend to fall in love during our time with our tiny friends. Fear of sending kittens to their forever homes is so daunting that the idea itself actually stops many animal-lovers from fostering to begin with! Having parted ways with hundreds of kittens, I am passionate about helping foster families learn how to frame adoption with a positive perspective, and to discover the joy of a kitten's graduation day.

When a student graduates from high school, it's a day filled with happy emotions such as pride and excitement, but it's also natural to feel a tinge of sadness for what is now in the past, or nervousness for the future that lies ahead. This is the day when all the hard work pays off, and the student is ready to launch into the real world. While we may shed a tear over the end of an era, we certainly don't question whether the student should stay in high school for four more years! We recognize that her future is bright and unwritten, and we move bravely ahead.

We look at graduation as a celebration, because it means the student has completed a big task, and has met her goal. As rescuers, we need to stay goal-oriented and remember that adoption day is a celebration, too! The goal of fostering is to help prepare kittens to be independent enough to enter a forever home, so once they've survived and made it to adoption day, we should feel an incredible sense of accomplishment as they launch into the first day of the rest of their lives.

Feeling emotional about parting with a foster kitten is perfectly natural and healthy. While I've handed off countless kittens to their new homes, I still do cry every once in a while, and that's absolutely normal. Bonding and connecting with an animal is to be expected, and crying simply means that you're alive and that you've loved. It's those of us with tender hearts who make the best rescuers! I cry not because I am sad, but because I am happy. Crying is cathartic. I cry because it's beautiful to know that my love has transported a kitten from hopeless to home. I cry because I'm grateful that I could give him immense love during his most vulnerable weeks, then lovingly part ways when he is in a safer place.

When we cling to the fear of good-bye, we occupy a space of doubt that can be counterproductive both for the kittens and for our own well-being. Fear is a nasty beast, and one that is worth challenging and defeating. We may fear that ours is the only home that can provide love, when in reality the world is filled with loving

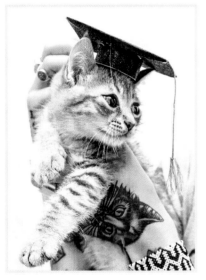

homes that may be even more suitable than ours. We may fear that this is the only kitten for us, when in reality, there are dozens of equally worthy kittens waiting for our help. We may fear detachment, when detaching is actually a critical aspect of sustainable rescue (see "Detach with Love," page 264).

By separating from the kitten, we give her the gift of a lifelong friend and caregiver, and we give future kittens the gift of a vacant spot in our home so that they can know the same triumph. It helps me to remember that without kitten foster parents, there wouldn't be kitten adopters, and we are therefore not just improving the lives of our kittens, but also spreading immeasurable joy to others. Good-bye is the goal!

WHAT IS LOVE?

I'm often told, "I wish I could foster kittens, but I can't, because I'd love them too much and never say good-bye." While I appreciate the expression of love, I find this sentiment to be a bizarre pretext for inaction. After all, love isn't about ownership; it's about meeting others exactly where they are. Love is about recognizing an opportunity to improve a life or prevent suffering, and seizing it. Love is about allowing yourself to see and accept others for who they are: their beauty, their pain, their potential. Love isn't just a noun; it's a verb. It's an action.

Imagine for a moment that you see a stranger with their arms full, struggling to open a door. Your hands are empty and you can easily give them assistance. Do you open the door to let them through, or do you stop to worry about what might happen if you fall in love? Does your mind flood with fears that you'll never be able to say good-bye to this human, and you'll have to marry them and stay together forever? Or do you simply recognize that they are struggling, help them open the door, and wish them a good day as you part ways? The answer is obvious: you don't think twice about opening the door. Being a loving human is simply about meeting others where they are and offering kindness as we are able.

Maybe it's a silly comparison, but it's really that simple. Kittens need us to open the door to the possibility that they might live. They don't need us to keep them; they just need us to keep them *alive* long enough to reach adoption age. When we meet them exactly where they are, we learn a valuable lesson about operating with a loving and generous heart. We discover that it feels good to hold the door open, and it feels good to save a life. We learn that compassion isn't measured by the love we keep, but by the love we give away.

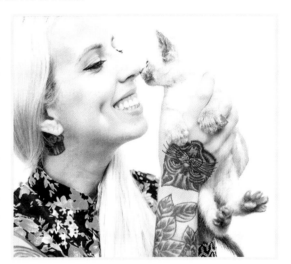

FOSTER WINNING

There's a term that's often used by pet parents: "foster fail." This term means that you fostered an animal but failed to actually adopt him out; to foster fail is therefore to keep your foster animal. This is usually said with a playful tone, joking about one's inability to part ways with the foster animal who became a forever friend. It's usually said to me in the context of "I just can't do what you do. I tried, but I foster failed, and now I have three cats!" or, even more commonly, "You love that kitten so much, I bet you're going to foster fail!"

So many pet parents proudly proclaim that their companions are "foster failures" that the term has become embedded in the vernacular of the animal-loving community. I'm going to state an unpopular opinion here: I believe that the term "foster fail" is antithetical to the goal of saving lives.

Hear me out.

The decision to adopt a cat or kitten is a beautiful, important one. It's a commitment to love, protect, and provide care to another being for twenty-plus years. But we already have a word for what it is to make this commitment, and the word is "adoption"! When I made the decisions to adopt Coco and Eloise, I wasn't doing so because I was failing at giving them up; I was doing so because I was succeeding at making a thoughtful commitment that I was ready to make. It's absolutely acceptable and wonderful to adopt a foster animal if you so desire, but it's important that this decision only be made with full consideration and a deliberate desire to take on this lifelong responsibility. It isn't something we ought to be guilting one another—or ourselves—into doing. A commitment of this magnitude should not be made without intention, and should not be born from the pressure of being afraid to say good-bye.

For many people, the idea of having an animal in their care is synonymous with ownership, so they feel that if they're giving up foster kittens for adoption, they must be *giving up* on them. In reality, adoption simply frees up space for more kittens to be saved! The kittens I rescue today are only alive because I said good-bye to those who came before them, and the future lives I will save are dependent on me thinking ahead and saving them a spot. As someone who cares deeply about being part of the solution for years to come, I'm a big believer in the importance of staying goal-oriented.

Yet people often have a challenging time focusing on their goal of saving lives, and many compassionate first-time foster parents thus never become second-time foster parents. In a 2016 survey I conducted, 41 percent of former kitten foster parents reported that the primary reason they were no longer fostering was "I adopted the kitten(s) and no longer have room to foster." Of course, you may someday encounter a foster kitten whom you'd like to adopt, and as long as that fits within your goals and abilities, that's great! But I encourage you to call this "adoption," a term that implies you've made an intentional decision after much consideration.

I'm told constantly that people feel guilty about adopting out their foster kittens. They feel pressured by friends to foster fail, and feel influenced to keep their foster animals, even if that was not part of the plan or their original intention. It breaks my heart to hear that a foster parent feels guilt; she should instead feel tremendous pride for her selfless act! I believe the language we use is impactful on our communities, and we should therefore be careful about how we talk about fostering. Rather than joke about failing at something so important, I think we should call "foster failing" what it is—adoption—and create new terms that empower foster parents to say good-bye.

Fostering saves lives. Why would we want to fail at that? Why foster fail when you can foster *win*? To foster win is to succeed at adopting out your foster animal(s) into a new home so that you can continue to save more lives. By fostering sustainably, we not only expand our impact, but we improve our skills, too. As we gain more experience, we're able to help with more challenging cases, to develop our abilities and grow more confident, and even to become mentors to others in the rescue community. To keep oneself open to saving lives is to make a commitment not to an individual kitten—but to kittens as a whole.

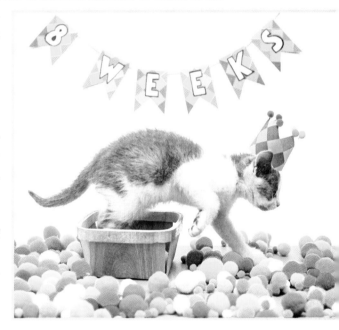

When hundreds of thousands of lives are at stake and fostering is the one opportunity they have to survive, we should be rooting for the brave people who have the compassion to foster. We should not be guilting them into failing; we should be encouraging them to succeed. I believe we need to create a culture of positivity around adoption day. Let's celebrate that when we say good-bye to our fosters, we get to say hello to more—and the kittens win!

THE BABY BEES

"Please help! Three newborn kittens found abandoned in window well!" read the message posted online. I stopped what I was doing and called the phone number to get more information, and before I knew it I was rushing out the door with my rescue bag. I arrived at the family's home, and as I knocked and waited for the door to open, the fall breeze swept through the chimes on the porch and filled the air with a twinkly tune.

I was welcomed into the home by two young children and their mother, who eagerly guided me over to the three little kittens. They were indeed very small newborns, no more than two days old, with their eyes closed and umbilical cords attached. The family had waited several hours for a mother cat before scooping the babies up, and had been caring for them in their living room until they could find a foster parent to help out.

"How did you know what to do?" I asked.

"I watched your videos!" the mother responded. I was overjoyed to hear that she'd researched syringe-feeding, and she'd done a great job of keeping them healthy so far. "Your video was helpful, especially how to get them to pee and poop," she continued.

With great excitement, the little girl chimed in: "I wiped the booty!" I couldn't help but grin ear to ear at this admirable family effort. It really does take a village! I packed the kittens up, thanked the family, and was on my way.

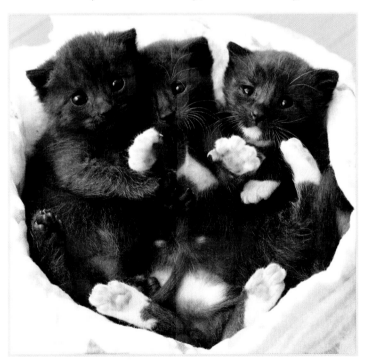

Back at the house, it was time to weigh them, help them go to the bathroom, syringe-feed them, and get them warm and cozy. I placed a big plastic tub containing a heated disk and a plush blanket on my coffee table, and Boomba, Bumble, and Bee curled up together like three little mice in a nest. For the first few weeks, they slept at all hours of the day, only waking to empty their bellies and fill them back up. Lucky for me, I wasn't without help; my friend Elena wanted to learn to bottle-feed, so she came over to help out with the babies periodically.

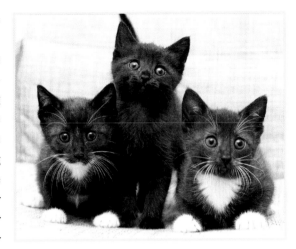

Before I knew it, my pint-sized mice were lengthening into sleek little lanky mini-jaguars, with lustrous silky coats and big green eyes. Having been hand-raised since they were born, these three grew into the most trusting, loving trio. After wearing themselves out from playing, they'd lounge belly-up on my legs, sleeping with their mouths open just enough to expose their adorable baby teeth. Once it was time for them to cuddle someone new, I started to post them for adoption—but Elena interjected. She and her girlfriend had talked it over, and they were in love with Bumble! Since I already knew how committed she was to her pets at home, hearing that she wanted to adopt him was music to my ears. Immediately I knew he'd be spoiled with toys, cat trees, and a family that was absolutely obsessed with their animals.

Boomba and Bee were adopted together, and Bumble was indeed given a home with my friend, who had known him from infancy. When I visit Bumble now, I lift his hefty twelve-pound body with two hands, and it's hard to believe that he used to fit curled up in my palm. It puts into perspective the incredible power that humans have on our hands, both figuratively and literally. By dedicating ourselves to the nourishment of the tiniest and most vulnerable felines, our hands can give the gift of more than just chin scratches—they can give the gift of a life well lived.

FINDING FOREVER FAMILIES

Adoption is the goal of fostering—so how do we achieve it? True adoption isn't about simply handing the kitten off; it's about having a thorough process in place that ensures the kitten will have a good life. The adoption process entails getting kittens ready both physically and behaviorally, and taking steps to find the perfect match to bring them home. As the kittens reach adoption age, it's time to start vetting adopters—and taking the kittens to the clinic for their "vetting," too!

Before adoption, make sure you've met the kitten's health needs so that you're giving her a head start at a healthy life. Plan to provide the adopter with the kitten's medical history, noting any issues the kitten has had, as well as records for her preventative care. Here are my recommended guidelines for pre-adoption veterinary care:

- FVRCP vaccine (plus as many boosters as age-appropriate)
- Rabies vaccine (if twelve weeks or older)
- FIV/FeLV test
- Dewormer
- Microchip
- Spay/neuter

Note that if you're fostering through an animal shelter or rescue, this care will be provided by the organization. Just make sure you're staying on top of appointments and meeting the kitten's needs as outlined by the group you are working with.

SPAY DAY

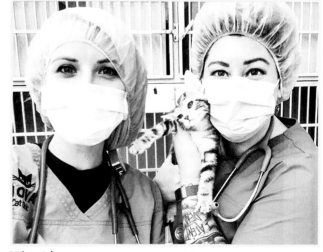

The last step before a kitten gets adopted is spay/neuter: the process of surgically sterilizing the kitten so that they cannot reproduce. Spaying and neutering are critically important tools for reducing the population and saving lives—we do not need cats having more babies while so many go without homes! On an anatomical level, a spay is an ovariohysterectomy in which the ovaries and

Velouria's spay surgery was a success!

uterus are removed, and a neuter is a castration surgery in which the testicles are removed; both surgeries result in permanent sterilization. But spaying or neutering isn't just important for the population as a whole; it's also helpful for the individual animal's health and well-being.

In recent years, there have been advances in veterinary medicine that allow kittens to be spayed and neutered at a younger age than was previously typical. In the US shelter system, spay/neuter is now typically conducted at two months/two pounds for pre-adoption kittens, just in time for the transition into their forever home. You may find that your private practice veterinarian will not spay until an older age, but I encourage you to explore other options in your area if you're fostering kittens. Some of the benefits of pediatric sterilization are:

- No teen moms! Female kittens can go into heat and become pregnant as young as four months of age, so in order to avoid pregnancy they should be spayed *no later* than fifteen weeks (unless there is a legitimate health reason for delaying surgery).

- Male kittens can begin to spray as they reach pubescence—a stinky, unpleasant behavior that no one wants in their home. Neutering greatly decreases or completely eliminates this behavior.

- Kittens recover quickly and have fewer postsurgical complications than older cats due to their decreased amount of fatty tissue and the smaller incision size.

- Sterilization at eight weeks allows kittens to be adopted quickly so that rescuers and shelters can save even more lives.

It's important to find a veterinarian who is comfortable with and trained to perform surgeries on pediatric patients so that the kittens can receive proper care before, during, and after the operation. Not all veterinary clinics are the same, so don't be scared to ask questions about the procedure and protocol. Kittens should receive a physical examination before surgery to ensure that they are in good health and can tolerate anesthesia. They should be given an IV catheter as part of their surgery, which acts as a safety net if something goes awry. Females, whose surgery is more intensive, should be intubated. All kittens should have a technician monitoring their vitals, including the kitten's respiration, blood pressure, and blood oxygen, for the duration of the operation. Additionally, they should have proper pain management after surgery to ensure a comfortable recovery. Talk with your clinic if you have questions about their practices so that you can feel comfortable knowing your kittens are in good hands.

Pediatric surgery varies from adult sterilization operations only slightly, mostly with regard to the dosing of anesthesia medications and the preoperative instructions for the caregiver. While adult cats are typically fasted after dinnertime the night before surgery to ensure an empty stomach, small kittens should not be fasted for nearly as long. Kittens' small bodies can become hypoglycemic if it's been too long since their last meal, so I always recommend being very intentional about their last meal before surgery. You'll want to time it so that the kitten has an empty stomach but isn't starving—ideally, they'll get surgery right around the time they would be ready for their next meal. For instance, if they are eight weeks old and eating four meals a day, they should have a small meal six to eight hours before surgery to keep their blood sugar up.

Once the surgery is complete and the kitten is awake, she will feel woozy from surgery and should stay at the clinic for at least an hour to be monitored. When she's back to her senses, the clinic should give her a nice rewarding meal that she's sure to gobble right up. Follow the clinic's postsurgical instructions, keeping an eye on the incision site and making sure it heals properly. At your home, give the kitten food and water, and monitor her for the evening to ensure she's recovering well. If you observe any bleeding, pus, irritation, or extended lethargy, call the veterinarian to follow up and bring her back in to be examined.

In my experience, male kittens tend to recover from surgery so fast it will make your head spin! Within a few hours they are typically back to their usual playful selves. But because spaying is a more invasive procedure, female kittens tend to feel a little more sensitive for a few days. Be sure that you're limiting jumping, playing, and any activity that might aggravate their incisions. If you find that they're roughhousing a little too hard, it's okay to separate them, but kittens can generally be housed together during recovery. Sterilization is an awesome rite of passage, and that shaved tummy is a sign of good things to come: adoption day!

MICROCHIPS: A LITTLE THING THAT GOES A LONG WAY

A microchip is a small, rice-sized implant that is inserted just under the skin in the scruff of the kitten's or cat's neck, typically during spay/neuter surgery or even during a routine vet exam. Just like kittens, microchips are tiny but mighty! Embedded in the tiny chip is a scannable code that is unique to the animal, allowing him to be traced back to his rescuer or adopter if lost. Microchips are a small thing that makes a huge difference if a cat goes missing, as they can sometimes be the one thing that helps bring a cat home.

I'm hugely passionate about microchip awareness, as there are many misconceptions about what microchips do and how they are used. It's important to know that a microchip is not a tracker—it does not allow you to locate the animal on a map like you would a lost smartphone. It is simply a code that, if scanned, can be looked up to search for the person who registered the chip. All adopters should register their microchips on adoption day.

A 2009 study found that while lost cats were reunited with their owners at a rate of just 1.8 percent, microchipped cats had a much higher rate of reunification—38.5 percent.[1] This same study found that only 58 percent of microchips were ever registered with the family's contact information, which is a devastating error. It is critically important that adopters register their microchips so that the code is associated with contact information for the animal's family. A microchip that is not registered is simply debris; a microchip that is registered can save a life.

Most important, adopters should know to keep the registration information up-to-date. Every time you move, change your phone number, or switch your email address, you should update that information in the microchip registry by adding it online or calling the microchip company. While the initial implantation of a microchip comes at a small cost, registering or changing the information on a chip can be done for free. I highly recommend microchipping as part of kittens' spay/neuter package so that they are set for life—just remember that whether you are the adopter or the foster parent, it's important for the forever home to be fully educated about how to register and update the chip!

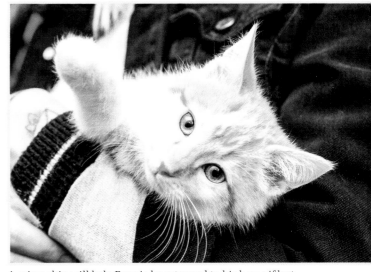

A microchip will help Beanie be returned to his home if lost.

They say the best things in life are free, so you might assume I'd be jumping for joy over a sign that reads FREE KITTENS. In reality, the concept of a kitten giveaway is absolute nightmare material to a rescuer like me! When it comes to finding a home for a kitten, there should always be a process that goes beyond simply handing them out like freebies.

Andrew and I were on a long seven-hour road trip from Connecticut to Washington, DC, and as we crossed the border into Maryland, we hit some truly gnarly traffic. The highway was at a standstill, and I decided to try taking a detour onto a country road for a few miles to pass by the gridlock. The country road was a welcome change of scenery: expansive greenery, vast cornfields, and small family farms. As we drove on the one-lane rural road, we passed a few small houses whose mailboxes lined the pavement. Against one mailbox was a bright green poster board with the handwritten words: FREE KITTENS.

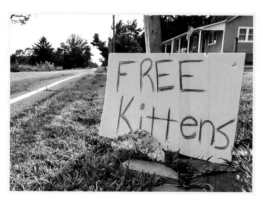

I slammed on the brakes. "Oh my god. Did you see that sign?"

I turned the car around and pulled into their driveway. Even knowing nothing about the situation, I knew there was nothing good about advertising free kittens on the side of the road. My heart raced—I had no plans of getting kittens that day, but I knew that if I wanted to ensure they would go somewhere safe, the right thing to do would be to offer to take them. I looked around the back of the car to see what I had on hand: a few cans of cat food, a baby blanket, and a humane trap I'd just used to teach a community cat class at a university. It would do.

We stepped onto the small porch and knocked on the rickety door. As the door cracked open, a shirtless man with a long, scraggly beard emerged.

"Hi, we're here to ask about the free kittens. I'm a cat rescuer, and I'd like to help. What's the situation?"

He looked us over with a furrowed brow, then called for his girlfriend to come to the door. She explained that they were cat-lovers, but their cats kept having babies that they couldn't afford to keep. She was familiar with spaying and neutering, but didn't have the means to pay for it . . . and so her cats were now on their third litter of kittens. To deal with the ongoing cycle, her routine was simply to put out a FREE KITTENS sign every time they had a litter.

Oof.

I breathed deeply and tried to really listen and assess the situation. The woman wasn't malicious; she just seemed exhausted and sad. She said how much she loved the kittens and hated that they couldn't keep them. She told me how she'd given them all baths, trimmed their nails, and tried her best to get them ready to go. She wasn't a bad person; she was just living on a low income in a very rural area, and didn't have access to the resources that would help her be a better advocate for the cats in her life.

In these situations, it's easy to judge, but it's more impactful to have a conversation and provide support. There is nothing effective about lecturing someone who doesn't have the resources or knowledge to do better. And so we had a conversation. I asked if they had the ability to call to make an appointment at a vet, and if they'd be able to transport the cats, and she said yes. It was a dream for her to have her cats spayed and neutered, but it had never seemed possible. We offered to cover the cost of her cats' surgeries, and she was stunned. She said it seemed too good to be true, and was overjoyed to have the support that would help them end this cycle.

Now for the kittens. She told us that there had been five kittens in this litter, but that right before we'd arrived, someone else had stopped and taken two. My heart sank—there was certainly nothing we could do for those two now, other than hope that they'd ended up with a good, stable home. The three remaining kittens were still available, and I told her we would love to take all three.

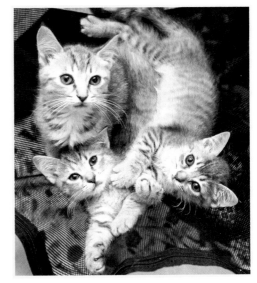

She walked into the other room and came back holding a bouquet of beautiful silver tabbies. Their fur was soft and icy-toned, and their green eyes were large and skeptical. They weren't feral, but they were confused and a bit scared to be meeting new people. She handed me the littlest one, a boy, and as I brought his fluffy head toward my face for a kiss, he smelled like shampoo and cigarette smoke.

I lined the trap with a blanket, and she said good-bye to the babies one by one as we placed them in the trap. We shook hands, and we told them how grateful we were that we could help the babies find good, loving homes, and to end the perpetual giveaways. As we walked toward the car, the woman picked up the FREE KITTENS sign from the yard and said, "I guess we won't be needing this anymore!" With their past disappearing into the rearview mirror, the kittens' future was brighter than ever.

FREE OR FEE?

It's all too common to see advertisements for kittens who are "free to a good home." People find themselves in a situation where there are kittens in their care, and they don't always know the best way to get them homes. While the intention might be

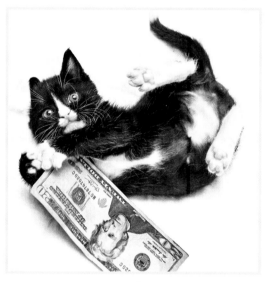

good, the fact is that a free giveaway tends to be a detrimental method. It's important for people in this situation to have the tools to help kittens find a home where they can be happy, healthy, and safe for the duration of their lives.

Due to the unstructured nature of a giveaway, freebie kittens will typically have received no veterinary care, and may have untreated medical conditions or underdeveloped immune systems due to lack of vaccination. Oftentimes, the kittens aren't even old enough to be eating independently, much less physically ready for an adoptive home. The majority of "free to a good home" kittens are not sterilized, and can go on to create even more accidental kittens in their new home.

Without due diligence on the part of the caregiver, the new home can turn out to be less than ideal. Many people warn that giving away free kittens is dangerous because they could be used in some extremely cruel way, like dogfighting, snake feeding, or other abuse. That is certainly true—when you're giving away kittens without vetting the homes, you really don't know where they're going, and you take the risk of something tragic happening—but while abuse is a possibility, the much more likely scenario is that they will simply be taken home by someone who made an impulsive decision and isn't aware of the kittens' needs or ready to make a life-long commitment to an animal. When you combine that with the fact that the kittens probably haven't had any medical care, that's a recipe for disaster.

This is why it's important that any time a kitten is going to a new home, there's an adoption process in place. This process consists of two things: vetting the kittens and vetting the adopters. That means providing important preventative care like vaccines, dewormer, and sterilization, and it also means checking out the adopters to make sure they're really ready for a kitten. Adoption applications and interviews allow us to understand who the adopter is, what the home is like, and whether they're a good fit for a commitment of twenty-plus years. When one of my kittens goes home, I can feel confident that this person intends to make a lifelong commitment to her, that she'll be treated with love, and that she'll continue having her health needs met.

So is it the financial transaction that makes an adoption a success? Not at all! In fact, many animal shelters will run occasional promotional events wherein they offer *fee-waived adoptions*: the opportunity to adopt an animal at no cost. Unlike a kitten giveaway, a fee-waived adoption is still a full adoption process. That means that the animal organization is providing medical support, preventative care, and sterilization to the kittens. They're still having people fill out an adoption application, complete an adoption interview or counseling session, and sign an adoption contract. The only difference with a fee-waived adoption is that there is no payment.

This might surprise you, but research shows that fee-waived adoptions do not have a negative impact on animals, and actually can save lives. A study in the *Journal of Applied Animal Welfare Science* showed that adopters are no less attached to their animals when fees are eliminated, and that free programs actually have the ability to save thousands of lives. The national initiative Clear the Shelters is a perfect example: every August, hundreds of participating shelters throughout the country waive their fees for one day, and over the first four years of the program, there were over 250,000 adoptions!

When it comes to effective adoptions, it isn't about money—it's about the process. Charging an adoption fee is often part of that process, as this helps rescues and rescuers recoup some of their expenses from providing the kittens care. If you've found yourself in a situation where you have kittens whom you can't care for, the best thing to do is reach out to your local animal welfare organizations and see what kind of support they offer. If you want to find the kittens homes by yourself, you can do that, but I highly recommend covering the expense of veterinary care to the kittens up front and then using an adoption fee as a way to recoup your costs. This way you ensure that the kittens are healthy and won't be having babies in their new home. Most important, never give away kittens without having a system in place for ensuring they're going somewhere safe.

SMILE FOR THE PAWPARAZZI

Finding an adopter is all about sharing your kittens with the world so that prospective adopters can find and connect with them. It sounds silly, but finding a forever home all boils down to marketing! By spreading the message throughout the community with stunning photos and thoughtfully written descriptions, we can generate widespread interest in adoption.

There's nothing more adorable than a kitten, so don't hog all their cuteness for yourself—share the wealth through photography! Photography is an important part of telling your kitten's story, whether for purposes of finding adopters, asking for donations, or even just making your friends say "aww." While having a dedicated camera does help, you don't have to have professional gear to snap a beautiful shot. With the incredible advances in smartphone camera technology, you can often get a fantastic photo right on your phone.

The photos in this book were taken by myself and my partner, Andrew Marttila, the professional photographer behind the photography books *Shop Cats of New York* and *Cats on Catnip*. Together, we've shared thousands of photos that have helped find homes for cats and kittens, and we have an absolute blast doing it! Using some simple tips, you can improve your skills and get crisp photos that truly showcase your kittens' personalities.

🐱 **Let there be light.** Natural lighting is an important key to making a photo appear soft and flattering, so try to focus your photography efforts around the time of day that your house gets the most sunlight. Our homes tend to have a "magic hour" when the light hits the room best, so find out when your magic hour is and aim to shoot then. You'll be able to capture the true color gradients and texture of the animal beautifully by working with the available light! In order to avoid unpleasant shadows, be sure that the light source is in front of the subject, not behind. You might also want to turn off any especially harsh overhead lights to avoid unpleasing shadows. Open up those curtains, and let the sun shine!

If you're using a digital camera or a smartphone, turn the flash off. As tempting as it is to add a light source, a direct flash will result in a harsh and unattractive photo, and might even cause an odd glow in the kitten's eyes. If you're struggling to find natural light but want to avoid using the direct flash, try an external light source like a ring light or a soft box. Or if you're shooting with a DSLR or mirrorless camera, an external flash bounced at a wall or ceiling can result in a studio-style photo and is my preferred way to photograph cats indoors; just avoid pointing the flash directly at the subject. Try playing with different angles and light sources until you find what works best for you.

Get on their level. No one wants to see a photo of the top of your kitten's head, so place your lens at eye level, whether that means putting him in a cat tree or lying down by his side. Andrew and I spend the majority of our photo shoots sprawled across the floor! This is part of the fun of connecting with the cat and really getting a visual sense of who he is. Meeting face-to-face will help you capture the kitten's expression, and help the viewer feel an immediate bond from looking at the photo. Anyone can take a photo from above, but seeing things from the kitten's vantage point will create a special connection with the lens that makes viewers fall in love.

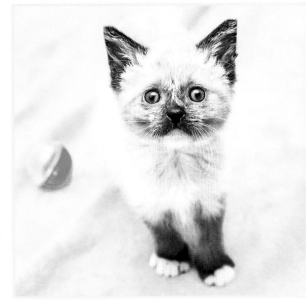

Keep it clean. The best kitten photos are those in which the animal is the centerpiece, so ideally you want to avoid any background clutter. A gorgeous image can be ruined by a pile of laundry in the background or a dirty carpet, so straighten up a bit before you start snapping photos. Clutter can be a real eyesore to potential adopters and might make it harder for them to envision the cat joining their home. Choose your placement and framing wisely, bearing in mind that the fewer colors and textures you see in the background, the more you'll be able to focus on the details of the kitten himself. Items like a cat bed or toy can make a great photo prop, but no one wants to see a pile of junk mail behind the subject. Pick a clean spot with a blank background and turn the kitten into a super-meowdel!

Keep it crisp. One common issue with amateur animal photography is that images are often blurred, which makes it harder to see the fine details of the face. This is especially common for photos of active little kittens, whose busy bodies can be too fast to capture with the automatic settings on a phone. If your camera roll looks anything like mine, then you know the struggle of having to scroll through tons of blurry photos to find a sharp shot. For every crisp kitten pic on my phone, there are dozens of unrecognizable furry blobs!

Don't fret. If you're shooting with a cell phone, you'll simply need to decrease the amount of movement happening with your subject (and with yourself) so that you can get an in-focus shot. Try to keep a steady hand, or if that's a challenge, place your camera on a sturdy surface to decrease motion. If you're using a DSLR or mirrorless camera, you can capture a crisp shot even if the kitten is moving by simply manually increasing your shutter speed or using an external bounced flash. Otherwise, you'll want to opt for moments of stillness such as right after a nap or while seated comfortably—or you'll have to create stillness by capturing their attention with noise and toys!

Noise and toys. Let's face it: cats don't always bow to our command. It can seem impossible to get a kitten to look at the camera for a photo, but it doesn't have to be a challenge. Once you're ready to snap your picture, you can easily get their eyes to focus on the lens by either showing them a favorite toy and then quickly placing it beside the camera, or by making a surprising sound!

If you're making a sound to get a kitten's attention, the stranger and more unfamiliar the better—cats quickly become bored with their paparazzi and will often stop looking once they know the source of the noise. For this reason it can be helpful to try many things: the sound of paper crinkling in your hand, the sound of a shaking bag of treats, or a wide range of vocalizations. Make a really new sound and you might even capture a cute expression of confusion or bewilderment! Just be sure to snap the photo quickly before the moment has passed.

But with all that excitement, be sure to be careful not to scare off the cat. Andrew says, "My favorite photos are those that are taken when the cat is most relaxed. First and foremost, let them be themselves, but if you can get their attention at the lens, it makes for a much better photo."

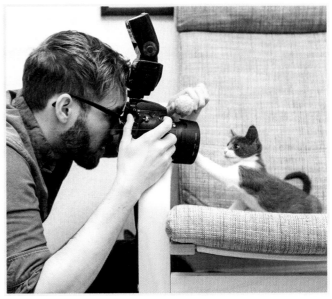

Andrew gets Small Fry's attention using a toy.

🐱 **No makeover necessary.** Social media may tempt you to use filters to edit photos, but try not to go overboard. Your finished product will look strongest if it's only minimally edited to enhance the natural qualities of the photo. Editing software is great for increasing the exposure of a photo that's a bit too dim, or bringing more cool tones to a warm image, but you don't want to rely too heavily on effects to make your image unique. Overediting can make a photo appear cheesy or odd, and makes the viewer feel less connected to the subject. Instead, let the cat's natural beauty come through, and you'll have a photograph that makes you want to reach right through the screen and boop him on the nose.

TELLING THE STORY

Whether you're creating an old-school flyer or a social media post, make sure that you're including a thoughtfully crafted biography of each kitten. You know that your kittens are superstars, but strangers don't (yet)—so this is your chance to help them shine! Here are some tips for writing a kitten bio:

🐱 **Capture their attention.** Write a title or intro sentence that makes readers stop in their tracks. "Cute Tabby Kitten" might be descriptive, but it isn't as eye-catching as "This Tiny Tabby Is the Queen of the World!" For your intro sentence, write an endearing note that grabs people by the heart and reels them in.

🐱 Example: "Velouria is her name, but her loyal subjects call her Queen V."

- 🐱 **Connect with your reader.** Try to imagine the ideal home for your kitten . . . then keep that home in mind as you write the kitten's bio. Envision speaking directly to the person you're hoping to find, and cater the ad to their desires and abilities. Build a bridge between the kitten and the prospective adopter.

  - 🐱 Example: "If you're a TV binge-watcher, Barnaby is your boy! This lil' snuggle-dumpling will cuddle you for hours while you catch up on your favorite show."

- 🐱 **Share what makes them special, physically and behaviorally.** Help the reader imagine seeing, touching, interacting with the kitten. Don't be scared to get creative or a little silly. Does her fur feel softer than a cotton candy cloud? Say so! Describe her skills. Does she make biscuits on blankets like she's a professional baker? Tell the world how sweet she is! Write from the heart, and others will be able to connect with the idiosyncrasies of your special kitten.

  - 🐱 Example: "Winston is a proud little hunter who likes to carry a stuffed bird in his tiny teeth. Between his superior fetch skills and his big puppy-dog eyes, we're not convinced he isn't a canine in disguise!"

- 🐱 **State the facts.** Share the kitten's age, sex, name, and color. If she has any medical conditions or special needs, explain what they are and what kind of home she will need. If she's part of a bonded pair, mention that. If you're posting online, make sure you indicate your city and state so you don't end up with inquiries from far away. Be sure to share the basic information that potential adopters need to know.

  - 🐱 Example: "Phillip is an 8-week-old male with beautiful brown tabby fur and a white tail tip. He's healthy, neutered, dewormed, microchipped, and up to date on his vaccines. This playful fella is looking for a home in the Washington, DC, area!"

- 🐱 **Urge readers to apply.** At the end, provide a call to action, encouraging people to reach out. Give instructions on how people can take the next step, and provide contact information such as a phone number, email, or website where applicants can submit an inquiry.

  - 🐱 Example: "If you've got the perfect lap for Margot's naps, we'd love to hear from you! Contact us by phone or email for more information about the adoption process."

Don't forget to keep your bio short and sweet, and to focus on the positive. People connect more with happy tales, so keep the sob stories to a minimum. If the kitten has an upsetting backstory, you'll do best to either omit it or frame it in an uplifting, hopeful light. Adoption should be a celebration, not a pity party! Write an upbeat and joyful bio, and keep it brief; it shouldn't take readers more than a minute to get to know the animal at this stage. Additional information can always be given once the applicants reach out!

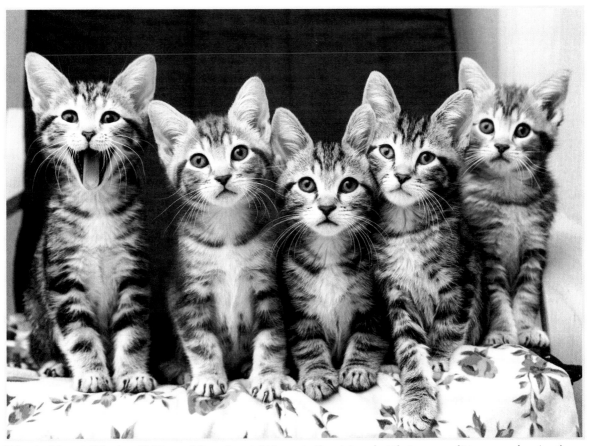

Velouria, Margot, Winston, Phillip, and Barnaby might have similar stripes, but their personalities are each unique!

I'm named after donuts
'Cause I'm round and sweet,
And I'm quite petite
Like a bite-sized treat.

—Jelly's rap

Listen, I've always been obsessed with donuts, so it was inevitable that I'd someday name a litter of kittens after my favorite dessert. I have a tradition that whenever I work in Las Vegas, I go to this tiny, hole-in-the-wall pastry shop that carries delicious vegan donuts, buy a massive bright pink box filled with sweets, and stuff my face until I can't stomach another bite. I'm so dedicated to my love of donuts that sometimes I even haul a dozen of the super sweet pastries on my flight home as a carry-on! Shortly after returning from one such Vegas trip, I was at home unpacking my bags and recovering from my donut-induced bellyache when I got a call from a shelter about three little orphans who needed my help.

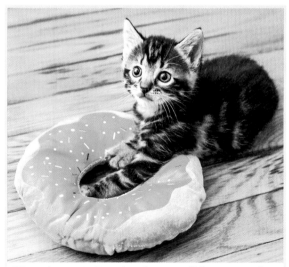

His real name is Bearclaw, but we call him Mr. Perfect because he is supermodel flawless. I'm pretty sure his parents were a Beanie Baby and a Lisa Frank drawing. If he were a high schooler, he'd be class president and captain of the football team.

I arrived at the shelter and was introduced to three tiny two-week-old tabbies. The first kitten was a beautiful, curious boy with bright eyes and smooth, silky fur. The second kitten was a raggedy mess, with disheveled fur and heavy eyes that begged for naptime. Last but not least, there was an itsy-bitsy girl with poofy fur and a scrunched miniature face. I lifted the little girl to my eyes, and she let out a powerful yell, as if to say, "I'm the smallest, but I'm the boss!" *What a funny trio*, I thought. I brought them home, got them fed, and started cleaning them up. As I wiped their faces clean, Andrew and I started to go through name ideas, when all of them started to purr in sync.

"Ugh, those purrs! They're so sweet, I could just eat them." I said. It immediately hit me: *They're donuts!*

The sleek, stripy boy would be named Bearclaw. The fluffy, sloppy boy would be named Fritter. And the scrappy, sassy girl would be called Jelly. The donut crew were hilariously entertaining and every bit as delightful as the treats they'd been named after. As they grew, so did their personalities—each one developing a distinct and hysterical character. They were like caricatures, and I couldn't help but giggle while sharing their photos and descriptions with the world . . .

By building a persona for each kitten, we helped onlookers discover their unique characteristics and idiosyncrasies, and they were a smash hit. Creating a character profile makes people laugh, smile, share, and get a glimpse at the individual and how he or she might fit into the family. Between the photos and the descriptions, people grew so connected to the kittens that they felt they already knew them . . . resulting in dozens of adoption applications!

Fluffy siblings Jelly and Fritter were adopted together, and handsome Bearclaw was adopted into a loving home with tabby playmates who became his best friends. It's been incredible to see them blossom into well-loved adult cats. They may have moved to their forever homes, but their striking personas remain.

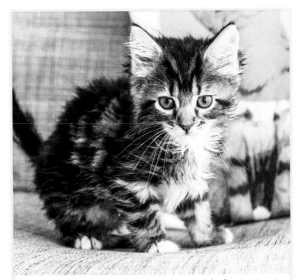

Fritter is a furry woodland creature with the most epic bedhead. This sloppy, happy dude has the appetite of a ravenous wildebeest and the purr of a Harley. If he were a high schooler, he'd be a hacky-sack-playing burnout with a serious case of the munchies.

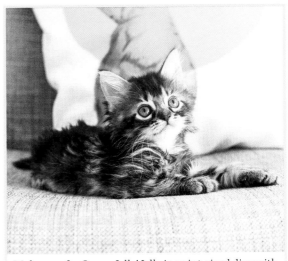

Make way for Queen Jelly! Jelly is a pint-sized diva with the confidence of a lion. She likes to strut her stuff, demand affection, and try to carry things that are way too big for her. If she were a high schooler, she'd be the prom queen and the coolest girl in school.

Now that you've got your photos and your bio, you're ready to start spreading the word to potential adopters. Woo-hoo! Don't be afraid to advertise your kittens far and wide. Cast a wide net by posting across multiple platforms and communities in order to increase the number of eyes looking at your kittens. Remember, just because you've shared their adoption profiles doesn't mean that you have to say yes to the first random person who picks up your flyer or responds to your listserv post; it just means you'll have lots of options while choosing an adopter. Here are some places you might consider sharing your kittens:

- Shelter adoption page
- Adoption websites
- Online listservs
- Community boards
- Social media
- Old-school flyers around town

If you're fostering through an organization, they'll manage the adoption process for you! They will likely even have public adoption events you can attend, and they'll guide you through meeting with applicants, or they may even have you simply bring the kittens back to the facility for adoption. Just make sure you chat with the shelter or rescue to find out what they'll need from you as your kittens prepare for their big day. You shouldn't have to do this alone, so I highly encourage you to reach out to local organizations about fostering through them so you have support. Rescue organizations and animal shelters help you out not just with veterinary care, supplies, and mentorship, but also with finding suitable adopters and placing the kittens into loving homes!

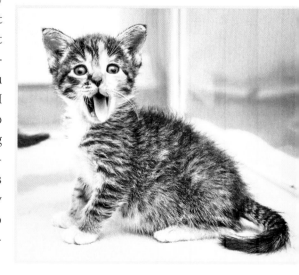

When it comes to picking a forever home for your kittens, it's natural to want the best for them. Whether you're personally finding a home for kittens or doing so through a shelter, there should be an adoption process in place that includes an application, a conversation, and an adoption agreement. This ensures that you (or the representatives of the organization) are doing your due diligence and placing the kittens into an appropriately safe and suitable home, and that there is a written agreement that outlines the expectations of the adoption.

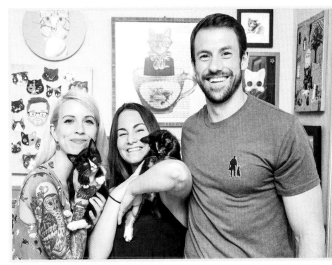

Badger and Leeni meet their wonderful new parents!

There are many philosophies about the right way to conduct an adoption process, and if you ask ten rescue organizations for their protocol, you're likely to get ten different answers! Many organizations used to believe that the process for adopting a pet should be lengthy and complex, with requirements for personal references, vet references, and even home visits. Nowadays, most organizations have discovered that increasing barriers to adoption doesn't actually achieve the intended goal of saving lives, as it drives people away from bringing home an animal. Researchers have found that "those that adopt through conversation based adoptions . . . provide similar high quality care and are just as likely to be highly bonded to their pet as those that adopt through policy based adoptions."[2] Consequently, many organizations have done away with the strict processes and have moved toward adoption processes based on conversation.

My adoption process is therefore less about checking boxes and more about communication, listening, and coaching. By having conversations with prospective adopters, I can learn about their motivations for adopting, their past experiences with pets, and their knowledge or lack of knowledge about cats' needs. This allows me to provide education rather than judgment, and to help applicants become more aware of the needs of cats and kittens, whether they end up adopting through me or not.

Here are some things you may want to consider when choosing an adopter:

🐱 **Applicant and family.** Who is applying, and who else lives in the home? Does the person have financial stability and a support network? Who will be responsible for the animal's care and well-being? If there are children in the home, it's a good idea to talk with the parent(s) and ensure that the children understand how to be gentle with animals.

🐱 **Home.** Is the adopter allowed to have animals in the home? Does everyone living in the home want to adopt? Ensure that the home is a stable environment where all roommates or family members are aware of and supportive of the decision to bring home an animal. Does the home pose any physical dangers to the kitten, such as balconies or windows without screens? Talk to the adopter about kitten-proofing and home safety.

🐱 **History with animals.** Has the applicant had pets in the past? If so, inquire about their experience. Did the animal pass away of old age? Were they taken to the vet when they were sick? Has the person abandoned a pet outdoors or surrendered a pet to an animal shelter? Talk to the person about their previous experiences. If they have rehomed an animal, you'll want to discuss the situation and determine if the issue has since been addressed. Keep in mind that we all experience changes and growth over the course of our lives.

🐱 **Current pets.** Does the applicant have other animals at this time? If so, are they friendly toward cats and small animals? Talk to them about introductions and the integration of a new kitten into a home with an existing pet. How will they handle the transition? If there are no other animals in the home, it's a good idea to recommend adopting two kittens (see "Buddy System: Forming Feline Friendships," page 141).

🐱 **Expectation.** What does the adopter anticipate having a kitten in the home will be like? How will they handle the transitional period? Are there behavioral, health, or other issues that would be a deal-breaker for the adopter? Are they prepared for the high energy of a young kitten, or might they do better with an adult cat? It's a good idea to determine if the person has a patient, realistic, and flexible attitude about adopting a kitten.

- 🐱 **Commitment.** What is the applicant's overall philosophy on being an animal guardian? Does the person understand that adopting a kitten is a twenty-plus-year commitment? Will they have a plan in place for their pet in case of the adopter's serious illness or death? While none of us can know where we will be in twenty years, it's still important to have a conversation about the future and how the applicant envisions their long-term relationship with the cat.

- 🐱 **Loving care.** Will the person provide humane, loving care to the cat? Have a conversation about what that looks like, including providing routine and emergency vet care, an enriching and safe home environment, and a healthy diet. Are they considering declawing? Talk to them about why that's unethical, and coach them about nail trims and scratching posts. Ensure that the kittens are going to a home where their bodily autonomy is respected and their well-being is prioritized. It's a wonderful idea to spend some time talking about what it truly means for a cat to live a good life.

By having a dialogue with prospective adopters, we can both gauge their mind-set as well as help them become more informed about animal care. Of course, you may encounter applicants who are not suitable for adoption, such as students living in dorm rooms or people with pets who are aggressive toward small animals. Have a gentle, thoughtful conversation with those who don't meet your requirements, and perhaps even guide them to other options. Just because someone isn't suited for adoption right now doesn't mean they won't be in the future, or that they wouldn't make a great volunteer. Just because kittens aren't right for a family doesn't mean an adult cat wouldn't be. Bear in mind that even in these situations, you're helping future animals by educating the applicant, so be patient, kind, and honest!

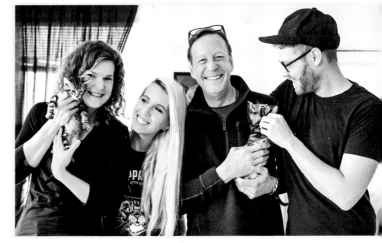

Phillip and Winston head to their forever home!

While it's a great idea to have an idea of your perfect adopter, you also want to be realistic and to know when good enough is good enough. Know where you're willing to budge and where you aren't, and don't be afraid to truly make it a conversation so that you can help steer the adopter in the right direction. After all, you're the expert! By listening, asking questions, and counseling, we can help adopters be the best cat guardians they can be.

YOU SAY GOOD-BYE, AND I SAY HELLO

Before you know it, it's the big day! On the day you say good-bye to your foster kittens, they say hello to the beginning of the rest of their lives. It's important to enter this day with a feeling of achievement and celebration—because of you, this tiny life can now grow! Because of you, some lucky human will have a new best friend. Because of a few weeks of your time, this kitten will now have the gift of twenty years of life. Congratulations, you lifesaving superhero!

Every organization handles adoptions differently, so if you're fostering through a group, make sure you know how the adoption process works. Sometimes you'll bring the kitten into the facility and drop her off, sometimes the adopter will come to your home, and sometimes you might even meet the adopter at an adoption

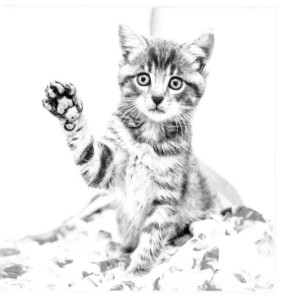

event. If you're handling the adoption on your own, you may choose to meet the adopter in your home or theirs, and facilitate a short playdate where you can get the new family up to speed on everything they need to know about the kitten.

I generally like to prepare my adopters ahead of time by letting them know what to expect in terms of the kittens' likes and dislikes so that they can do a shopping spree for all the things that will help the kittens feel at home. For instance, I'll recommend the kittens' preferred food and litter, favorite toys, and any other considerations that can help the adopter prepare. In some cases, I'll even send kittens to their new home with a beloved toy or blanket from their time with me, which helps ease the transition. I've had kittens leave the house with everything from mouse toys to wicker baskets to a stuffed donut!

Know that it's okay to feel emotional when you say good-bye, and do whatever it takes to help yourself feel triumphant. Tell your friends about your achievement and feel good when they congratulate you. Celebrate with an ice cream party. Sleep in the following day—you deserve it! You should be so proud of yourself for your foster win. Know that I am so proud of you, too!

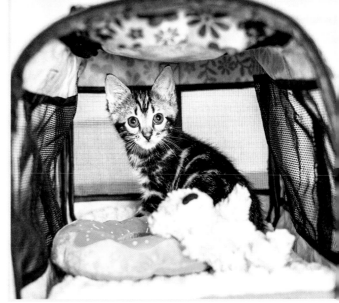

Bearclaw goes home with his donut toy!

NEW KIT ON THE BLOCK

Once the kitten or kittens have made it to their forever home, adopters should be prepared for an adjustment period. Just like with any move or new relationship, adoption is a major life transition that will take a bit of time for the kitten(s) to get used to. Fortunately, kittens are pretty flexible and tend to be a bit of a blank slate; cats can adjust to new surroundings very quickly if adopted young. But first impressions can make a big difference, so it's important to have a plan of action for bringing home newly adopted kittens.

🐱 If possible, adopt on a day when you will have a few days to spend with the kittens. For instance, if you work a nine-to-five job, aim to pick up your kittens on Friday evening or Saturday morning to ensure that you'll be able to spend time getting them comfortable and set up.

🐱 Start the kittens out in a small room for the first twenty-four to forty-eight hours. In this room, place at least one litter box, a cat bed, food, water, and toys. During this time, you want to help them get used to the fact that they're in a new environment, but are safe and have everything they need. Be sure to show them their food and litter several times to ensure that they know where everything is. This is their new home base.

🐱 Once the kittens are feeling comfortable and confident in their home base, start allowing them to explore other parts of the home with supervision. Over the next forty-eight hours, monitor how they're doing with the new territory, but return them to the home base when unsupervised. Once you feel that they're ready to take on the full space, you can acclimate them to their full home range.

🐱 I recommend always placing a litter box within eyesight of any room the kittens explore during the first weeks in a new home so that there are no accidents. After the kittens have become more comfortable with the layout of the home, you can remove the extra boxes.

🐱 If there is another animal in the home, get him and the new kittens used to each other through scent swapping: switching their blankets or bedding so they can start to process the unfamiliar animal through smell. Take it slow. Introduce the kittens to other animals in a safe manner for a short period of time. Meeting under a doorway or through a baby gate can allow them to look at one another or even touch paws without feeling threatened. Having treats or mealtime on separate sides of the same room can help them observe one another from a safe distance. Keep introductions short and sweet until they begin to feel more comfortable.

🐱 Be patient. It's absolutely normal for kittens to feel a little freaked out during their first days in a new home, so don't feel discouraged if they want to hide or if they hiss at the resident cat. Challenge them to spend time playing and cuddling with you, but do so in a way that is calm and loving. Takes things slow and steady, and you'll find that they will slowly get used to their new digs!

CHAPTER EIGHT

TAKING CARE OF YOURSELF (SO YOU CAN TAKE CARE OF THEM)

AN INVITATION

aving lives is an extremely joyful, deeply rewarding experience, but it can also be a double-edged sword. By dedicating ourselves to the protection of those who are vulnerable, we make ourselves vulnerable, too. We sacrifice our time and energy; we lose sleep to care for a neonate or a sick animal; we witness suffering or death; we open ourselves up to challenging ethical situations that wear on the heart and mind. For this reason, a critical part of learning to take care of animals is learning to take care of ourselves.

My personal journey in kitten rescue has been one of tremendous self-development, and I could never have anticipated that by committing myself to helping kittens grow up, I'd also experience growth. Caring for animals has taught me to stay hopeful, to practice gratitude, to collaborate with others, and to love myself. Living in a culture where insecurity, fear, and hopelessness are rampant, I'm grateful that I've been able to create a life that feels meaningful and positive.

I believe animal care offers an invitation to become better at caring for ourselves and one another, and we can

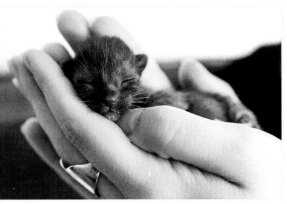

We must learn to care for ourselves as much as we care for others.

either accept the invitation, or ignore it at the cost of our own well-being. Animal advocacy provides a framework in which we can experience tremendous emotional growth and healing, build deeper relationships with ourselves and others, and feel pride in the contribution we make. Rescue can unite us or tear us apart, and can help us feel fulfilled or defeated. This chapter seeks to invite you on a journey of personal development, and it's an invitation I hope you will accept. By caring for not just animals but also ourselves, we create a sustainable movement that is built to last.

KEEP YOUR FIRE: COMPASSION FATIGUE AND BURNOUT

Those of us who work in the trenches of animal rescue carry a heavy weight. We may be faced with unending volumes of animals in need or bear witness to unpreventable pain and suffering. This highly emotional work can take a toll on the caregiver over time, sometimes leading to a condition called "compassion fatigue." Compassion fatigue is a secondary form of post-traumatic stress disorder (PTSD), also called secondary traumatic stress disorder. With nearly identical symptoms to PTSD, compassion fatigue is different in that it happens not to the suffering individuals but to the people who are helping. We absorb trauma, and it becomes our own.

Having graduated with a degree in psychology in 2008, I spent some of the most formative years of my career working with adolescent trauma survivors and helping them strengthen their coping skills. I feel deeply passionate about mental health and believe that we must bring this awareness into the animal-caring space as well, where so many suffer in silence, unaware of the risk of secondary traumatic stress. Whether you've been involved in animal welfare for a long time or are just starting out, it's important to know about compassion fatigue, how to prevent it, and what to do if it occurs.

By acknowledging the emotional, mental, and physical impact that prolonged exposure to animal suffering can have on us, we can set into motion a plan of action to keep ourselves healthy and resilient. "If you don't learn to manage the stress associated with helping others, then your compassion satisfaction can slowly fade, leaving you feeling angry, depressed, anxious, physically exhausted, and emotionally drained," says Jennifer A. Blough, LPC, in her book on compassion fatigue in the animal welfare community, *To Save a Starfish*.[1] Compassion fatigue ultimately leads to burnout, a condition marked by exhaustion, feelings of failure, and withdrawal. Knowing that empathetic caregiving is a risk factor for traumatic stress and burnout, we must develop healthy coping skills in order to protect ourselves and our important work.

If you've experienced compassion fatigue or burnout, you are not alone—it happens to many of us who are heavily involved. It isn't a sign of weakness; it's a sign of deep and prolonged empathy. Over the years I've had to navigate periods of extreme stress and anxiety myself. A few years ago, I really hit a wall after taking on multiple extremely stressful sick-kitten cases back-to-back without a break, without a lot of support. After several kittens passed away in my care, I reached a very low point. I would lie on the couch and stare at the ceiling with tears in my eyes. My heart would physically ache when I'd think of the kittens who had passed. My feet dragged underneath me as I'd walk to my office; I dreaded going in to work, and each step felt like a heavy weight. I felt emotionally raw and unprepared to take on new kittens, but simultaneously guilty about wanting to take a break, so I kept going and going at my own expense.

I remember having this horrible recurring nightmare about standing between two conveyor belts, with a line of kittens coming toward me, one after the next. In the nightmare I'd have to pick the kittens up off one conveyor belt and put them on the other, one by one, in order to get them to safety; otherwise they'd fall into a deep, dark pit. I'd feel overcome by anxiousness about the unending assembly line,

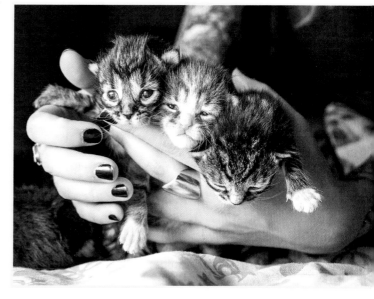

and I'd wake feeling absolutely drained. It was a warning sign— a reflection of what was happening in my real life. I wasn't giving myself any time to rest or unwind. I wasn't listening to my body as it was telling me, through physical exhaustion, tears, and upsetting dreams, that something had to change.

Compassion stress grows when empathetic individuals are overexposed to traumatic experiences, triggered by trauma memories, and dealing with other stressful life events.[2] These risk factors accumulated in my life, and eventually I realized I was at the bottom of a deep pit myself. I was experiencing compassion fatigue, and I needed to arm myself with coping strategies so that I wouldn't burn out. Nothing felt more important to me than developing healthy habits and equilibrium so that I could be a strong rescuer for years to come. As I began to learn more about compassion fatigue, I began to value the knowledge as an essential component of sustainable animal care. With intention and effort, we can develop strategies that let us keep our fiery passion without burning out.

The first step to preventing compassion fatigue and burnout is to know and acknowledge the signs. Intrusive thoughts, shortened temper, numbness, disillusionment, guilt, and anxiety are indications that it might be time to step back and take care of yourself. It's important to recognize this not as a failure, but as a sign of a beautifully empathetic heart—one that is worthy of protection, and of healing when it is injured. We have to find ways to keep the fire in our hearts without letting it destroy us.

Researchers have found that there are four primary variables that can protect caregivers and reduce the risk of compassion fatigue: *self-care*, *detachment*, *sense of satisfaction*, and *social support*.[3] These protective factors are associated with high resiliency in people who work in compassionate fields. My belief is that we must treat these protective factors the same way we would treat the factors that protect animals, such as food and water: they are not an option; they are a necessity. Let's dive into each of these variables and learn how we can integrate them into our lives.

SELF-CARE IS ANIMAL CARE

Imagine that kittens' lives are in peril, and they need to be driven to safety on a hot summer day. What kind of vehicle would you like them to be driven in? A clean car with functional brakes, an air conditioner, and a tank full of gas, or one that hasn't had an oil change in three years, is overheating, and has the side-view mirror duct-taped on? This is the scenario we are faced with as advocates, except that it's not a literal car that's saving cats: it's us. Self-care *is* animal care! When we are the vehicle responsible for protecting someone else, we must practice essential self-maintenance to ensure that we're able to function properly.

Self-care means meeting our basic physical and psychological needs, including maintaining proper nutrition and hydration, getting enough rest and exercise, caring for our emotional needs, and participating in fulfilling relationships and activities. When you consider that many kitten caregivers are waking up throughout the night or dedicating large portions of time to animal care, it's easy to see how even basic needs can begin to fall by the wayside. This means we need to be especially mindful about putting our own care on the to-do list, too! Don't forget that we have to feel good in order to do good.

Unfortunately, so many of us almost take pride in our lack of self-care. We joke about never finding time to eat a good meal or get a full night's sleep. I've found that lack of self-care is reinforced in our culture because we often celebrate those who sacrifice their own wellness in order to protect others. When we help others at the expense of our well-being, we are like burning martyrs—our fiery passion destroying us from the inside out. Over time, I've come to believe that our martyrdom helps no one if it burns us out prematurely.

Research shows that self-care is inversely correlated with stress in general, and secondary traumatic stress specifically.[4] When we care for ourselves, we are able to sustainably care for others. Ever since I learned to put on my own oxygen mask first, I've found that I'm much better equipped to be of service to others. Now when I feed a kitten, I make sure I'm eating a snack, too—so I can keep fuel in the engine that's driving the kitten to safety. Each of us has our own path to self-care, and the only way we each can know what we need is to learn to listen to ourselves, and to respond with the same loving empathy that we would give to an animal. Here are some ideas for meeting your basic self-care needs:

- Plan your meals for the week. Ensure that you're getting three healthy, balanced meals a day.
- Take a catnap if you need to. Spoon your cat and enjoy the stillness.
- Scan your body for tension and focus on releasing it. Unclench your jaw.
- Take a long bubble bath.
- Buy a big water bottle in a color you love. Cover it in your favorite stickers. Fill it with fresh water and drink liberally throughout the day.
- Go to the doctor for that issue you've been avoiding. Your health is so important!
- Throw out your gross old socks. You're better than that.
- Change your sheets and make your bed. It'll feel great.

- Set aside a chunk of time each week to run errands and take care of your personal affairs. You'll feel relieved knowing you have it off your plate.
- Deep-clean and declutter your bedroom or workspace.
- Go to therapy. It really helps.

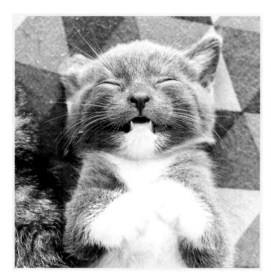

Take a catnap!

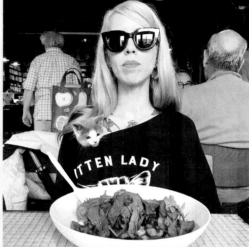

Remember to feed yourself, too!

DETACH WITH LOVE

The sun is sparkling on the sea, gently warming my skin as I lie on a surfboard. Floating in the ocean, I realize that I haven't seen a kitten in four whole days. While the thought of this once would have filled me with guilt, it now fills me with pride. In this moment, I am doing the work of sustainable animal advocacy because I have chosen to step back and take some time to reenergize.

Sometimes we need to do more than just get a full night of sleep to protect ourselves from compassion fatigue. We also need to establish a healthy detachment by occasionally taking a physical or mental break from rescue work. Research finds that individuals with higher levels of detachment have greater life satisfaction and decreased emotional exhaustion.[5] This means that taking time away from the constant pressure of rescue can actually increase our effectiveness over time, because it gives us the emotional space to decompress, but then safely dive back in again.

It's important to establish hobbies and interests outside of animal care in order to stay balanced and healthy. This is easier said than done, especially when we know that there's an endless supply of kittens in need (à la my conveyor belt nightmare), so we should be intentional about carving out time to take a breather. When I take time to do activities I enjoy, like hiking, rock climbing, swimming, drawing, sewing, baking, playing music, or even engaging in advocacy for other social justice issues, it helps me to zoom out on my life and see things from a different perspective. Engaging in other movements, expressing ourselves through creative outlets, and taking short breaks help us stay refreshed and capable.

Detachment isn't about not caring; it's about self-preservation. In fact, by allowing ourselves to attend to other activities and interests, we actually decrease our chances of emotional numbness or depression, allowing us to do our compassionate work with a stronger heart than ever before.[6] Now when I take a break, I try to feel impactful rather than guilty. I recognize that as an animal caregiver, I'm still helping animals even by going for a walk in the woods or dipping my feet in the ocean because I'm doing the personal work that will keep me saving lives for years to come.

Here are some of my personal ideas for stepping back and detaching, but find what works best for you!

- Practice yoga.
- Read a book that has nothing to do with animal welfare.
- Speak up when you need a break. Feel proud of yourself for doing so.
- Go outside. Ride your bike, go for a run, or go rock climbing. Go hiking and try to identify the trees and plants you see. Isn't it amazing out there?
- Make art. Color in a coloring book. Paint a picture. Take a pottery class, or learn an instrument you don't usually play. Knit a scarf for your grandma; she'll love it.
- Detach from your cell phone at night. Let yourself truly unwind before bed.
- Put an autoresponder on your email for a day. Maybe two days. People can wait.
- Plant something and watch it grow.
- Volunteer for a project unrelated to animals.
- Watch a favorite movie from your childhood.
- Make a playlist of your favorite songs from high school.
- Take a walk down memory lane by looking at old photos or keepsakes. Remember who you are and where you're from. Be proud of how far you've come.

- Bake a pie. Eat the pie while it's still warm. Preferably with coconut milk ice cream.
- Learn something new. Dive deep into an issue you're interested in but don't know a lot about.
- Plan a vacation. You deserve one.

WE GOT THAT PMA

Another factor that has the ability to decrease compassion fatigue is keeping a positive mental attitude (PMA) and building a framework within which your rescue work can feel satisfying. By approaching rescue with a spirit of positivity and sincerity, we are better prepared to get through the inevitable challenges that accompany the work. In their book *Compassion Fatigue in the Animal-Care Community*, Drs. Charles R. Figley and Robert G. Roop state that "understanding the 'calling' of animal care . . . is a critical factor in predicting and managing compassion stress, because no matter how bad the medical emergency, no matter how distressing or upsetting the event at the time, the animal professional's attitude and sense of motivation are a critical salve for the traumatic wound."[7]

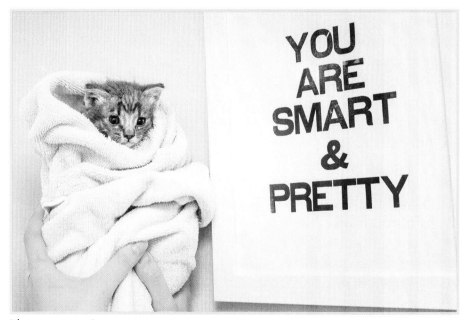

It's true—you are!

When I first got involved in animal advocacy as a teenager, you couldn't have found a more negative person than me. I was brooding and short-tempered, and I looked the part, too! If my tense shoulders and funeral-home-inspired wardrobe weren't enough of an indicator about how I viewed the world, my I've-got-two-black-eyes makeup style and refusal to smile certainly were. Underneath the tough exterior I'd built were deep sadness and hopelessness. I saw so much suffering in the world, and being just a teenager, I felt helpless to do anything about it.

As I got older and found the punk community, my views began to shift. I found that you can be both countercultural *and* hopeful—that you can be angry *and* proactive at the same time. I began to understand that life itself is a DIY project, and you build the world you want to live in through your actions and your attitude. Coming from this perspective, I learned to frame everything I do with a positive and productive outlook, and keep chugging ahead toward a better world.

Staying positive may be easier said than done, but there are important steps we can take to make our rescue efforts feel both joyful and emotionally gratifying. I find that I feel most fulfilled when I am able to focus on the positive impact I've made, and to see that my work matters and I'm making a difference. Here are some ideas for increasing your satisfaction and keeping that PMA:

- Create a scrapbook with before/after photos of your foster kittens. Marvel at the impact you've made. You're amazing.
- Use kind, empowering, self-affirming words when talking about yourself and your rescue work. Verbally acknowledge that you are a superhero.
- Make a list of ten things you admire about yourself.
- Set small, specific, achievable goals that allow you to feel a sense of accomplishment on a frequent basis.
- Focus on the things you can change, and accept the things you can't. Apply your energy where you can make a positive impact, and don't sweat the rest.
- Celebrate minor and major victories. Do happy dances when your kitten poops in the litter box for the first time. Throw a small party when your kitten recovers from an illness.
- Surround yourself with other positive people.
- When you're sad, don't judge yourself for that feeling—love yourself. Have a good cathartic cry. It's healthy to cry and it's totally normal.
- Accept compliments. Really allow yourself to hear when someone tells you you're awesome. You totally are.

🐱 Make a list of ten things you are grateful for, big and small.

🐱 Do away with perfectionism. You are enough, and you are doing great.

WE'RE ALL IN THIS TOGETHER

"I love animals, but I hate humans."

It's a phrase you'll hear a lot in the animal advocacy community. The statement generally falls somewhere on the spectrum between jest and sincerity, and while it's one I've been guilty of saying a few times myself, it's a sentiment I believe we should challenge. Working with other people is essential to our success as a movement, and we do our best work when we are able to communicate, collaborate, and problem-solve as a team.

Social support is also directly linked with resilience against compassion fatigue.[8] The social climate in which we save lives has a major impact on our ability

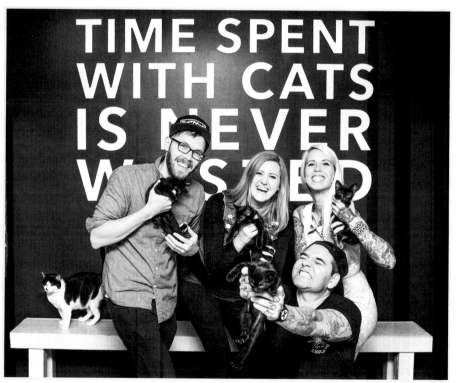

The rescue community is full of wonderful people—like Chris and Shelly, who run the Catcade in Chicago!

to do so sustainably, without burning out. Having healthy relationships allows us to experience joy and laughter, to feel safe expressing ourselves, to have tangible assistance in times of need, and to feel a sense of encouragement. Having a healthy community makes all the difference in both our personal experience and our effectiveness as advocates.

Collaboration will always be a part of animal rescue, because it requires engaging with people such as foster coordinators, veterinary professionals, and other rescuers. Yet one of the biggest challenges of a life devoted to animal welfare can be navigating the social landscape of a community that often struggles to work cohesively. When we're engaged in such an emotional effort, there are bound to be differences in perspectives and personalities, and even in the way we cope with stress and communicate with others. We must therefore be intentional about our social relationships and make every effort to collaborate in the spirit of mutual support.

Throughout my advocacy career, I've worked alongside some of the most selfless, badass, intelligent, supportive individuals in the world, and I can't imagine where I'd be today without them. People like Ellen, who has taught me more about neonatal health than anyone I know. People like Adam, who always brings a healthy dose of silliness into the seriousness of rescue work. People like Erin, whom I can count on for TNR inspiration and inside jokes. People like Christina, whose limitless advocacy efforts inspire me to stay active and creative. The list goes on and on.

I've also worked with people whose behavior has been problematic. We must remember that many in the rescue community have deep wounds, and that occasionally we will encounter people who have difficulty working with others. We should treat others with kindness to the extent that we are able without exposing ourselves to toxic situations, and remove ourselves from relationships that perpetually cause us grief. Remember that even this can be done gracefully and with love.

We should be aware of not just the impact others make on us, but also the impact we make on others. When we experience emotional pain, we often harden ourselves and become angry, judgmental, and oppositional—the very qualities that make it harder for us to thrive in our relationships and in our work. It might sound paradoxical, but our instinct tends to be to withdraw or to lash out, when social support is precisely the antidote we need for our sorrows. For this reason, I'm a major advocate for intentional community building and encourage all advocates to carefully consider how we treat one another, even when times are tough.

How do we find great communities? We build them! Here are some ideas for building a healthy social community:

- Share your knowledge, and ask others to share theirs. Skill sharing is essential for growth, and there is so much we can learn from one another! Knowledge is meant to be shared, not hoarded.
- Offer a hand to other rescuers when you can. Spread the support and goodwill.
- Avoid gossip. Leave the cattiness to the cats!
- Address complicated situations with an open heart and mind, acknowledging that ethical decision making requires context. Be open to growing.
- Apologize to someone you hurt, or forgive someone who hurt you.
- Communicate your emotional needs to your close loved ones.
- Check yourself if you feel jealousy, and recognize that others in the movement are not a threat. There's enough room at the table for every single person to make an important impact!
- Lift up those you admire! These are the people you will stand alongside as you craft a safer community for cats.
- Delegate. Ask others to help you out. You don't have to do everything alone.
- Give hugs. It's good for you.
- Say "no" to something you don't want to do. Cancel plans that are stressing you out.
- Remove chronically toxic individuals from your life. Your energy is best spent elsewhere.
- Surround yourself with people who fan your flames. Figure out who fuels you with love and support, and put your energy into cultivating those relationships.

SPOTLIGHT: WHEN NO OPTION IS A GOOD OPTION

Occasionally, you may encounter very challenging ethical situations and be forced to make a decision when every option sucks. From decisions about medical procedures to judgment calls about euthanasia, it can be absolutely brutal to find yourself caught in the middle of an ethical conundrum. If you've found yourself in such a situation, my best advice is to talk to other rescuers who have experience with the issue you're facing rather than to seek advice from bystanders who mean well but may not fully understand all that you are going through. Listen to others who have been where you are, and do your best to operate with a steady balance of head and heart. No matter what, be kind to yourself about the choices you make; it takes so much courage and strength of character to stand where you do, practicing compassion as best you can with the resources available to you.

ON LOSS AND GRIEVING

Occasionally, you may encounter a kitten who is not viable and cannot survive no matter how hard you try to save her. Losing a kitten is without a doubt the most painful part of animal rescue, and is something you may occasionally experience if you're fostering very young or very sick kittens. Navigating grief mindfully is critical to our emotional health and our sustainability as rescuers. While nothing can undo the sadness we feel, there are ways we can help ourselves process grief, honor the kitten, and remain emotionally grounded so that we can continue to save more lives.

Everyone processes death differently, and it's important to grieve in the way that feels right for you. Be gentle with yourself and listen to what your heart needs in order to process what has happened. Allow yourself to feel sorrow, but challenge any feelings of guilt or regret that may pop up. Recognize that you are the best thing that ever happened to the kitten and your compassionate action was deeply valuable. The reason we feel grief is because we also feel great love, and that love is what makes us fantastic advocates for the little guys. This is how you know you are alive and that you have a big, beautiful heart.

I've lost many kittens in my rescue career, and while it doesn't get easier, I have learned how to be more resilient. When I lose a kitten, I allow myself to feel deeply mournful in the immediate aftermath. I have a long cathartic cry if I need to, I cancel my plans if I am able, and I give myself permission to be a bit of a mess for the rest of the evening. Sitting in my sadness for a moment helps me feel like I'm confronting head-on the inevitability of grief. Once I've gotten through the initial guttural pain, I say good-bye to the kitten, either at the vet's office or through a burial ritual. I say some words to honor her life, and I stay at the site as long as I need to, then try to wipe my eyes, breathe, and move forward.

Central to my grief-processing strategy is the belief that sadness is good fuel, and should be channeled as such. I don't allow myself to wallow for more than twenty-four hours without getting proactive. I find it very healing to do something positive in the kitten's memory, like ask for donations to a rescue organization in his honor. While this doesn't lessen the sadness of loss, it comforts me to know that the kitten's life can inspire support that saves the life of a future kitten.

I also do a deep dive into researching the kitten's specific condition and become ravenous for information that can help me be better prepared next time. I channel my emotional energy into becoming a more knowledgeable rescuer and springing into compassionate action. After all, it's those of us who have experienced loss who become the experts on saving similar kittens in the future. By collecting information and moving bravely ahead, I've become stronger in my ability to save lives. I let my grief fuel my love.

Another component of a healthy grieving process, for me, is meaningful community support. Many people don't know what to say, or may not relate to the emotions we feel when we lose a small kitten, so I find it helpful to focus on talking to other people who have shared my experience. I let my friends know what is and is not helpful so that they can support me better. When we communicate our needs to others, they know if we want to be hugged, consoled, distracted, or left alone. At the end of the day, we get to decide how we grieve—so it's up to us to let people know how to support us.

While we all experience loss a little differently, many of us do share similar coping mechanisms. I've spoken with hundreds of foster parents about grief processing, and I've compiled information about approaches that are often helpful in times of bereavement. Here are some common helpful strategies I've found:

- Take the rest of the day off from all responsibilities. Rest and reflect.
- Snuggle your cats. Sob if you need to. It's perfectly healthy to cry.
- Have a ritual to help you say good-bye. This could be a burial, getting back the ashes of the kitten, or even planting some wildflowers in his memory. Many people report that a ritual helps them process grief.
- Talk to other foster parents. It can be helpful to speak with someone who can validate your heartache and experience. Acknowledge feelings of guilt, anger, or sadness, and work through it with someone who understands. Being part of the community helps us feel less alone.
- Allow yourself to feel sad, but don't dwell for too long. Most people report feeling worse if they don't pull themselves out of their sorrow and direct their energy toward something productive.

- Research the disease that caused the kitten's death, and learn something new that you can try in the future. Take a workshop or sign up for a webinar. Buy a new book about cat health. Talk to your vet. Knowledge is empowering.
- Take action through TNR or volunteering at a spay/neuter clinic. This can help you feel proactive about preventing suffering.
- Honor the kitten by donating or asking your friends to donate in his or her memory.
- Spend the evening doing something that feels comforting to you. If it helps you to make a collage of photos or write a poem, do that. If it helps you to put on fuzzy pajama pants and watch cartoons, do that.
- Focus on pouring love into remaining fosters, if you have others. Nothing heals a heart quite like a purring kitten.
- When you're ready, help more animals. Many people report that they feel the healing process begins when they successfully help another kitten. You may choose to boost your spirits by fostering a different population, such as older or healthier kittens, or nursing moms with babies.
- Focus on the lives you have saved. Thank yourself for how much good work you have done, and all the good work you will do in the future.

THE LOGISTICS OF LOSS

If you've lost a kitten, the first step is to deal with the immediate situation, which can feel overwhelming when your head is spinning and your heart is imploding with sadness. Here's a quick list to help you in the immediate aftermath of a loss:

- Wrap the kitten in a sheet or blanket.
- Give yourself a moment to process. Cry. Call a friend. Scream. Wash your face.
- Call the organization you're fostering for and let them know the kitten has passed. Breathe.
- Are there other kittens? Make sure you're still caring for them, or ask someone to help you if you need a break.
- Determine what you need to do with the kitten's remains.
  - If you are fostering for an organization, they may require you to bring the remains back to them, so find out what they want you to do.
  - If you aren't bringing the remains to an organization, you may choose to

surrender them to your local shelter or veterinarian, or dig a grave that is three feet deep and have a burial.

🐱 If the kitten passed away at the veterinarian's office, they will generally offer cremation.

🐱 If you want to get more information about the cause of death, you may consider opting for a necropsy. Put the remains in a plastic bag, place them in a cooler or refrigerator, and call your vet to make arrangements.

🐱 Did the kitten die of an infectious disease? Don't forget to sanitize the space and supplies to avoid future transmission.

🐱 Be kind to yourself. You've just gone through trauma. Love yourself like you would love your friend after a loss. Be gentle and patient with yourself.

MY FIRST LOSS

The first time I lost a kitten, I was in my early twenties. I had a few years of fostering under my belt, but I'd never dealt with a truly critical kitten before. Bramble and Mulberry came to me at about three weeks old, completely covered in fleas and very thin. After I had removed the fleas and cared for them for a few days, Bramble began crashing before my eyes. He suddenly couldn't stand or lift his head. He was weak and frail. I rushed to a vet, who simply gave him fluids and sent us home.

The rest of the night was a disaster. He got worse and worse, and I stood over him panicking, knowing that no amount of comfort I offered him would change whatever was physically harming him . . . and to make matters worse, I didn't have any idea *what* was harming him or how to handle it. My heart physically ached in my chest. When he started to show signs of suffering and dying, I was in an absolute state of panic—an emotional wreck. I'd never seen a kitten die.

I drove to the emergency hospital hardly able to think. I recall being such a mess that I hadn't even remembered to put on shoes! Barefoot, I ran into the hospital in tears and was told what the other vet couldn't tell me: Bramble was completely anemic from blood loss due to fleabites, and he was dying. In what felt like a whirlwind moment, they euthanized him and returned his lifeless body to me in a box. I can still remember the complete shock to my system in that moment—a sickening combination of outer blankness and inner devastation that tore through my chest. It felt like part of my heart died with him.

I did not handle my first loss gracefully. I cried for days. I held a burial for him, and my friends stood by as I lay in the dirt and wept like a baby. I buried him alongside the brambly berry bushes for which he was named. I hated myself for not being able to save him and retraced the experience in my mind over and over, wishing I'd done something differently. But I was young and I was inexperienced; though I'd rescued many kittens, I'd never dealt with one who was so sick. I had the heart for rescuing critical kittens, but not the experience. I felt like I'd failed him.

Thinking back, this first loss had a huge impact on my life. This early experience is what drove me to become deeply invested in understanding critical kittens and how to save them. Throughout the grieving process, I kept my hands busy by sewing a hand-bound book filled with blank pages, which I pledged to fill with as much knowledge as I possibly could about kitten health, and by the time it was complete, my eyes were dry and I was ready to learn. I titled it "Cat-astrophe! DIY Guide to Kitten Health," and I started reading every study I could get my hands on, watching videos, and talking to veterinarians. I scribbled any new knowledge I obtained into the pages and studied it daily. Looking back, this was the moment I transitioned from being a kitten babysitter to being a dedicated lifesaver.

I still have this relic from my past, and its pages are filled with information that I have subsequently used to save hundreds of lives. It's got doodles of different parasites, medication dosing charts, and tons of handwritten information about viruses and infections common in kittens. Seeing this DIY book on my shelf reminds me how far I've come, and how far I hope to keep going in the future. Knowledge is something you gain through time and experience; knowing that it is cumulative gives me the motivation to keep forging ahead and picking up information as I go. I know that by not giving up after losing Bramble, I have been able to save so many kittens I would never have had the skills to save before. I see his face in so many little lives today, and I will never forget him.

LIGHT AND LEVITY

As heavy as rescue can sometimes be, we should create levity at every opportunity we can, celebrating the moments when things are light and joyful. Rescue can (and should) be a fun, rewarding experience that creates far more smiles than tears! It's important to balance the hard work we do with a little laughter and playfulness.

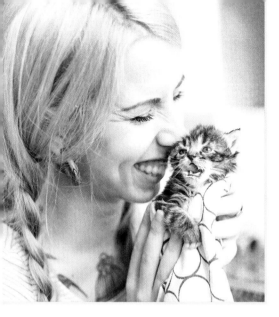

As children, we're taught to express our creativity through art, to use our imaginations, and to laugh and play, but as adults we sometimes focus so much on the serious nature of life's responsibilities that we forget to have fun, too. This is especially true when doing something as serious as rescue!

When we keep our hearts open to the happy moments, we are fortified with love and lightheartedness that help us stay strong through the trials and tribulations. We are able to experience the full range of what it means to love and to live. There's no one right way to bring levity into your rescue life, but here are some ideas to get you started:

- Take adorable photographs of your fosters, maybe even with some cute props. Weekly themed photos can be a fun way to track their progress!
- Write a song or rap for your kittens. I do this all the time! Don't be ashamed to get silly with your rhymes.
- Invite your friends over for a kitten cuddle party! There will be no shortage of happiness between your friends, the kittens, and you.
- Make a cardboard-box castle for your kittens. They'll be feline royalty in no time!
- Go to kitten therapy: Lie on the ground and let the kittens climb all over you. Breathe deeply and be in the moment. Aren't they great little healers?
- Try making some cute paper hats for them—the fancier, the better!

At the risk of sounding totally cheesy, I truly believe that happiness is a choice we make. Happiness is the little moment of bliss we have when a kitten falls asleep in our hands, purring. It's the hearty belly laugh we have when a kitten hops sideways while learning to play and hunt. It's the pride we feel when they reach a new milestone. We should cherish these positive moments and seek to build as many of them as we can, for the emotional well-being of our kittens, our communities, and ourselves.

Step 1: Prepare your supplies.

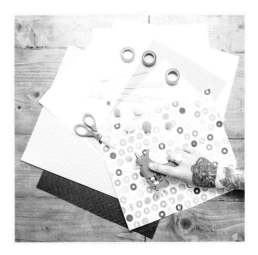

- Scissors
- Hot glue gun and glue
- Glue stick
- Double-sided tape
- Pen or pencil
- Paper in various colors and patterns
- Anything else you'd like to add: poofballs, glitter, stickers . . . get creative!

Step 2: Make the cylinder of the hat.

- To make the cylindrical top of the hat, cut a rectangular shape. Curl the two short ends to meet, and glue them together to make a tube.
- Try different widths and heights until you find a size and shape you like!
- To make a contrasting ribbon, use washi tape, or cut a thin slice of paper and glue it around the base of the tube.

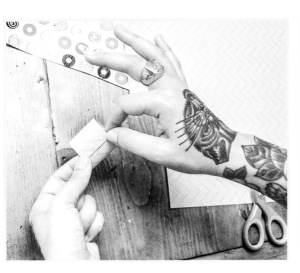
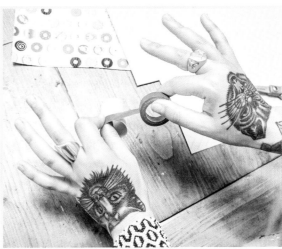

Step 3: Make the top of the hat.

🐱 Take the paper you'd like for the top of the hat and cut it into a square that is larger than the width of the tube. Flip the paper upside down.

🐱 Using your glue gun, drizzle a line of hot glue on the inside rim of the top of your cylinder.

🐱 Place the top end of the cylinder upside down, against the square of paper.

🐱 Once the glue has dried, trim the excess paper from the square, leaving only enough paper to create the top of your top hat.

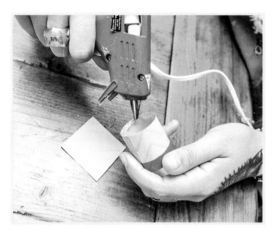
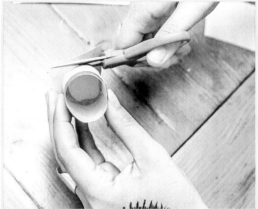

Step 4: Make the brim of the hat.

🐱 Choose the paper you'd like to use for the brim. Bear in mind that you'll be able to see both sides of this paper, so you can either choose a double-sided print or use a glue stick to fix the paper to another sheet so that a pattern/color is visible on both sides. Cut it into a square that is larger than your cylinder.

🐱 Using your glue gun, drizzle a line of hot glue on the inside rim of the bottom of your cylinder.

🐱 Place the cylinder against the square of paper.

🐱 Once the glue has dried, trim the paper in a circle that exceeds the width of the cylinder, creating the brim of the hat.

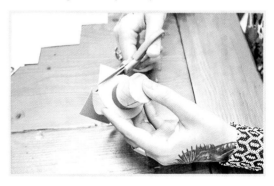

Step 5: Add final touches, and you're ready to go!

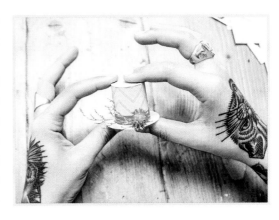

- Now that you have your top hat, add any other details you'd like, such as a feather or a button.
- Place a small strip of double-sided tape on the underside of the hat. This will help the hat gently stick to the kitten's fur without hurting the kitten. Never glue a hat to a kitten's head, and never force a kitten to wear a hat if she isn't feeling up for it. Always supervise kittens when using any sort of prop.
- Place the hat on the kitten's head, and get ready to snap a cute photo, or simply revel in the perfection that is a little cat in a little hat. Excellent work!

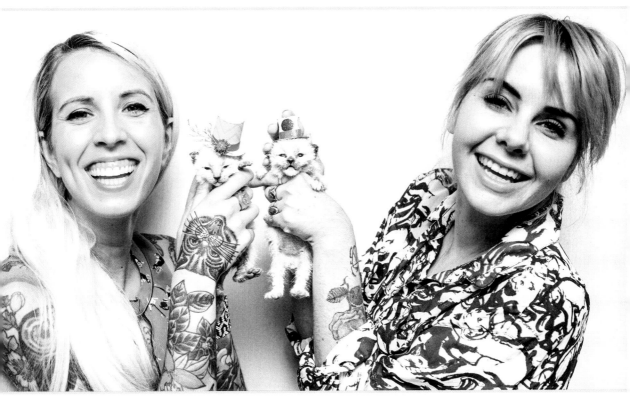

Want more paper hat inspiration? Check out Adam Ellis's super fun book *Tiny Hats on Cats!*

CHAPTER NINE

CHANGING THE WORLD FOR THE TINIEST FELINES

THE FUTURE IS FELINE-FRIENDLY

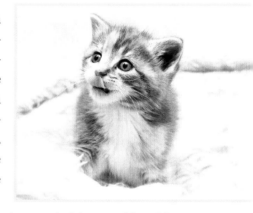

We can't change the past, but we can change the future—and we are. Every morning I wake up feeling inspired to march ahead toward a day when the killing of kittens is a thing of the past. The path is lit by the incredible shelter leaders, researchers, policy makers, industry professionals, and, most important, individual advocates who are building a movement to change the world for the tiniest felines. This is happening!

There are so many exciting and innovative advances in kitten welfare. More shelters than ever before are expanding their foster programs to meet the needs of the vulnerable kitten population. More than six hundred communities in the United States now have TNR-friendly ordinances or policies, and new community cat programs are being developed all over the country to reduce the numbers of kittens being born outdoors. Researchers are beginning to turn their attention toward neonatal kittens so that we can have more scientific data about their needs and care. Large national nonprofits are developing kitten campaigns to raise awareness about the need for foster homes. The public is becoming more aware of the issues, and at the same time, the industry is starting to turn its eye toward strategically saving kittens' lives.

Some organizations are now putting their resources toward creating an on-site kitten nursery: a dedicated 24-hour facility that is designed specifically for the care of kittens too young for adoption. Volunteers and staff are scheduled at all hours to feed, stimulate, medicate, and otherwise care for dozens or even hundreds of unweaned kittens at a time. Nurseries are saving the lives of thousands of previously underserved kittens in cities like San Diego, Austin, New York, Los Angeles, and Salt Lake City. For those communities that have the ability to develop a nursery facility, the impact is incredible!

But even organizations that don't have the funding or capacity to create a kitten nursery are increasing their lifesaving efforts for kittens. In Jacksonville, Florida, a group of kitten rescuers formed a "Kitten Army" with the sole purpose of recruiting and educating more kitten foster parents for multiple local shelters. By focusing on awareness and education of the entire community as a whole, they've been able to make a massive impact on not only the numbers of kittens being saved but also the quality of care being provided to them by caregivers.

Ramping up community participation is the key to saving lives, and there are so many ways that organizations are doing just that. Many shelters are now enacting kitten intervention programs, wherein people attempting to surrender found kittens are invited to foster the kittens instead. Instead of being a place for people to *drop off* kittens, these shelters are becoming a place for people to *pick up* support! By offering training, supplies, and free medical care, shelters are able to turn kitten finders into kitten fosterers—and shelters are succeeding at a rate of about 40 percent. This innovative approach creates a community-based solution to a community-wide problem, and the response is clear: when people have the knowledge and resources to save lives, they want to pitch in!

Every community has its own path to saving the lives of kittens, but one thing is for sure: getting each community to solve the kitten crisis on a local level will be an essential component of achieving a truly no-kill nation. I believe that the protection of kittens will be one of the final puzzle pieces to place as we build a feline-friendly future. We must be aspirational in our efforts and be daring enough to include kittens of *all ages* and *all needs* when we talk about what it means to be "no-kill." We must create and participate in these critical programs. We must recognize that if an animal can be saved, we have a duty to try to save her—and believe that when we show the world what it is possible to do, the world will take notice and be inspired to save lives, too.

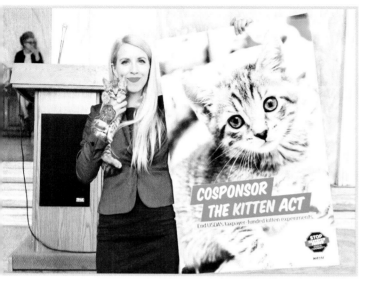

If you're feeling pumped to make change for cats and kittens in your community, then welcome to the wonderful world of advocacy! Kittens can't speak for themselves, so they need strong advocates like us to lift our voices and speak up for them. There may be programs, policies, or protocol that you'd like to influence locally, but before you go grabbing your megaphone, let's talk about how to advocate for policy change effectively. Here are my ten tips for effective advocacy for cats:

Be a participant, not a spectator. It's easy to stand on the outside and criticize what a shelter is doing, but it's much more impactful to get actively involved. By volunteering, you'll get to know the organization more intimately, and gain a greater understanding of the issues you'd like to see addressed. You'll also begin to understand what changes may be feasible to make and what may not be possible at this time. You'll make a bigger difference as a trusted and informed collaborator than as an outside observer, so rather than pointing a finger, start by lending a hand.

Identify the issue. You can't change something you can't identify, so get the lay of the land and discover what life is like for the cats and kittens in your community. Read up on your local animal ordinances and find out if they support TNR. Learn about what programs are available for kittens and which populations still need support.

Do your research. Your community isn't the only one that has had to address these issues, so try looking at other cities for model programs and policies. Gather information about what has worked well in communities like yours, and reach out to people from those programs to get advice on how to start. You may even benefit from attending a national conference where you can share ideas and meet like-minded advocates from other regions!

🐱 **Identify the gatekeeper.** Who is in charge of the policy you want to change? Who holds the key to the door you'd like to open? It could be a shelter administrator or program director, a city council, a county commission, a state board, or even a member of Congress. Understand what agency has the power to make the change you want to accomplish, and be sure you're addressing the issue with the right person.

🐱 **Start small and specific.** Be specific and realistic about the changes you'd like to see made. Instead of trying to change the entire system, try to influence one component, such as a specific protocol or policy. Keep your eyes on the big picture, but zoom in on the incremental steps it takes to get where you're trying to go.

🐱 **Offer support, not judgment.** Rather than saying, "You need to start a neonatal kitten program," offer tangible assistance, such as, "I'd like to organize a kitten shower to raise funding and awareness about neonatal kittens." Offer to play a role in the change you'd like to see, and be willing and able to do the follow-up work.

🐱 **Be kind and pleasant to work with.** People don't want to be around someone with a rotten attitude any more than they want to eat a rotten apple. Try to keep a warm, open, friendly disposition, even (and especially!) when navigating complex situations. Be grateful for others' time, and listen to other perspectives, too. You'll find that it's much easier to influence people if they like being around you!

🐱 **Find common ground.** When working with policy makers, don't start from where you're standing—start from where *they* are standing. What is their motivation to enact the change? Perhaps it's a political representative who wants to defend public health, so rather than explaining TNR as a kitten-prevention program, you focus on the fact that it provides rabies vaccinations. Perhaps it's a shelter that struggles with a tight budget, so you bring them funding ideas or cost-saving strategies that would also help them save more lives. Meet them where they are, and it'll be easier to walk together toward the change you hope to achieve.

🐱 **Take off the cat ears.** There's a time and a place for everything, but when trying to enact social change, we need to be the most professional version of ourselves. It's not that wearing cat-themed apparel is *bad* (trust me, I have a closet filled to the brim with cat-print dresses!), but it's important to know your audience when picking out your clothing, especially when meeting with public officials. Get out the lint roller, put on a nice blazer, and don't show off your collection of cat photos at a public meeting. Be relatable and calm, and stay focused on the facts rather than the emotions.

🐱 **Be persistent.** Keep showing up. Whether it's for a volunteer shift at the shelter or a monthly city council meeting, keep showing up in support. Take a deep breath and recognize that change doesn't happen overnight—it takes time and effort. Thank you for being a change maker in your community!

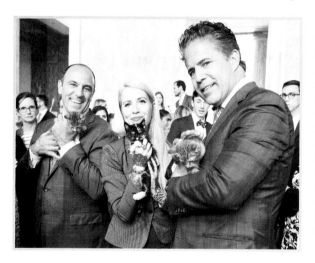

When it was uncovered that the United States Department of Agriculture was conducting deadly taxpayer-funded experiments on kittens, I visited Capitol Hill with a group of eight-week-old felines to advocate on their behalf. After more than fifty members of Congress on both sides of the aisle added their support to the campaign, the USDA finally announced it would halt all experiments on kittens—and never use cats in its labs again! Representatives Jimmy Panetta (D-CA) and Mike Bishop (R-MI) agree: saving kittens' lives is a bipartisan effort.

RETIRING THE "CRAZY CAT LADY"

Our culture has a lot of preconceived notions of what it is to be a cat person, but are these stereotypes really accurate, and do they help cats or hurt them? You know the type: a lonely, disheveled old lady with messy curlers in her hair, donning a bathrobe and living in a stinky house full of felines. This image shows up in everything from television shows to action figures, from Halloween costumes to board games. With all the hard work that the rescue community does, it's both belittling and totally erroneous to reduce the effort to save cats to simply being a "crazy cat lady." I believe that this stereotype is not just harmful to people; it's actually damaging to the cause of saving cats' lives.

Let's break it down, starting with the term "crazy"—a rude, derogatory term for a person struggling with a mental health condition. Crazy cat ladies are depicted as struggling with everything from social connection and personal hygiene to emotional regulation and animal hoarding. It's problematic enough that these very real conditions are made into fodder for humor and ridicule, but it's even more problematic when we create the impression that these conditions have anything *at all* to do with cats. Associating cats with mental illness doesn't help anyone . . . least of all cats!

I'm told all the time, "If I got involved in kitten rescue, I'd probably end up with thirty cats." I'm always surprised by this bizarre projection. Where do people get the idea that if you save cats, you become a cat hoarder? To me, the answer is clear: they got this idea from pop culture. When we have no recognizable model of a person who saves cats and also lives a balanced life, it results in an assumption that one who saves cats inadvertently becomes unstable. Representation is so critical to getting people invested in a cause and helping them aspire to be involved, and when we have no positive role models, people will assume this is a losing team. No one aspires to be the cat lady from *The Simpsons*.

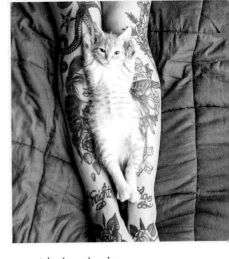

I don't consider myself to be crazy, and while some people may proudly claim this term, I do not. I believe that what my colleagues and I do is an extremely measured, compassionate effort. We dedicate our lives to building strategic change. We stay focused on our goal to create a nation where no cat or kitten is needlessly killed. It isn't crazy at all—it's social justice work! It has nothing to do with mental health. I think it's important to push back against this stereotype and show that loving cats and being balanced are not mutually exclusive options.

It isn't just that people are scared that they will become crazy—it's that they're scared that they will be *perceived* as crazy. That's what negative stereotyping does: it creates false associations and discourages people from being associated with something neutral, lest they be classified as something unfavorable. And when it comes to the crazy-cat-lady stereotype, it isn't just associating cats with mental illness; it's also associating cats with femininity.

Kids are encouraged from a very young age to stay within the confines of a strict gender identity. Our culture arbitrarily assigns a gender to various interests, products, jobs, clothing items, and even colors, then polices our activities to ensure we don't stray from these cultural norms. Completely random items become coded as male or female, and it's very clear what happens when we fail to conform to the expectation of our gender: we're ridiculed and told to get back in our box. Men who wear nail polish are shamed. Women with body hair are shamed. Shame is a cultural tool that we use to keep people in their place—and shame is therefore damaging to the process of becoming a fully self-actualized, authentic individual.

Somehow, cats ended up being coded as female, and that's a big problem. When hundreds of thousands of cats are being killed in the United States, we need to invest as many people in their protection as possible—yet our very culture discourages the participation of half the human population! This is evidenced by the hugely disproportionate number of women who work or volunteer in cat welfare, and the relatively absent male population. Even attendees at my workshops and on my educational platforms are, on average, about 81 percent female.

Shame and fear keep good, compassionate people from getting active for cats because they don't want to be associated with being crazy or feminine. But the cats desperately need these people to be their advocates, too. I believe that if we want an effective movement, we have to have a diverse movement. We have to have a movement that looks and feels welcoming to people from all backgrounds. We need to be inclusive and show that there are endless possibilities for what it looks like to be a cat or kitten rescuer. We need men to know that it's more than okay to adopt a cat—that it's awesome to do so.

So how can we undermine the crazy-cat-lady stereotype? We can start with setting a good example. We can show people what being a modern cat person is about: being a socially conscious, compassionate advocate who is helping protect a vulnerable population. We can create rad events where we can socialize and share ideas. We can set goals and reach them. We can engage politically and be a positive force in the larger community. We can maintain balance in our lives through self-care. We can lift up the work of other advocates and show that cat welfare is an inviting space for everyone. When we do these things, we create a winning team—a team that people want to join!

Cat and kitten rescue is for *everyone*, regardless of who you are or what you look like. Let's dismantle the tired old crazy-cat-lady trope and show the world that anyone can make a difference for felines!

When I pierced my own nose with an earring at age fourteen, my mother was pale with shock. I don't think the average parent dreams of her child turning into a punk rocker, but looking back, my discovery of the punk community as a young teenager actually had an unquestionably positive influence on me that directed the course of my life. Growing up in a community of self-made weirdos, I've always been surrounded by a DIY ethic that empowered me to create the world I want to live in.

Whatever our interests or skills, my friends and I always shared a similar vision: if you want something to exist, make it exist. Want an all-ages venue? Hold a show in your basement. Want people to hear your music? Record your own songs, create your own flyers, and design your own merchandise. Want a cute dress? Cut up some fabric and sew it. Want to share your ideas and skills? Put out a zine or hold a workshop. Want to live in a kinder world? Build it.

Maybe it sounds silly to trace my determination to save animals all the way back to dying my hair pink as an angsty teen, but the root of what I do grew from a seed that was planted when I discovered that a little creativity, independence, and defiance go a long way. My approach to animal welfare has therefore always been one of stubbornness and hope, of positivity and determination. I refuse to accept that animals must die if they can be saved, and I refuse to believe that the animal-loving community can't work together to solve this issue. With enough hard work, we can. We will!

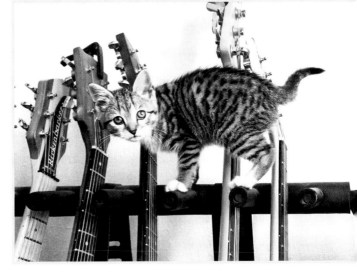

You don't have to study at a conservatory to be a musician, and you don't have to go to vet school to save animals. Anyone can learn how to do either by trying hard, practicing, soaking up knowledge, staying passionate, and simply making the time to do it. While becoming a veterinarian is one of many admirable paths, there is so much work that *anyone*

can do to help animals, regardless of career path or educational background. We don't have to wait until we're perfect to start. We just have to be stubborn enough to figure it out.

This DIY mentality has led me on some crazy rescue adventures, and pushed me to involve myself in things that were new and unknown. A few years ago, I learned about six black bears who were set to be euthanized, and I suddenly found myself spearheading a monthlong campaign to rescue them from a dilapidated roadside zoo. Having no experience with black bears at all, I became overwhelmed with the conviction that I wanted to save them. Once I had it in my mind that I could do something about it, I was determined. I did everything I could: I filed for an extension on their euthanasia so that I had time to coordinate a plan, I worked with the state's Department of Environmental Conservation, I fund-raised, and I collaborated with two animal sanctuaries, Lions, Tigers & Bears and Wild Animal Sanctuary, that would ultimately help conduct the rescue and provide a permanent sanctuary to the animals. At the end of a long day of transferring the six black bears out of their tiny, filthy roadside enclosure into the transport vehicle, I lay in their empty concrete pen and cried. I couldn't believe that my pipe dream had been actualized.

I didn't know that was something I could do, but I was willing to suspend my disbelief in order to try. Now I know that with enough effort . . . I am capable of saving bears! I try to let this awareness propel me: the awareness that even though I'm one small person, I can make big things happen.

Many of us feel powerless when we witness injustice, or doubt our ability to make an impact. But what if we start with the premise that we in fact have *incredible* power to make a positive difference? I believe that whatever we feel passionately about, we should work toward without delay; we have only one lifetime to make our impact. For me, this has meant finding a way to make rescue fit into my life no matter what so that I can save the maximum number of lives possible. It has meant working hard even when people think an animal can't be saved . . . and proving them wrong.

Start small. Each of us can change something, and together we can change the world. We have to get creative, get determined, and take matters into our own hands. We have to live with a DIY heart and a burning passion. We have to stop looking for reasons we *can't* save lives, and start looking for ways that we can.

MEOWCHU PICCHU: MY PERUVIAN KITTEN RESCUE ADVENTURE

There's a running joke that I can't go anywhere without coming home with a kitten. Being a full-time rescuer means that in order to take time off, I usually have to go *pretty far* from home. So when Andrew and I booked a vacation to Peru, we thought that we were taking a break from kitten care . . . never expecting that we were actually embarking on one of our most adventurous kitten rescues yet.

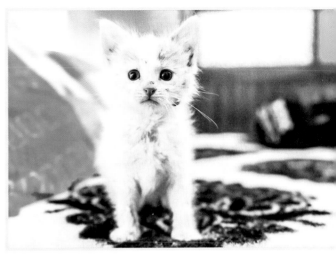

It was our last day in Peru, and we had just come down the mountain from Machu Picchu to begin our long trip home. With just forty minutes until our train departed, I suddenly found myself running, almost reflexively, toward the sound of a screaming kitten. Scanning the area, I located the source of the sound—a terrified little kitten being passed around by local children. The children meant her no harm, but being young and unsupervised, they squeezed her and fought over who could hold her, and by the time I got close enough to see her face, she was visibly trembling.

There she was: a one-pound, emaciated, flea-covered kitten with filthy dreadlocks in her fur, looking up at me with bright blue eyes. I approached the kids and began to ask questions using the little Spanish I knew—"*Es tu gatita? Tiene una madre?*" One of the boys had found her all alone and brought her to a football field to show his friends, but she didn't belong to anyone and was barely surviving on the street. I pulled cat food from my backpack (don't laugh . . . rescuers always come prepared!) and offered it in my palm, and the kitten began to scarf it down immediately.

Unfortunately, there are almost no resources for cats in Peru. While I typically work in the United States, where we have municipal animal shelters and a dozen rescue groups in nearly every county, Peru does not have these resources available. With the clock ticking, our only options were to leave the kitten on the street or take

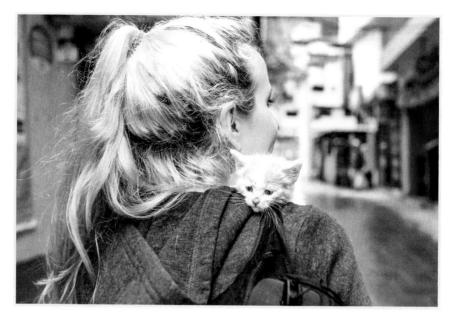

her with us. Andrew looked at me with a knowing expression, and without a thought the words escaped my mouth: "Let's just take her. We'll figure it out."

On the walk back to the train station, we were both frantically asking questions. How would we sneak her on this train? Was it even possible to bring a kitten back to the United States on a plane, and with just twenty-four hours' notice? Could we find a veterinarian who would help us? If none of this worked, was there somewhere safe we could bring her? I placed her in my hoodie, and as we boarded the train I felt her first purrs vibrate against my belly. She was already learning to trust us.

My rescue philosophy has always been to take action first and figure out the details later. With enough willpower, I've found myself able to overcome impossible odds to save an animal's life . . . and so with great determination we began an evening of research to work out the logistics of travel. We learned that in order to board an international flight with a kitten, you need a health certificate and proof of vaccination from a certified vet, a carrier that meets the airline's requirements, and a reservation on the flight for the animal. Andrew and I divided up our duties, and after a few hours we were prepared for the day ahead.

When we got to the apartment we were renting, it was time to clean the kitten up. With gentle dish soap and warm sudsy water, I washed away her fleas and the grime from the street. Next I trimmed her dreadlocks and cleaned out her ears. She emerged a new kitten—fluffy and soft, purring and cuddly. We decided to name her Munay Michi (pronounced "moon-eye mee-chee"), which means "lovely cat" in Quechua, the beautiful native language spoken in the Andes. We tucked Munay in, and after just a few hours of sleep, the sun was up and we began our big day.

We would need to be at the airport at ten for a flight from Cuzco to Lima, so we showed up bright and early for a walk-in vet clinic that opened at eight and hoped for the best. We purchased a carrier, waited our turn, and excitedly received our Certificado de Salud with just enough time to catch a cab to the airport. Sitting in the back of the cab, my heart pounding, I thumbed through the paperwork, anxiously checking it against the requirements to ensure that we had done everything correctly.

At the airport, we showed Munay's paperwork to the airline agent, paid her ticket fee, and made it through security with no issues. Breathing a huge sigh of relief, we celebrated as the wheels lifted and we took off for our first leg of the trip. Andrew and I kept looking at each other in awe, saying, "Oh my god, this is happening!" This was a small victory, but the big challenge would be making it from Lima into the United States.

Our second flight was much the same. An examination of paperwork, a ticket fee, and a look of disbelief on both of our faces when we made it onto the airplane with relative ease. Munay did a beautiful job of staying happy and relaxed while I obsessively monitored her throughout the long international flight, taking bathroom breaks to help her pee, providing extra hydration and nutrients to ensure that she stayed healthy on the flight, and brushing her with a toothbrush to help her feel at ease.

The flight landed in the US and it was time for the final challenge: Customs and Border Protection. I filled out my customs declaration form, indicating that I was indeed bringing "(b) meats, animals, animal/wildlife products." Accepting my form, the customs agent asked, "What food item are you declaring?" I nervously responded: "Well, I have a cat . . . but she isn't a food item." He laughed, I laughed, and he stamped the form. I couldn't believe it. Munay was officially a US citizen!

In less than thirty-six hours she'd gone from dreadlocked and hungry on the streets of Aguas Caliente to fluffy and full in my Washington, DC, bedroom. The experience was as transformative for me as it was for Munay. We had done something incredible together, and truly, no one was as shocked as I was! Munay's story taught me that with enough determination, resourcefulness, and love, anything is possible. We figure it out. When faced with impossible odds, the difference between

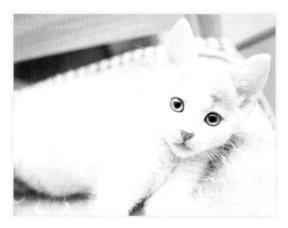

success and defeat just might be the willingness to throw your hat in the ring—to believe that you have what it takes.

The Peruvian princess adjusted immediately to her new life in our home, where she was afforded every feline luxury imaginable: fun toys, soft beds, expert vet care, and new feline friends! For a month she thrived in our nursery, where she played with other kittens in our care, became healthy and well-fed, and soaked up lots of love and affection.

Munay was adopted into a home with a friend in Philadelphia, where she lives a happy life with her American brother, a former street cat named Grendel. Although her journey brought her out of Peru, she still left a huge mark on the country she used to call home. Through her story, I raised several thousand dollars to send to one of the only cat shelters in Peru, and now her impact has touched the lives of dozens of cats and kittens in her home country.

For a two-pound furball, she had more adventures and impact than many cats have during their entire nine lives. Munay traveled the world, raised money for cats in need, and inspired people around the globe to believe in the importance of helping those who are vulnerable, even against all odds.

YOU CAN DO WHAT YOU BELIEVE YOU CAN DO

My experience of saving Munay taught me an important lesson, which is that you learn what you're capable of doing by trying to do it. I had no idea if it was possible to bring back a kitten from Peru with twenty-four hours' notice, but I was bold enough to try. It's this boldness of heart that is sometimes required in order for us to discover what we're capable of, and since Munay's international adventure, I can honestly say I've become more daring than ever in my willingness to give scary things a chance.

There's a famous quote by Wayne Gretzky: "You miss 100 percent of the shots you don't take." It's a platitude scrolled across motivational posters that is easily overlooked, and it never meant anything to me until I started taking on such challenging kitten cases. Now I feel the power of this sentiment in my bones. Having been faced with severely sick or injured animals, challenging rescue scenarios, and tiny neonates who I was told had no chance at all, I've come to find that my outlook has a huge impact on the outcome. If I don't believe they have a chance, then it's true. But if I do believe they have a chance . . . there's a chance they do!

If you look for reasons that you can't save lives, you will find them. But for the animals, this is urgent. They need our help now. Animal rescue is an opportunity for us to discover that within each of us is an incredible superhero capable of swooping in and saving lives. Finding your inner superhero starts with a mental framework that says, *I think I can.* After all, the one thing that unites all people who do amazing things is that they first had to believe they could do it. Believe you can, and you'll shock yourself with what you can achieve.

FIND YOUR FELINE SUPERPOWER

When it comes to saving lives, there's truly something for everyone! There is no shortage of ways that individuals like me and you can get active to make the world a safer place for cats and kittens. Any time I hear someone lament that they *can't* do something, I always encourage them to instead think about what it is they *can* do. After all, we each have our own skill sets, schedules, connections, and abilities that make us uniquely situated

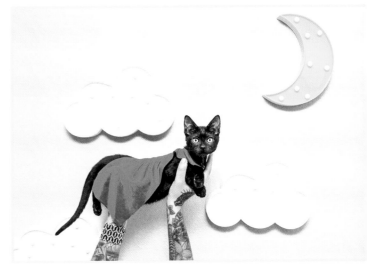

to make a difference in our own way. So put on your superhero cape and discover your feline superpower! Here are some ideas to get you started:

- 🐱 Volunteer on-site at your local shelter. You can help with things like socializing the cats, feeding, cleaning, and more.
- 🐱 Trap community cats for TNR.
- 🐱 Volunteer at a TNR clinic or spay/neuter clinic.

- Donate money to a nonprofit rescue organization. It's tax-deductible, and each dollar helps save lives!
- Transport cats for your local rescue group.
- Use your photography skills to take great photos of adoptable cats at your shelter.
- Skilled at graphic or web design? Find a nonprofit that can use your help!
- Educate your community about the needs of cats and kittens.
- Attend a fund-raising event.
- Donate supplies to your local organizations. Think beyond cat food—how about office and cleaning supplies? Ask them what they need!
- Got schmoozing skills? Help out by finding local sponsors to support your shelter's fund-raising events.
- Volunteer as an adoption counselor at local adoption events.
- Educate yourself! Read books and watch videos about cat and kitten welfare.
- Offer your skills as a grant writer to a local nonprofit organization.
- Attend county and city council meetings to support policies that save cats' lives.
- Make winter shelters for the community cats in your neighborhood.
- Be a community cat colony caregiver.
- Host a workshop to teach other rescuers a specific skill.
- Foster orphaned neonatal kittens.
- Got construction skills? Your animal shelter will love having your help.
- Hold a bake sale or craft sale and donate the proceeds to a group of your choice.
- If you're multilingual, help by translating educational materials into other languages.
- Sponsor the adoption fee for a cat who needs a little boost.
- Volunteer at a kitten nursery.
- Foster adult cats and help their personalities blossom.
- Offer to do laundry for shelters and rescue organizations—you will be their new best friend!
- Got social media skills? Find local organizations that need a hand and offer to help out.
- Share educational videos and articles on social media.
- Foster senior kitties and give them a wonderful, relaxing home environment.
- Got writing skills? Your local nonprofit organizations may need your help writing cat adoption profiles or fund-raising appeals!

- Get active legislatively at the federal, state, and local level. Support candidates and campaigns that push for progressive policies for animals.
- Work with children? Create a kid-friendly curriculum to teach them all about how to be kind to cats!
- Foster mama cats and their babies.
- Own a business? Consider sponsoring a local fund-raising or adoption event.
- Share this book with a friend!
- Have legal or accounting expertise? Use your skills and knowledge to support your local organizations. Join a nonprofit board or sit on an advisory board.
- Foster feral kittens who need socialization support.
- Plan an event to support your local shelter or rescue.
- Adopt a cat or kitten in need, and spread the word about adoption to friends and family!
- Make crafts for the cats! Blankets, cat beds, and cat-safe toys are always appreciated.
- Build kits of kitten supplies and donate them for your local foster program to hand out.
- Do a cat food drive at your work, school, or community center.
- Ask for donations to your favorite rescue organization for your birthday!
- Dream big. Ask yourself what skills you possess and how you can apply them toward saving animals. Get active and you'll discover how valuable, impactful, and needed you truly are.

SPOTLIGHT: STRENGTH AND BRAVERY

It takes strength to be gentle and kind.

—The Smiths

Kindness and compassionate action require strength, but if there's one lesson I've learned from saving little lives, it's that acts of kindness actually *give* you strength, too. If I pour my strong heart into little lives, they don't deplete my reserves—they make my compassion grow even stronger. When we allow ourselves to experience empathy and caring, we are in turn rewarded with love and gratitude. This circuitous love is transmitted back and forth between the caregiver and the animal—an incredible gift of connection.

Although tiny kittens may appear hopeless to the undiscerning eye, the truth is

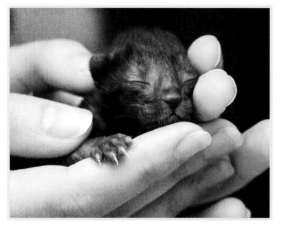

that everything inside them is calling out that they want to live. They want to recover from their wounds. They want to be nourished with food that helps them grow into mighty cats. They want to discover the sunny spot on the floor and to know what it is to be safe—to be loved. They are brave, and they need us to be brave by their side. If a kitten is brave enough to have hope for her future, I want to dignify her hopefulness with hope of my own.

PERFECTLY IMPERFECT CHLOE

For the first day I had Chloe, all I could do was cry.

I'd never met a paralyzed kitten before, and I had no idea what to do. I'd gone to the shelter to pick up a two-week-old orphan named Tetley, but when I got there, I was asked, "Would you also like to take home a four-week-old whose back legs don't work?" I looked in the back of the metal kennel, where a small peach-colored kitten with big blue eyes was huddled on a blanket with her legs sprawled behind her. I took one look at her, and that was it.

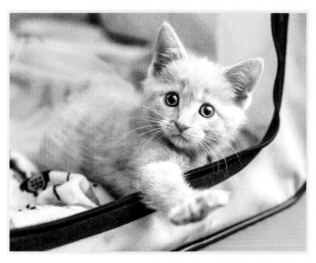

Next thing I knew, we were back at my house and I was lying on the floor next to her with tears in my eyes. I didn't know where to start. In my mind, I imagined that she must be suffering, scared, and in pain. I wondered if she could ever be happy in a body like hers, and if anyone would ever be willing to adopt a kitten in her condition. I looked at her sweet, innocent face, and she let out a silent "meow" as if to try to introduce herself. I wept. I wanted her to have a name I could call her—a beautiful, lovely name that you'd give to a child. "Chloe?" I said, and she responded with another silent "meow."

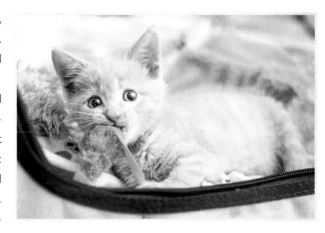

I reached out to other friends and rescuers who had worked with paralyzed cats in search of support. Right away, the response was encouraging: I was told that cats like Chloe can, and do, live wonderful, normal lives . . . They just get around a little differently. Still, I looked at her and I wanted so badly to change her situation, so I forged ahead with my mission to get her on her feet.

Over the next three months, she would go to more than two dozen vet appointments—my most excessive case to date. I took her to three neurologists, an orthopedic specialist, cold laser therapy, acupuncture, and physical therapy. Some doctors told me she would never walk again, but that if I was willing to raise her as a paralyzed cat, I could. Other doctors told me she would never walk again, and to euthanize her. But when I looked at her, she looked bright-eyed, aware, intelligent, and, aside from her dangling hind limbs, healthy. Nothing about her seemed hopeless.

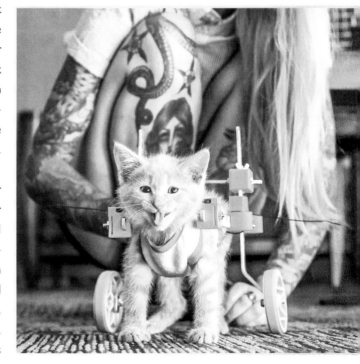

Accepting that she wouldn't ever walk again, I then set out to help her walk with an assistive device. I reached out to a 3-D printing engineer, who helped me design a custom wheelchair just for Chloe. We worked together to design the most epic, adorable, super-fly set of wheels, complete with Malibu Barbie colors and a cozy harness I sewed myself. I was convinced that this would be the ticket to her happiness, and envisioned that she would hop into it and feel liberated and free.

On the day that her wheelchair was finally complete, we placed her into it, and she squirmed frantically, trying to escape. I patiently calmed her and tried to ease her nerves, but she was miserable. Finally, she tried it out, taking some steps . . . but she was still miserable. We made alterations to it and tried again, and as I placed her into it, she cried to be set free. Strapped into a metal and plastic unit, she hung suspended in the air, trapped. She looked up at me with the biggest, saddest eyes, and it suddenly dawned on me that this wheelchair wasn't liberating at all.

All this time, I'd imagined that she was unhappy in her body, but I'd never stopped to consider what happiness looked like for Chloe. I'd projected my own expectations onto her—that she couldn't be fulfilled unless she could walk—instead of pausing and imagining myself in her position. See, kittens want to be able to play, pounce, slink around, hide, climb, and curl up . . . *none of which* you can do while strapped into a heavy-duty piece of machinery! What I thought would be liberating was in fact restricting.

I began to reframe my perspective. Instead of comparing her to other cats, I started to ask myself what a full, meaningful life would look like for her. Instantly, I became more aware of slight alterations I could make to the home so that she would be more comfortable in her body, such as mats on the floor she could easily access, padded steps by the side of the bed, and a runner for the stairs that would allow her to pull herself up. I began to imagine life from her standpoint, and the more I did, the more empathetic a caregiver I became. As I stopped trying to change her and simply accepted her for who she was, she began to open up more and more, and our bond grew.

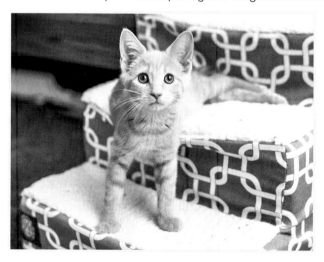

This little cat wasn't imperfect at all—she was already perfect. She could catch a feather toy like a fearsome beast (as long as you kept it close to the floor!). She could climb a cat tree using her buff forearms; she'd just have her legs dangling adorably off the end of it as she lounged. She could get herself up and into the bed, where she'd sleep with me at night, gently kneading the soft blanket. She wasn't just capable of living . . . She actually lived one of the most enthusiastic, full lives ever. She thrived.

Chloe helped me to drastically reframe the way I understand even the most hopeless of situations, to step outside my fears and see the individual looking back, softly meowing. Chloe isn't a sob story or a case number to file away. She isn't a statistic or a lost cause. She is just a happy little baby who wants, and who deserves, to live and know acceptance, care, and love.

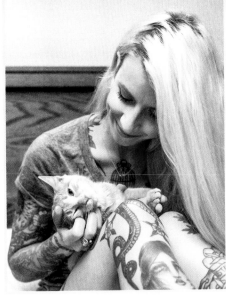

One of my last moments at home with Chloe.

Parting ways with Chloe was hands down the most difficult good-bye I've ever experienced. The two of us had gone through so much growth together, and she had impacted me emotionally to an unquantifiable degree. When it was time for her to go to her forever home, I spent hours on the phone with her incredible new family, talking about her special care needs, her likes and dislikes, and my hopes and dreams for her. Soon, she and I would take a cross-country flight to bring her to her new mom and dad.

As we drove to the airport, I was raw with emotion. The route took us past the shelter where I'd first seen her, so small and all alone. It hit me that in that moment, sitting in that cage, her life had been hanging by a thread. Her fate was completely intertwined with the outlook of those who peered in at her from the outside. Would they see hopelessness, or would they see hope? For this little girl, the path to her success was paved with hope—the hope of the shelter employees who kept her alive, the hope of the veterinarians who treated her, and the hope of her foster family, who dreamt of a day where she'd be safe and happy in a home of her own.

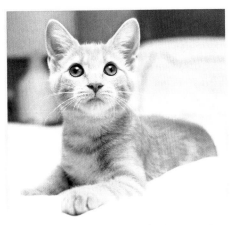

When her new mom and dad met her, they beamed with joy. I slept on their couch for two nights, and we spent three days all getting to know one another and, most important, helping Chloe settle in. In her San Francisco home, Chloe enthusiastically slid around the floors like a race car, eager to check out every nook and cranny of her new kingdom. She flew up the new hallway at high speed, gripping the runner beneath her. She lay in the sunny spot in the kitchen. She tried out the bath mat—so plush and cozy. She met her new brother, a massive orange tabby named Doogie, and shared a handful of treats with him. She had made it all this way, and finally, she was home.

MIGHTY

As animal advocates, we sometimes stay zoomed out on the big picture, and it overwhelms us. To know that so many kittens are dying in the United States every year, although nearly all of them are in a condition where they could be saved, is a monolithic weight on our hearts. But when we stay zoomed out on the devastating volume of suffering, we sometimes forget that those big statistics are made up of much smaller parts—that the hundreds of thousands of lives who need our help are nothing more than a series of ones.

It's not often that the path is clear, but when it comes to the welfare of kittens, the future is bright as long as enough people take the first steps to get involved. Each of us may be only an individual, but together we are a movement, and movements can change the course of history. When we see ourselves as part of something bigger, we realize that we don't have to do *everything*; we just have to do *something*—that each act of kindness counts toward the bigger picture.

By volunteering our time and opening our homes, we can make a big impact for little kittens. My hope for the future is that cat- and kitten-lovers will feel empowered to take their love a step further. To stop saying, "I wish someone would save them," and to instead look into the mirror and realize: *I am someone*. One person can do only so much, but what each of us is able to contribute is perfect. Every individual contribution is deeply critical to the success of the whole.

Little lives aren't saved by big actions; they're saved by small, individual acts of compassion. Those tiny actions add up, and together we can make a mighty difference.

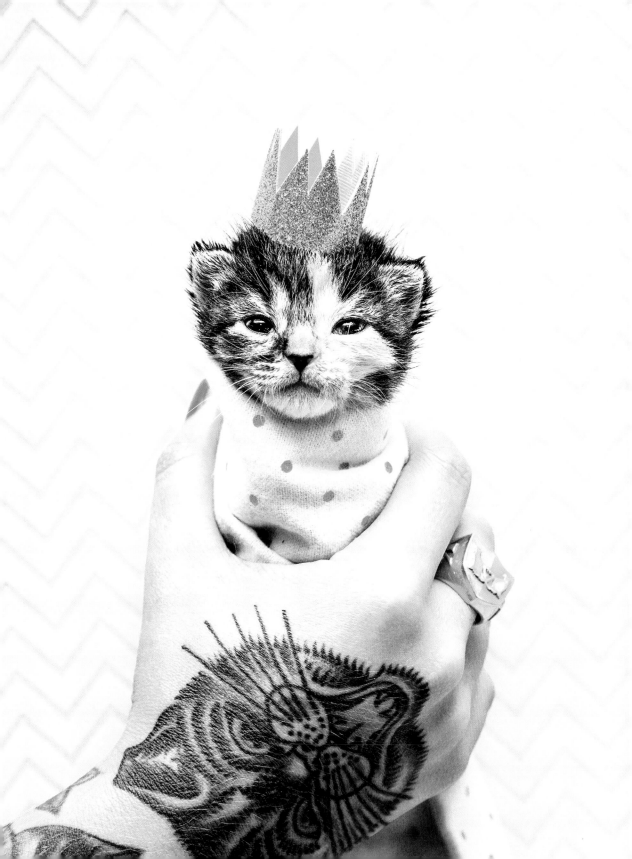

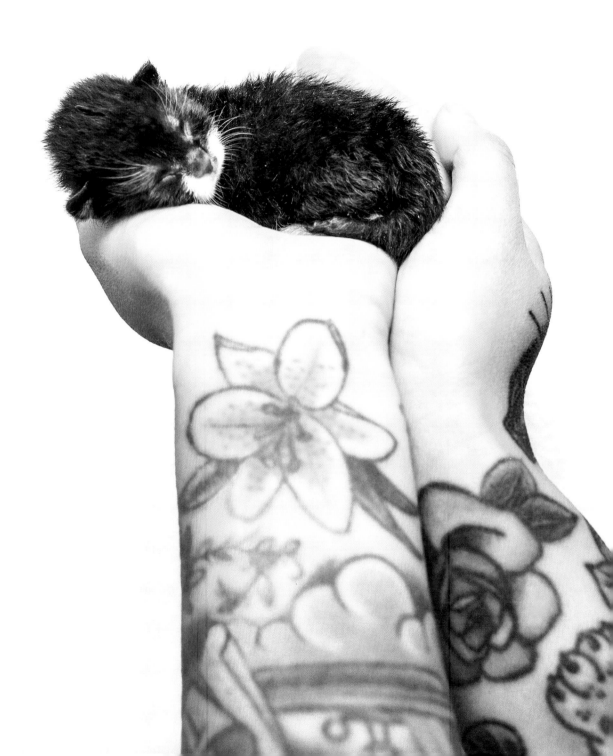

KITTEN NAME:

Date	Time	Pre-Feeding Weight	Post-Feeding Weight	Notes

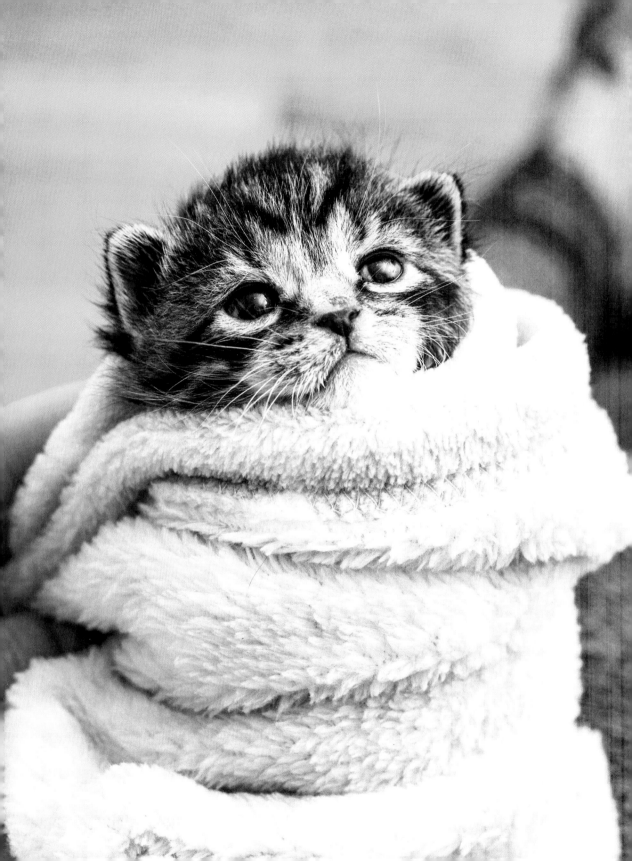

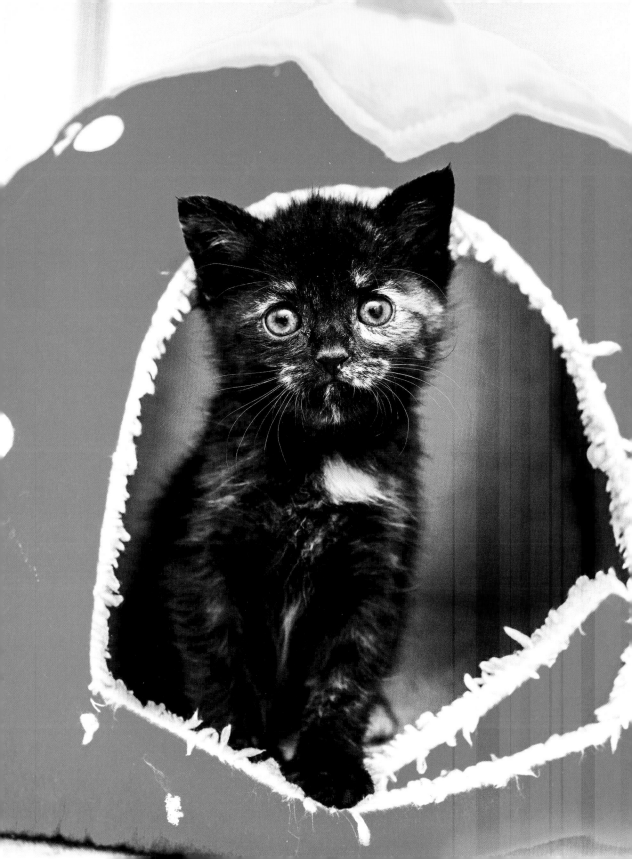

ACKNOWLEDGMENTS

Creating this book has been a dream come true, and I am wholeheartedly grateful to the people who helped me along the way.

First and foremost, I'd like to thank Andrew for being the most loving partner, friend, and kitten papa on the planet. Thank you, Andrew, for lending your immense talent to this project and for being on this wonderfully weird ride with me.

To my literary agent, Myrsini, thank you for seeing the potential in me and working so passionately by my side. Your love of books (and cats!) is contagious, and I'm thankful for the literary fire you've sparked in me.

To the entire team at Plume, especially my incredible editor, Stephanie—thank you. Stephanie, I'm so grateful to you for helping this book come to life.

To the friends and colleagues who have supported me along this journey, thank you. Jackson, Ellen, Rachel, Michelle, Sonja, Jackie, Kendra, David, Eliana, Neal, Adam, Christina, Candace, Mel, Christy, Kate, Ingrid, Wendel, Erin, Lena, Brie, Elena, Sharon, Alaina, Katherine, and so many others—I absolutely cherish our friendship and collaboration.

To my mom, thank you for showing me what it means to be a passionate and brave woman.

To my dad, thank you for being proud of me—it means so much.

To all the little lives who inspired this book, thank you. You've changed my life. I hope I've changed yours, too.

NOTES

Chapter One: State of the Kitten

1. "Pet Statistics," ASPCA, https://www.aspca.org/animal-homelessness/shelter-intake-and -surrender/pet-statistics.
2. "Euthanasia," Merriam-Webster, https://www.merriam-webster.com/dictionary/euthanasia.

Chapter Two: It's Raining Kittens

1. Sara White, "The Case for Low-Cost, High-Quality, High-Volume Spay and Neuter," Humane Society Veterinary Medical Association, August 11, 2011, http://www.hsvma.org/case_for _low_cost_high_quality_high_volume_spay_neuter_081111#.W4g9p5NKhN0.
2. Julie K. Levy and P. Cynda Crawford, "Humane Strategies for Controlling Feral Cat Populations," *Journal of the American Veterinary Medical Association* 225, no. 9 (November 2004): 1354–60.
3. "Return to Owner," Table 8, "2016 Animal Sheltering Statistics," Shelter Animals Count, https://shelteranimalscount.org/docs/default-source/DataResources/2016animalsheltering statistics.pdf?sfvrsn=12.
4. Julie Levy, Natalie M. Isaza, and Karen C. Scott, "Effect of High-Impact Targeted Trap-Neuter-Return and Adoption of Community Cats on Cat Intake to a Shelter," *Veterinary Journal* 201, no. 3 (September 2014): 269–74, https://www.sciencedirect.com/science/article /pii/S1090023314001841.
5. Levy, Isaza, and Scott, "Effect of High-Impact Targeted Trap-Neuter-Return."
6. Fairfax County Police Department, "Trap, Neuter, Return Program Decreases Homeless Feral Cat Population," WUSA9, January 19, 2012, http://springfield.wusa9.com/news/news/89821 -trap-neuter-return-program-decreases-homeless-feral-cat-population.
7. ASPCA, "A Closer Look at Community Cats," https://www.aspca.org/animal-homelessness /shelter-intake-and-surrender/closer-look-community-cats.

Chapter Six: In Sickness and in Health

1. Sylvie Chastant-Maillard, Charlotte Aggouni, Amélie Albaret, Aurélie Fournier, and Hanna Mila, "Canine and Feline Colostrum," *Reproduction in Domestic Animals* 52, no. 52 (April 2017): 148–52, https://onlinelibrary.wiley.com/doi/pdf/10.1111/rda.12830.
2. "The 2006 American Association of Feline Practitioners Feline Vaccine Advisory Panel Report," *Journal of the American Veterinary Medical Association* 229, no. 9 (November 2006): 1405–41, https://www.catvets.com/public/PDFs/PracticeGuidelines/VaccinationGLS.pdf.
3. American Veterinary Medical Association, "Feline Panleukopenia," https://www.avma.org /public/petcare/pages/Feline-Panleukopenia.aspx.

4. American Veterinary Medical Association, "Feline Panleukopenia."

5. Mohamed Abd-Eldaim, Melissa J. Beall, and Melissa A. Kennedy, "Detection of Feline Panleukopenia Virus Using a Commercial ELISA for Canine Parvovirus," *Veterinary Therapeutics* 10, no. 4 (Winter 2009): E1–6, https://www.ncbi.nlm.nih.gov/pubmed/20425728.

6. American Veterinary Medical Association, "Administration of Rabies Vaccination State Laws," last updated September 2017, https://www.avma.org/Advocacy/StateAndLocal/Pages /rabies-vaccination.aspx.

7. Janet K. Yamamoto, Missa P. Sanou, Jeffrey R. Abbott, and James K. Coleman, "Feline Immunodeficiency Virus Model for Designing HIV/AIDS Vaccines," *Current HIV Research* 8, no. 1 (January 2010): 14–25, https://www.ncbi.nlm.nih.gov/pmc/articles/PMC3721975/.

8. American Association of Feline Practitioners, *Feline Retrovirus Management Guidelines* (Hillsborough, NJ: 2009), https://www.catvets.com/public/PDFs/PracticeGuidelines /RetrovirusGLS-Summary.pdf.

9. Julie K. Levy and Staci Hutsell, "Overview of Feline Infectious Peritonitis," *Merck Veterinary Manual*, https://www.merckvetmanual.com/generalized-conditions/feline-infectious -peritonitis/overview-of-feline-infectious-peritonitis.

10. "Feline Infectious Peritonitis Therapeutics/Clinical Trials Team," UC Davis Veterinary Medicine, last updated September 25, 2018, http://www.vetmed.ucdavis.edu/ccah/cats /feline-infectious-peritonitis-clinical-trials.cfm; Niels C. Pedersen et al., "Efficacy of a 3C -Like Protease Inhibitor in Treating Various Forms of Acquired Feline Infectious Peritonitis," *Journal of Feline Medicine and Surgery* 20, no. 4 (April 2018): 378–92, http://journals.sagepub .com/doi/abs/10.1177/1098612X17729626?url_ver=Z39.88-2003&rfr_id=ori%3Arid%3Acrossref .org&rfr_dat=cr_pub%3Dpubmed&.

11. Cornell Feline Health Center, "Gastrointestinal Parasites of Cats," last updated June 2018, https://www2.vet.cornell.edu/departments-centers-and-institutes/cornell-feline-health-center /health-information/feline-health-topics/gastrointestinal-parasites-cats.

12. Lihua Xiao and Ronald Fayer, "Molecular Characterisation of Species and Genotypes of *Cryptosporidium* and *Giardia* and Assessment of Zoonotic Transmission," *International Journal of Parasitology* 38, no. 11 (September 2008): 1239–55, https://www.ncbi.nlm.nih.gov /pubmed/18479685.

13. "Dehydration in Animals," Infovets, http://www.infovets.com/books/smrm/f/F145.htm.

14. Royal Canin, "Curiosity Can Save the Cat: Royal Canin Rallies Cat Owners to See the Vet This Year as Part of a National Take Your Cat to the Vet Day Campaign," news release, August 18, 2016, https://www.royalcanin.com/newsroom/2016/08/18/TYCTTV.

Chapter Seven: Preparing for Takeoff

1. Linda K. Lord, Walter Ingwersen, Janet L. Gray, and David J. Wintz, "Characterization of Animals with Microchips Entering Animal Shelters," *Journal of the American Veterinary Medical Association* 235, no. 2 (August 2009): 160–67.

2. Emily Weiss, Emily D. Dolan, Jamie E. Scotto, Margaret R. Slater, and Shannon Gramann, "Do Policy Based Adoptions Increase the Care a Pet Receives? An Exploration of a Shift to Conversation Based Adoptions at One Shelter," American Society for the Prevention of Cruelty to Animals via IssueLab, October 20, 2014, https://www.issuelab.org/resource/do-policy-based -adoptions-increase-the-care-a-pet-receives-an-exploration-of-a-shift-to-conversation-based -adoptions-at-one-shelter.html.

Chapter Eight: Taking Care of Yourself (So You Can Take Care of Them)

1. Jennifer Blough, *To Save a Starfish: A Compassion-Fatigue Workbook for the Animal-Welfare Warrior* (New Boston, MI: Deepwater Books, 2016), 4.

2. Charles R. Figley and Kathleen Regan Figley, "Compassion Fatigue Resilience," in *The Oxford Handbook of Compassion Science*, eds. Emma M. Seppälä, Emiliana Simon-Thomas, Stephanie

L. Brown, Monica C. Worline, C. Daryl Cameron, and James R. Doty (New York, NY: Oxford University Press, 2017).

3. Figley and Figley, "Compassion Fatigue Resilience."
4. Sandy Newsome, Michael Waldo, and Clare Gruszka, "Mindfulness Group Work: Preventing Stress and Increasing Self-Compassion among Helping Professionals in Training," *Journal for Specialists in Group Work*, 37, no. 4 (2012): 292–311, http://dx.doi.org/10.1080/01933922.2012.690832.
5. Charlotte Fritz, Maya Yankelevich, Anna Zarubin, and Patricia Barger, "Happy, Healthy, and Productive: The Role of Detachment from Work during Nonwork Time," *Journal of Applied Psychology* 95, no. 5 (September 2010): 977–83, http://dx.doi.org/10.1037/a0019462.
6. Figley and Figley, "Compassion Fatigue Resilience."
7. Charles R. Figley and Robert G. Roop, *Compassion Fatigue in the Animal-Care Community* (Washington, DC: Humane Society Press, 2006).
8. Figley and Figley, "Compassion Fatigue Resilience."

INDEX

Note: Page numbers in *italics* refer to illustrations.

weaning
    about, 115
    and age of kittens, 79
    and emotional adaptability, 152
    messiness of, 120–121, *121*
    premature, 117, 118–119, 211
    and rejection of food, 121–122
    and slurry transition, 119–120
    and space of mother cat, 117–118
and supplemental feedings, 79, 122
    supplies required for, 115
    and teeth of kittens, 117
    timing of, 116–118
weight of kittens
    loss of weight, 217–218
    recording, *98*, 98–99
work, providing kitten care at, 67–68
worms, 194, 196, 201–204

HANNAH SHAW is an award-winning kitten rescuer, humane educator, and unwavering animal advocate who has dedicated her life to protecting the tiniest and most vulnerable felines. Her project, Kitten Lady, provides educational media, training resources, and instructional workshops that help individuals and animal shelters learn how to save the lives of kittens—in a fun and engaging format. Hannah is the author of the forthcoming children's book *Kitten Lady's Big Book of Little Kittens*, and she has been featured as a guest expert on Animal Planet's *My Cat from Hell*. She is also the founder of Orphan Kitten Club, a 501(c)(3) charitable organization, which provides rescue and adoption services to orphaned kittens in the San Diego area. Visit her at KittenLady.org, YouTube.com/KittenLady, Facebook.com/kittenxlady, and Instagram at @kittenxlady.

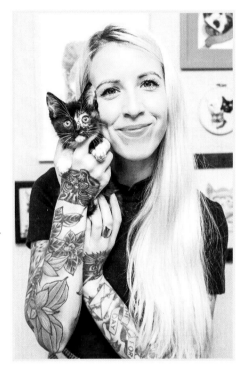